DEDICATION

For Annette, Sandra, and Vivian

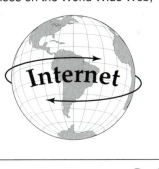

AMBULATORY CARE MANAGEMENT

THIRD EDITION

AMBULATORY CARE MANAGEMENT
THIRD EDITION

Austin Ross, M.P.H., FACMPE
Professor
Department of Health Services
School of Public Health and Community Medicine
University of Washington
Seattle, Washington

Ernest J. Pavlock, Ph.D., C.P.A.
Professor of Accounting
Virginia Polytechnic Institute and
  State University
Falls Church, Virginia

Stephen J. Williams, Sc.D.
Professor and Head
Division of Health Services Administration
Graduate School of Public Health
San Diego State University
San Diego, California

Foreword by
James S. Todd, M.D.
Executive Vice President
American Medical Association
Chicago, Illinois

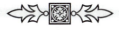

Delmar Publishers

I(T)P® **International Thomson Publishing**

Albany • Bonn • Boston • Cincinnati • Detroit • London • Madrid
Melbourne • Mexico City • New York • Pacific Grove • Paris • San Francisco
Singapore • Tokyo • Toronto • Washington

NOTICE TO THE READER

Cover Design: Carol D. Keohane

Delmar Staff
Publisher: William Brottmiller
Assistant Editor: Hilary Schrauf
Project Editor: Marah Bellegarde
Production Coordinator: Sandra Woods
Art/Design Coordinator: Carol D. Keohane

Printed in the United States of America
4 5 6 7 8 9 10 XXX 03 02 01 00

For more information, contact Delmar, 3 Columbia Circle, PO Box 15015, Albany, NY 12212-0515; or find us on the World Wide Web at http://www.delmar.com

International Division List

Japan:
Thomson Learning
Palaceside Building 5F
1-1-1 Hitotsubashi, Chiyoda-ku
Tokyo 100 0003 Japan
Tel: 813 5218 6544
Fax: 813 5218 6551

Australia/New Zealand
Nelson/Thomson Learning
102 Dodds Street
South Melbourne, Victoria 3205
Australia
Tel: 61 39 685 4111
Fax: 61 39 685 4199

UK/Europe/Middle East:
Thomson Learning
Berkshire House
168-173 High Holborn
London
WC1V 7AA United Kingdom
Tel: 44 171 497 1422
Fax: 44 171 497 1426

Latin America:
Thomson Learning
Seneca, 53
Colonia Polanco
11560 Mexico D.F. Mexico
Tel: 525-281-2906
Fax: 525-281-2656

Canada:
Nelson/Thomson Learning
1120 Birchmount Road
Scarborough, Ontario
Canada M1K 5G4
Tel: 416-752-9100
Fax: 416-752-8102

Asia:
Thomson Learning
60 Albert Street, #15-01
Albert Complex
Singapore 189969
Tel: 65 336 6411
Fax: 65 336 7411

Library of Congress Cataloging-in-Publication Data:
Ross, Austin.
    Ambulatory care management / Austin Ross, Jr., Stephen J.
Williams, Ernest J. Pavlock. — 3rd ed.
        p. cm. — (Delmar series in health services administration)
    Includes bibliographical references and index.
    ISBN 0-8273-7664-2
    1. Ambulatory medical care—Administration. I. Williams, Stephen
J. (Stephen Joseph), 1948-   II. Pavlock, Ernest J.   III. Title.
IV. Series.
    [DNLM: 1. Ambulatory Care—organization & administration. WX 205
R823a 1998
RA974.R67 1998
362.1'2'068—dc21   96-47935
DNLM/DLC for Library of Congress   CIP

INTRODUCTION TO THE SERIES

This series in health services is now in its second decade of providing top-quality teaching materials to the health administration/public health field. Each year has witnessed further strengthening of the market position of each of the principal books in the series, also reflecting the continued excellence of the products. Each author, book editor, and contributor to the series has helped build what is widely recognized as one of the top collections of professional health services books available today.

But we have achieved only a beginning. Everyone involved in the series is committed to further expansion of the scope, technical excellence, and useability of the series. Our goal is to do more for you, the reader. We will add new books in important areas, seek out more excellent authors, and increase the physical attributes of the books to make them easier for you to use.

We thank everyone, the authors and users in particular, who have made this series so successful and so widely used. And we promise that this second decade will be dedicated to further expansion of the series and to enhancement of the books it contains to provide still greater value to you, our constituency.

Stephen J. Williams
Series Editor

DELMAR SERIES IN HEALTH SERVICES ADMINISTRATION

Stephen J. Williams, Sc.D., Series Editor

CONTRIBUTORS

Jeanine L. Barlow, M.P.H.
Project Director
Center for Research in Ambulatory Health Care
  Administration
Englewood, Colorado

Dean C. Coddington
Managing Director
BBC Research and Consulting
Denver, Colorado

Doran A. Dunaway
Senior Associate Consultant
Tidewater Consulting Group
Ambler, Pennsylvania

Deborah Duncan
Director, Consulting Services
Medical Group Management Association
Englewood, Colorado

Barry R. Greene, Ph.D.
Associate Executive Director
Center for Research in Ambulatory Health Care
  Administration
Medical Group Management Association
Englewood, Colorado

Phillip A. Kieburtz
Kieburtz & Co.
Bellevue, Washington

Meryl D. Luallin
Sullivan/Luallin, Inc.
San Diego, California

Jeffrey B. Milburn, CMPE
Vice President of Finance
Colorado Springs Health Partners
Colorado Springs, Colorado

Steven P. Nohe, Sr., CMC
Managing Partner
Tidewater Consulting Group
Ambler, Pennsylvania

Mitchell J. Olejko, J.D.
Legacy Health System
Portland, Oregon

Ernest J. Pavlock, Ph.D., C.P.A.
Professor of Accounting
Virginia Polytechnic Institute and State University
Falls Church, Virginia

Austin Ross, M.P.H., FACMPE
Professor
Department of Health Services
University of Washington
Seattle, Washington
Emeritus Vice President and Executive
  Administrator
Virginia Mason Medical Center
Seattle, Washington

Thomas C. Royer, M.D.
Senior Vice President, Medical Affairs
Chairman, HFMG Board of Governors
Henry Ford Health System
Detroit, Michigan

Vinod K. Sahney, Ph.D.
Senior Vice President
Planning and Strategic Development
Henry Ford Health System
Detroit, Michigan

Kevin W. Sullivan
Sullivan/Luallin, Inc.
San Diego, California

Bette A. Waddington
Consultant
Medical Group Management Association
Englewood, Colorado

Frederick J. Wenzel
Formerly, Executive Director and
  Chief Executive Officer
Medical Group Management Association
Englewood, Colorado

Suzanne S. White
Research Project Director
MGMA/CRAHCA
Englewood, Colorado

Stephen J. Williams, Sc.D.
Professor and Head
Division of Health Services Administration
Graduate School of Public Health
San Diego State University
San Diego, California

CONTENTS

PART THREE

OPERATIONS MANAGEMENT   155

PART FOUR

HUMAN RESOURCES MANAGEMENT   227

PART FIVE

PLANNING FOR AND MARKETING THE GROUP PRACTICE   271

PART SIX

FOREWORD

Our nation's health care system presents us with tremendous challenges and opportunities in our quest for improved health and well-being. Increasingly, those managing the ambulatory care resources of the system are in the forefront of those challenges, seeking a more effective provision of health care for all Americans. The rapid rate of change in medicine and the underlying strengths of our technology and knowledge mandate that we efficiently deliver services throughout our nation. The education of those who assume this responsibility, the ambulatory care administrators, is of vital importance to our overall success in health care.

The third edition of this book delivers the knowledge and management techniques that our health care administrators need in today's challenging world. The contributors to this edition have succeeded in bringing together a thoroughly up-to-date collection of integrated topics, all of which are of vital importance in assisting administrators to perform their challenging and central role in the provision of health care.

New material on managed health care, financial management, integrated systems, the law, and research augment the book's content. Case studies help the reader think pragmatically about the challenges of ambulatory care management. Taken together, the chapters of this book present perhaps the most complete yet concise treatment of management information available for the practitioner and student alike.

I am pleased to recognize the participation of the contributors to this third edition, of the Medical Group Management Association, cosponsor of the book, and of the editors in bringing this publication to the field of practice. I hope that the information contained in the book will be of assistance to those who bear the burdens of managing our increasingly complex, but vitally important, health care system.

James S. Todd, M.D.
Executive Vice President
American Medical Association
Chicago, IL

PREFACE

How dramatically our nation's health care system has changed since the last edition of this book was published! Continued growth in group practice and technological and delivery system innovations have accelerated the shift of services from the inpatient to the outpatient arena. Indeed, the entire landscape of health care has changed nationwide with the rapid growth of managed care.

Ambulatory care services have assumed a central role in the operation of the health care system, promoted by managed care as a key control point for health services delivery. No longer only a modality for delivering care, but now also a means of controlling care, ambulatory care services have moved to center stage.

Now everyone wants to get into the act. Institutional providers, who used to view outpatient services as an afterthought, now realize the error of their ways. Health care networks, employers, insurers, and providers themselves realize the power of control inherent in the doctor's office.

While we may not be happy with all the fundamental changes occurring, there is no doubt that the organization of health care services will not return to that of days gone by. While the pendulum is always in motion, cost pressures and a quest for greater efficiency and efficacy in the system suggest that the pendulum will remain tilted toward the side of greater integration and control.

Although the dramatic changes in ambulatory care services that have occurred since the previous edition of this book was published mandate considerable changes in the book's content, the purposes of the book remain the same. This book is intended to serve two primary markets. The first is the practitioner seeking to gain insight and up-to-date knowledge about the function of the ambulatory care practice and the key duties of the administrator. The second is the student of health services administration or a related field, seeking an in-depth and comprehensive introduction to the field and to the principles of management, information that is necessary for an administrator to be successful. The knowledge base necessary to function in this field becomes more encyclopedic every year. As a result, the scope of topics and depth of coverage in the chapters that follow are now greater than ever.

As in the past, this book continues to be oriented more toward the field of practice than to academia. The book represents a practical guide to the issues faced every day by ambulatory care administrators throughout our nation. Taking an analytical approach, the chapters of this book are designed to provoke thoughtful appraisal of the many issues that challenge the administrator, as well as to provide practical information useful to the daily tasks at hand. The book is geared to all ambulatory care administrators regardless of setting, particularly as the challenges become more common across all institutional settings. The book is also designed for use by all administrators, including physicians and other clinicians.

The content of the book is divided into six functional areas. Part One sets the scene. Chapter 1 provides an historical overview of the development of health services and ambulatory care in the United States, including quantitative data that reflect the growth of the nation's health care system. Chapter 2 describes the legal and organizational environment within which ambulatory care services are provided. Part Two of the book, presented in five chapters, lays out in detail the components of the financial management of ambulatory care. Chapter 3 presents the basic principles of financial management, Chapter 4 deals with financial planning for operations, Chapter 5 focuses on evaluating and controlling operations, Chapter 6 covers short-term and long-term financial decision making, and Chapter 7 discusses physician compensation systems, an important topic in today's world of financial incentives. This entire section of the book is completely new and reflects the realities of the increasingly competitive health care market and of managed care.

Part Three discusses the operational issues of running a practice. Chapter 8 presents an updated overview of the design and operation of physical facilities, Chapter 9 addresses important issues relating to communication systems, and Chapter 10 presents critical information on management support systems. The increasingly important issues related to information and computer systems are the subject of Chapter 11. All four of these chapters are completely revised or new contributions.

Part Four of the book addresses human resources management issues that are key to employee supervision and management, physician involvement, and other important aspects of managing the people side of the business. Chapter 12 examines physician issues, and Chapter 13 focuses on the administrative roles of the administrator and the physician executive. Chapter 14 addresses managing the employee, and Chapter 15 covers managing the patient and patient relations.

Part Five focuses on issues of planning for and marketing the group practice. Chapter 16 addresses strategic planning issues, and Chapter 17 focuses on marketing.

Part Six, the concluding section, addresses issues of policy and other institutional matters. Chapter 18 discusses many of the institutional issues that confront ambulatory care administrators today. Chapter 19 is an essential look at managed care and its implications for ambulatory care administrators. In the same vein, Chapter 20 addresses the issues of integrated health care systems as they pertain to the role of group practice administrators and the need for alliances to promote practice survival. Finally, Chapter 21 examines the role of health services research in ambulatory care practice and the potential contributions of various forms of research to the increasingly analytical content of the administrator's job.

As in previous editions, case studies are presented throughout the text where useful to illustrate the issues and problems faced in day-to-day management. The case studies are intended to educate the student, further prepare the administrator, place the textbook in a realistic context, and offer opportunities to readers to think about how they would react if faced with various problems. To assure that the case studies are realistic, they were drawn from the authors' personal experiences as administrators or consultants. The case studies also form the basis for useful dialogue between administrators and students.

Although the book provides a tremendous amount of information regarding the field of ambulatory care management, it is in reality only a starting point. Each individual must work to develop the skills and expertise required to survive and prosper in an increasingly competitive environment. Professional administrators must constantly seek out new knowledge and information, improve their own performance, and gain a personal and professional competitive advantage for their physicians and their practices.

Now more than ever, the challenge of being an administrator in the field of ambulatory care is growing dramatically. We hope that our readers, due to the contributions in this book, will enter the fray better prepared to promote their own professional growth and help improve health care services for all Americans.

Austin Ross
Stephen J. Williams
Ernest J. Pavlock

ACKNOWLEDGMENTS

This book has been prepared with the invaluable assistance of the Medical Group Management Association (MGMA) of Denver, Colorado. MGMA is the national professional association of ambulatory care administrators, and it has been a leader in developing the field of practice. The authors of this book have worked with MGMA for many years and in a number of capacities, and they encourage all administrators to become familiar with the services that MGMA provides.

Many of our colleagues and students have helped in the preparation of this book by reviewing and commenting on portions of the text. We thank them for their time and their expertise. In a sense, this book is a synthesis of their knowledge as well as that of the editors and contributors.

Portions of Chapters 3 through 6 were adapted with permission from Ernest J. Pavlock's book, *Financial Management for Medical Groups,* published by MGMA. Chapter 9 includes material reprinted with permission from Sandra Matherly and Shannon Hodges, *Telephone Nursing: The Process* (1992), published by the Center for Research in Ambulatory Care Administration, 104 Inverness Terrace East, Englewood, CO 80112-5306 (303-799-1111).

Finally, although many people helped in preparing the manuscript, we are especially appreciative of the assistance of Dru Jepperson for manuscript preparation.

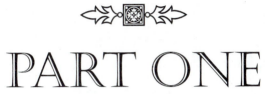

PART ONE

THE ENVIRONMENTAL CONTEXT FOR AMBULATORY CARE

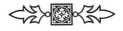

CHAPTER

1

An Overview of Health Care

Stephen J. Williams

CHAPTER TOPICS

Overview of Health Services
Overview of Ambulatory Care
Group Practice
Institutionally Based Ambulatory Services
The Management Role in Organizing and Operating
the System
Alternative Challenges for the Future

LEARNING OBJECTIVES

Upon completing this chapter, the reader should be able to:

- Appreciate the principal trends in health care in the United States during this century
- Understand the role of ambulatory care services in health care
- Understand the scope of group practice
- Appreciate the tremendous role of management in ambulatory care

Ambulatory services, or services for the "walking patient" (Roemer, 1981), are the backbone of the health care system. Although inpatient hospital services receive more public attention, most people have contact with the health care system through the highly diverse and widely distributed system of ambulatory care providers.

The health care delivery system, and ambulatory services especially, have changed dramatically over the past few years. Major trends include the development of new and often less invasive technologies, increasing consolidation of the health care system, greater emphasis on ambulatory as opposed to inpatient services, and dramatic expansion in the types and extent of use of managed care. This book addresses the way these changes affect the management of ambulatory care services. Historical trends in, and current status of, the nation's health care system, and ambulatory care services in particular, introduce this chapter, which sets the stage for the rest of the book.

This chapter outlines ambulatory care services in the United States and the managing and organizing roles of the administrator of ambulatory care services. The first part of the chapter provides an overview of ambulatory care services in the United States. The second part presents a parallel overview of the administrator's role in organizing and managing these services. The management functions reviewed here are expanded upon in the chapters that follow.

This chapter pays particular attention to quantitative measures of trends in health services delivery, especially those involving system performance and allocation of resources. An analytical approach is essential for making rational public policy decisions and assessing an individual institution's appropriate response to its marketplace. Only through an understanding of the whole system of health care can one hope to organize and efficiently manage the individual parts of the system. Thus, the administrator must keep the "big picture" in mind when applying the detailed technical skills that constitute the management role in health care.

OVERVIEW OF HEALTH SERVICES

It is difficult to understand the role of ambulatory care services without knowledge of the historical development of the health care system. The health care system in the United States evolved over many years, most dramatically since the Second World War. Perhaps the period of most startling change was the 1980s (Iglehart, 1992), although the future may be even more exciting and challenging than the past.

Part of the evolution of the health care system reflects changes in the role of the physician. The physician's role used to be predominantly one of patient supporter, occasionally including palliative therapy and very occasionally effective curative interventions. Today, due to medical advances, the physician's role is primarily to treat symptoms and cure diseases.

The health care system has also been affected by changes in the nature of disease in human populations. In the past, infectious diseases afflicted humans on a worldwide scale. The great epidemic diseases included bubonic plague, smallpox, diphtheria, typhoid, and syphilis. It has been estimated that during the 1300s alone, bubonic plague killed more than 13 million people in China, much of the population of India, 50,000 people in Paris, up to 90 percent of the population of some parts of France, and half the population of England.

The North American continent during these years had a rural and dispersed native population that was, therefore, less susceptible to the spread of disease. North America was also relatively protected from contamination by its geographic isolation. The United States has not been immune to epidemics of infectious disease, however. In the nineteenth and early twentieth centuries, the country was faced with epidemics of sizable proportions from a variety of diseases. For example, during the middle 1800s, cholera took more than 5,000 lives in New York, and yellow fever killed more than 15,000 people in New Orleans (Torrens, 1993).

The most significant factor in the control of infectious disease for most of our recent history has not been the fantastic technological advances in medical science of the twentieth century but the public health and environmental interventions of the late nineteenth and early twentieth centuries. These interventions remain a vital contributor to human health today.

Chronic diseases gained in prominence during the second half of the twentieth century. Whereas the major causes of death in 1900 were pneumonia, influenza, tuberculosis, and diarrhea, the major causes of death in recent years have been diseases of the heart, followed by malignancies, cerebrovascular disease, and accidents. Other causes include influenza, pneumonia, suicide, homicide, diabetes mellitus, certain diseases of infancy, arteriosclerosis, cirrhosis of the liver, bronchitis, emphysema, and asthma. Acquired immunodeficiency syndrome (AIDS) is also an important cause of death today in some age groups.

The dramatic changes that have occurred in health care in the United States since 1850 are summarized in Table 1–1. Increasing use of technology has meant that physicians can no longer carry their full complement of tools in a little black bag. More and more, care providers need the types of institutional support available in either the office or the hospital.

National Health Expenditures

The increasing use of technology and new types of health care personnel have led, in combination with the increasing size of the population, to a rapid growth in the costs of medical care. Table 1–2 shows the dramatic growth in national health expenditures since 1960. Note the increasing cost to federal, state, and local governments of health care services, which started with the

TABLE 1–1 Major Trends in the Development of Health Care in the United States, 1850 to Present

Trends	1850–1900	1900 to World War II	World War II to Present	Future
Predominant health problems of the American people	Epidemics of acute infections	Acute events, trauma, or infections affecting individuals, not groups	Chronic diseases such as heart disease, cancer, and stroke	Chronic diseases, particularly emotional and behaviorally related conditions
Technology available to handle predominant health problems	Virtually none	Beginning and rapid growth of basic medical sciences and technology	Explosive growth of medical sciences; technology captures the health care system	Continued growth and expansion of technology, with attempts to repersonalize the technology
Social organization for the use of technology	None; individuals left to their own resources or charity	Beginning societal and governmental efforts to care for those who could not care for themselves	Health care as a right; governmental responsibility to organize and monitor health care for everyone	Greater centralization of responsibility and control in federal government; greater use of organized systems of health insurance and financing to shape and control developments within the health care system

SOURCE: P.R. Torrens (1993). Historical evolution and overview of health services in the United States. In *Introduction to health services*, 4th ed., ed by S.J. Williams & P.R. Torrens. New York: Delmar Publishers, Inc.

TABLE 1–2 Gross Domestic Product, National Health Expenditures, and Federal, State, and Local Government Health Expenditures: United States, Selected Years

Year	Gross Domestic Product (in billions)	National Health Expenditures			Federal Government Expenditures		State and Local Government Expenditures	
		Amount (in billions)	% of Gross Domestic Product	Amount per Capita	Health (in billions)	Health (as a % of total)	Health (in billions)	Health (as a % of total)
1960	$ 513.4	$ 27.1	5.3	$ 43	$ .9	3.1	$ 3.7	7.8
1970	1,010.7	74.3	7.4	346	17.8	8.5	9.9	7.8
1980	2,708.0	251.1	9.3	1,068	72.0	11.7	33.3	9.9
1994	6,931.3	949.4	13.7	3,510	303.6	19.4	117.2	13.8

SOURCE: National Center for Health Statistics, Health, United States, 1995. Hyattsville, MD: Public Health Service, 1996.

TABLE 1–3 Personal Health Care Expenditures and Percent Distribution, According to Source of Funds: United States, Selected Years

Year	Total (in billions)	Per Capita	Out-of-pocket Payments	Private Health Insurance	Other Private Funds	Federal Government	State and Local Governments
				Percent Distribution			
1950	10.9	70	65.5	9.1	2.9	10.4	12.0
1960	23.9	126	55.9	21.0	1.8	8.9	12.5
1970	64.8	302	39.1	23.6	2.5	22.7	12.0
1980	220.1	936	27.8	29.1	3.5	28.8	10.7
1994	831.7	3,074	21.0	32.1	3.4	33.7	9.8

SOURCE: National Center for Health Statistics, Health, United States, 1995. Hyattsville, MD: Public Health Service, 1996.

passage of the Great Society legislation in the 1960s. National health expenditures have increased both in absolute dollars and as a percentage of total gross domestic product. National health expenditures now total approximately one trillion dollars and over 14 percent of the gross domestic product, a world record.

Personal health expenditures, which include only direct costs for the provision of health care to individuals and exclude public health service, research, and construction costs, are shown in Table 1–3. The increasing health care burden on government is again illustrated by this table. Patient out-of-pocket payments account for only about one-fifth of all personal health care expenditures, and private health insurance accounts for only about one-third. Other private funds, such as

philanthropy, account for an even smaller percentage of expenditures.

Significant increases in the costs of health services have occurred in many areas, but especially in nursing home care, as shown in Table 1–4. Ambulatory care accounts for somewhat more than half of all health care expenditures. The percentage spent for drugs has declined, and recently costs for hospital care have dropped. Dental services expenditures also declined between 1960 and 1994.

Recent Trends in Disease and Longevity

Table 1–5 reflects the age-adjusted causes of death for the United States in 1950 and 1993. Significant

TABLE1–4 Percent Distribution of National Health Expenditures, According to Type of Expenditure: United States, Selected Years

Type of Expenditure	1960	1970	1980	1994
	Percent Distribution			
All expenditures	100.0	100.0	100.0	100.0
Health services and supplies	93.7	92.8	95.4	96.8
Personal health care	88.1	87.2	87.7	87.6
Hospital care	34.2	37.7	40.9	35.7
Physician services	19.5	18.3	18.0	19.9
Dentist services	7.2	6.3	5.3	4.4
Nursing home care	3.6	6.5	8.2	7.6
Other professional services	2.2	1.9	2.5	5.2
Home health care	0.2	0.2	0.8	2.8
Drugs, other medical durables	15.6	11.9	8.6	8.3
Vision products, other medical durables	3.0	2.7	1.8	1.4
Other personal health care	2.6	1.7	1.6	2.3
Program administration and net cost of health insurance	4.3	3.7	4.8	6.2
Government public health activities	1.4	1.9	2.9	3.0
Research and construction	6.3	7.2	4.6	3.2
Noncommercial research	2.6	2.6	2.2	1.7
Construction	3.7	4.6	2.5	1.5

SOURCE: National Center for Health Statistics. Health, United States, 1995. Hyattsville, MD: Public Health Service, 1996.

declines in death rates attributable to heart and cerebrovascular diseases, particularly stroke, are evident. On the other hand, mortality attributable to malignant neoplasms has not significantly improved in over 40 years, and new causes of death, particularly AIDS-related infections, have appeared. Our nation also experiences significant mortality due to motor vehicle accidents, suicide, and homicide.

Although overall age-adjusted death rates have dropped dramatically for the United States, there are numerous causes of mortality that do not respond to modern medical intervention, including mortality attributable to vehicular accidents, tobacco product consumption, and other behavioral and social causes. These causes of mortality are more difficult to tackle than those that are the subjects of most of our biomedical research.

Table 1–6 presents national mortality data as life expectancy from 1900 to 1994 for males and females and

for whites and blacks. Life expectancy at birth has increased significantly since the turn of the century and somewhat since World War II. Interestingly, life expectancy at age 65 has increased only somewhat over the past 25 years.

Life expectancy in Table 1–6 is computed as a total cohort experience, incorporating mortality at all ages of life. Reductions in infant and childhood mortality can greatly increase a population's overall life expectancy. Reductions in mortality at older ages, on the other hand, have far less effect on overall population life expectancy.

Allocation decisions regarding national health expenditures should target population subgroups that need improved health outcomes. Increases in infectious disease, particularly due to AIDS, and in violent deaths, including homicide, and vehicular accidents have had a tremendous adverse impact on life expectancy, particularly for middle-aged individuals, blacks, and males. Targeting these populations and their health and social

TABLE 1–5 Age Adjusted Death Rates for Selected Causes of Death, United States, 1950 and 1993

Cause of Death	1950	1993
	Deaths per 1,000 Resident Population	
All causes	840.5	513.3
Natural causes	766.6	459.7
Diseases of heart	307.2	145.3
Cerebrovascular diseases	88.6	26.5
Malignant neoplasms	125.3	132.6
Respiratory system	12.8	40.8
Colorectal	19.0	12.9
Prostate	13.4	16.4
Breast	22.2	21.5
Chronic obstructive pulmonary diseases	4.4	21.4
Pneumonia and influenza	26.2	13.5
Chronic liver disease and cirrhosis	8.5	7.9
Diabetes mellitus	14.3	12.4
Nephritis, nephrotic syndrome, and nephrosis	—	4.5
Septicemia	—	4.1
Human immuno-deficiency virus infection	—	13.8
External causes	73.9	53.6
Unintentional injuries	57.5	30.3
Motor vehicle crashes	23.3	16.0
Suicide	11.0	11.3
Homicide and legal intervention	5.4	10.7
Drug-induced causes	—	4.8
Alcohol-induced causes	—	6.7

SOURCE: National Center for Health Statistics, Health, United States, 1995. Hyattsville, MD: Public Health Service, 1996.

problems requires a broad public health perspective and an emphasis on education and population-based prevention programs.

OVERVIEW OF AMBULATORY CARE

There is no single, uniform definition for ambulatory care. Ambulatory care is difficult to define largely because of the diversity of practitioners, settings, and services that are included under this rubric. Some people refer to ambulatory care as all services for the walking patient. A working definition might be: ambulatory care encompasses all services provided to the noninstitutionalized patient.

Ambulatory care services are important because of their central role as the initial and continuing point of contact with the health care system for most people. Ambulatory care services are the major source of intake for patients who need health care. They also serve as the continuing point of contact for follow-up, routine, and ongoing care, and they perform a broker function by being the center of the referral network for more specialized services. These roles are especially visible in managed-care programs. In addition, ambulatory care services include most of the psychological support available for psychiatric, emotional, and social problems, except for the most severe cases.

An especially important component of ambulatory care is primary care. Primary care, especially in some managed-care programs, serves to provide coordination, rationalization, and rationing of health care (Starfield, 1992). The role of the primary care provider, while always central to the care process, has been increasing with an evolving responsibility for gatekeeping and coordinating care. Primary care is also typically provided to patients as a source of initial contact with the health care system and for ongoing maintenance. When properly organized, especially in more structured forms of managed care, primary care promotes continuity of care and allows for comprehensive services, with the primary care provider coordinating care for specialty services.

Historical Perspective on Ambulatory Care

Throughout history until the advent of institutional care, most "medical care" was provided on an ambulatory basis. Remarkable levels of medicine were practiced in Greece and Rome, and even tribal societies had their own indigenous practitioners. In more recent times in Europe and later in the United States, poor people were cared for in dispensaries and public clinics,

TABLE 1–6   Life Expectancy at Birth and at 65 Years of Age, According to Race and Sex: United States, Selected Years

Specified Age and Year	All races		White		Black	
	Male	*Female*	*Male*	*Female*	*Male*	*Female*
	Remaining Life Expectancy in Years					
At Birth						
1900	46.3	48.3	46.6	48.7	32.5	33.5
1950	65.6	71.1	66.5	72.2	58.9	62.7
1970	67.1	74.7	68.0	75.6	60.0	68.3
1994	72.3	79.0	73.0	79.6	64.7	74.1
At 65 Years						
1900	11.5	12.2	11.5	12.2	10.4	11.4
1950	12.8	15.0	12.8	15.1	12.9	14.9
1970	13.1	17.0	13.1	17.1	12.5	15.7
1994	15.5	18.9	—	—	—	—

SOURCE: National Center for Health Statistics. Health, United States, 1994. Hyattsville, MD: Public Health Service, 1995.

whereas wealthier people received care at home. As hospital care and the associated technology improved, patients of all social classes increasingly received both inpatient and outpatient care in hospital settings.

In the United States, ambulatory care services traditionally were provided by individual medical practitioners in their offices, patients' homes, and clinics. Physicians' offices often were located in their homes, as opposed to today's medical office building or large medical center. The general practitioner who made house calls, provided guidance, and offered whatever treatment was available was typical of the ambulatory care provider before the Second World War.

Since World War II, medical knowledge and specialization have changed both how and where services are provided. The explosion in technological advances in medicine, which started in the 1980s and continues today, probably represents a new era of biomedical progress. For ambulatory care managers, recent years are notable for the increasing emphasis on less invasive technologies and the dramatic shift from inpatient to outpatient services in many arenas of health care. Well over 60 percent of all surgical procedures are now performed on an outpatient basis, many drug therapies are provided at home, and postsurgical follow-up often consists of home care after discharge rather than longer hospital stays. The use of fiber-optic equipment in surgical procedures, for example, is expanding at an incredibly rapid rate, now extending even to experimental use in coronary artery surgery. These trends are likely to continue, fueled by managed care.

Use of Ambulatory Care Services

The measurement and analysis of the use of ambulatory care resources are extremely important in defining the scope and content of this field. To the extent that quantitative data are available, planning for ambulatory care and analysis of patterns of use are essential for strategic planning, managed-care bidding, and other purposes. The availability of certain data bases and the relevance of health services research to practice management are addressed in detail in a later chapter.

Based on the most recent federal data available from the National Health Interview Survey, which involves a national random sample of Americans, the average citizen experiences approximately six physician contacts annually, with the highest usage occurring for children

TABLE 1–7 Physician Contacts, According to Age: United States, 1994

	Physician Contacts per Person
Total	6.0
Age Group	
Under 15 years	4.6
Under 5 years	6.8
5–14 years	3.4
15–44 years	5.0
45–64 years	7.3
65 years and over	11.3
65–74 years	10.3
75 years and over	12.7

SOURCE: National Center for Health Statistics. Health, United States, 1995. Hyattsville, MD: Public Health Service, 1996.

and older Americans. These data are shown in Table 1–7. Over all ages, as well as for most individual age categories, females utilize more physician services than males do. The aging of the United States population suggests a trend toward higher utilization of these and other health care services in the future.

Additional data from the same survey indicate that most Americans, and particularly those in the middle and older ages and females, contact a physician at least once per year. As shown in Table 1–8, the majority of physician contacts occurs in offices. Lower income people and minorities obtain more care in emergency rooms, a reflection of access and income differentials.

National Ambulatory Care Survey

Although there is limited information available on the practice patterns of solo practitioners in the United States, on ongoing national study of all private office-based physicians, the National Ambulatory Medical Care Survey (NAMCS), is conducted by the federal government. The study reflects the nature of office-based practice.

The NAMCS involves a random sample of the nation's office-based, nonfederal physicians, who are asked to complete a data collection form for each patient treated during a two-week period. The principal reasons for physician visits in this survey include general

medical exams, well-mother and well-baby exams, post-operative visits, and upper respiratory infections. The high ranking of routine care, follow-up or ongoing care, and care for relatively simple problems is striking, reflecting the predominance of these types of care in office-based practice. Overall, more than half the visits require a follow-up visit. Nearly all the visits last less than 30 minutes, and almost half the visits last 15 minutes or less.

GROUP PRACTICE

Group practice is an affiliation of providers, usually physicians, who share incomes, expenses, facilities, equipment, medical records, and support personnel in the provision of services through a formal, legally constituted organization. Traditionally, group practice has primarily involved physicians. Increasingly, dentists, optometrists, and other specialized personnel are also developing group practices.

History of Group Practice

Some of the earliest group practices in the United States were started by businesses to provide care to employees at rural sites where medical care was unavailable. For example, the Northern Pacific Railroad organized a practice in 1883 to provide care for its employees who were building the Transcontinental Railroad.

Even more significant was the establishment of the Mayo Clinic in Rochester, Minnesota. This was the first successful nonindustrial group practice. The Mayo Clinic, originally organized as a single-specialty practice in 1887 and later broadened into a multispecialty practice, demonstrated that group practice was feasible in the private sector. The Mayo Clinic also represented a reputable model for group practice in a national atmosphere of fierce independence, where group practice was viewed with skepticism and distrust. By the early 1930s, there were approximately 150 medical groups throughout the United States, with many located in the Midwest. Most included, or were started by, someone who had practiced or trained at the Mayo Clinic.

In 1931, a national committee that was established to assess medical care needs for the United States, the

TABLE 1–8   Physician Contacts, According to Place of Contact and Selected Patient Characteristics: United States, 1994

	Place of Contact (percentage of visits)				
Characteristic	*Doctor's Office*	*Hospital Outpatient Department*	*Telephone*	*Home*	*Other*
Total	56.8	13.6	13.2	3.5	12.8
Age Group					
Under 15 years	60.6	13.1	14.3	0.8	11.1
Under 5 years	59.2	12.7	15.4	0.9	11.8
5–14 years	62.1	13.5	13.1	0.8	10.5
15–44 years	55.7	14.1	13.1	1.8	15.2
45–64 years	55.1	15.0	14.2	3.6	12.2
65 years and over	53.4	10.1	8.6	18.6	9.3
65–74 years	55.4	11.9	9.4	12.4	10.9
75 years and over	51.1	7.9	7.8	25.8	7.4
Sex					
Male	55.4	15.6	11.7	3.5	13.9
Female	57.7	12.2	14.3	3.5	12.2
Race					
White	58.4	12.2	14.1	3.3	11.8
Black	47.9	20.3	8.1	4.2	19.4
Family income					
Less than $14,000	43.9	19.0	11.9	5.7	19.5
$14,000–$24,999	53.8	16.6	13.0	3.9	12.7
$25,000–$34,999	61.5	12.1	12.7	2.0	11.6
$35,000–$49,999	56.9	11.6	16.3	3.9	11.2
$50,000 or more	63.8	9.4	15.5	1.6	9.8
Geographic region					
Northeast	59.0	13.0	12.8	4.0	11.2
Midwest	55.8	14.0	15.1	2.2	12.9
South	58.4	14.0	12.5	4.3	10.8
West	54.1	13.5	12.8	3.2	16.5

SOURCE: National Center for Health Statistics. Health, United States, 1995. Hyattsville, MD: Public Health Service, 1996.

Committee on the Costs of Medical Care, issued a report suggesting a major role for group practice in the provision of medical care. This committee recommended that group practices be associated with hospitals to provide comprehensive care and that all services be prepaid.

Other constituencies, including some unions, also developed group practices. After World War II especially, a number of pioneering groups were established. In New York City, the Health Insurance Plan of New York was organized to provide prepaid medical care to the employees of the city, an idea promoted by Mayor Fiorello La Guardia. In the West, the Kaiser Foundation Health Plans were established to provide health care to employees of Kaiser Industries; Kaiser is now an affiliation of plans and providers that serves millions of

Americans. In Seattle, a revolutionary development was the establishment of Group Health Cooperative of Puget Sound, a consumer-owned, cooperative, prepaid group practice. It was founded in the late 1940s by progressive individuals who were dissatisfied with the private medical care available to them.

Developments in medical practice also spurred on the group practice movement. Perhaps most notable were the increasing specialization of medicine and the rapid expansion of technology. Increasing sophistication meant that no individual practitioner could provide all the expertise that patients required. It also meant that more complex and expensive facilities, equipment, and personnel were needed to care for patients. Group practice provided a formal structure for sharing these costs among providers. Many people felt that resources would be used more efficiently in groups. Multispecialty groups could also provide patients with more of their health care under one roof and thus reduce problems of physical access to care.

Group practice was thought to promote high-quality care, because most of the different specialists that a person required would be practicing together, giving the specialists the opportunity to discuss patient problems among themselves, share a common medical record, and assure the quality and continuity of care. Group practice also offered advantages to the physician, such as easily developed referral arrangements, sharing of after-hours coverage, more flexibility in working hours, and less financial risk.

Despite these advantages, group practice was not without opponents. Opposition to group practice was mostly for political and philosophical reasons. The American Medical Association and local medical societies, for example, have at times opposed group practice. In addition, many early group practices had difficulties when physicians were denied privileges in local hospitals.

Survey of Group Practice

Since 1965, the American Medical Association has periodically conducted surveys of physician group practices in the United States. These surveys represent the most comprehensive data available concerning the growth and characteristics of group practice in this country. The most recent survey was conducted in 1992. Group practices meeting the American Medical Association's definition are identified from a variety of data sources and then surveyed by mail with a data-collection instrument. Numerous items of information are collected regarding the nature of the practice and its facilities.

The dramatic increase in the popularity of group practice is reflected in Tables 1–9 and 1–10. The number of group practices nearly doubled from 1975 to 1995. There are now more than 16,000 group practices

TABLE 1–9 Number of Medical Groups and Number of Physicians in Group Practice: United States, Selected Years

Year	Number of Groups	Number of Physicians in Group Practice
1969	6,371	40,093
1975	8,483	66,842
1980	10,762	88,290
1984	15,485	140,392
1988	16,579	155,628
1991	16,576	184,358
1995	19,478	210,811

SOURCE: P.L. Havlicek (1996). *Medical groups in the U.S., 1996 Edition: A survey of practice characteristics.* Chicago: American Medical Association.

TABLE 1–10 Total Number of Groups and Group Physicians by Size of Group, 1995

Group Size	Groups Number	Group Physicians Number
3–4	8,926	13,641
5–6	4,451	23,929
7–9	2,453	19,001
10–15	1,714	20,337
16–25	943	18,576
26–49	527	18,063
50–75	157	9,378
76–99	69	5,815
100 or more	238	64,770

SOURCE: P.L. Havlicek (1996). *Medical groups in the U.S., 1996 Edition: A survey of practice characteristics.* Chicago: American Medical Association.

in the United States, two-thirds of which are single-specialty groups.

Managed Care and Group Practice

Table 1–11 reflects the growth in health maintenance organizations from 1980 through 1995. Significant growth in almost all types of plans has occurred, with dramatic increases in the number of individuals currently enrolled in these plans (Nelson, 1987). Other forms of managed care add to the total numbers enrolled in managed care.

The development of managed care and its impact on group practice operations are the subjects of many chapters in this book. Managed care, strategic alliances, various forms of contracting, and other market-driven changes in the health care system form the fundamental impetus for new approaches to the operation of ambulatory care services in the future. With the great variety of managed-care alternatives, as discussed in other chapters of this book, specific strategies and operational considerations may vary greatly from practice to practice. Furthermore, the specific combination of alliances, partnerships, managed-care contracts, and other arrangements in which a practice engages can increase the complexity of the ambulatory care environment for the administrator. All of these considerations are discussed in detail in subsequent chapters of this book.

TABLE 1–11 Health Maintenance Organizations and Enrollment According to Model Type, Geographic Region, and Federal Program: United States, Selected Years

Plans and Enrollment	1980	1990	1995
Plans (number by type)			
All plans	235	572	550
Model type			
Individual practice assn.	97	360	323
Group	138	212	107
Mixed	—	—	120
Geographic region			
Northeast	55	115	99
Midwest	72	160	154
South	45	176	190
West	63	121	107
Enrollment (millions)			
Total	9.1	33.0	46.2
Model type			
Individual practice assn.	1.7	13.7	17.4
Group	7.4	19.3	12.9
Mixed	—	—	15.9
Federal program			
Medicaid	0.3	1.2	3.5
Medicare	0.4	1.8	2.9

SOURCE: National Center for Health Statistics, Health, United States, 1995. Hyattsville, MD: Public Health Service, 1996.

INSTITUTIONALLY BASED AMBULATORY SERVICES

The hospital has evolved from an institution for poor people who could not be cared for at home to a provider of a full range of health services, from primary to tertiary care. As technological advances have brought more services into the hospital and expanded the scope of care provided, the hospital has assumed an especially important role in providing highly complex health services (Stevens, 1989). At the same time, an increasing number of people have sought primary care from hospitals, sometimes as a result of lack of access to other sources of care.

The increased demands for care placed on hospitals taxed the ability of many facilities to respond with appropriate and adequate resources. This resulted in overcrowded facilities; the wrong mix of services, equipment, and personnel to respond to patient needs; and extremely dissatisfied consumers and providers. Most hospitals have now successfully responded to these demands by expanding outpatient services and hiring full-time providers to staff redesigned hospital ambulatory facilities. Hospitals with ambulatory care resources can negotiate contracts to provide a wide range of both inpatient and outpatient services. They are also able to control the use of services, and thus costs, more effectively. Competition in ambulatory care has led to integration of services, construction of medical office buildings, joint ventures, development of health plans, purchases of medical practices, and other activities.

Ambulatory Surgery Centers

An important innovation has been the development of ambulatory surgery centers. Originating in hospitals in Rhode Island, Washington, D.C., Los Angeles, and elsewhere, these organized hospital units provide one-day surgical care. Patients are usually first screened for acceptability by their personal surgeons and then asked to report at an assigned date and time for surgery. The surgeon is supported by the unit's facilities, equipment, and personnel, and the patient is discharged from one to three hours after surgery, when recovery from anesthesia is sufficiently complete.

In the early 1970s, freestanding ambulatory surgery centers were opened, of which one of the first was in Phoenix, Arizona. These facilities are independent of hospitals and usually provide a full range of services for the types of surgery that can be performed on an out-patient basis. Community surgeons are granted operating privileges and can perform surgery in these facilities when the patient agrees and when there are no medical contraindications.

Other facilities are also used for ambulatory or out-patient surgery. In the past, many physicians performed surgery in their offices, although this practice has declined in some specialties as a result of malpractice concerns and the increasingly availability of better equipped and better staffed facilities. Physicians in some specialties, however, such as oral surgery, plastic surgery, and ophthalmology, still use office-based facilities extensively.

The shift of health services to the ambulatory care arena, which has accelerated in recent years, enhances the critical role of group practice management in putting together an increasingly integrated health care system for managed care and other contracting arrangements. Surgical services and other related care, such as home infusion services, are increasingly provided outside the inpatient arena, shifting control to the ambu-

latory care practice. Surgical technology is continuing to advance with wider application of fiber-optic equipment, suggesting that, in the future, more and more care will be provided outside of hospitals.

Experimental approaches to coronary bypass surgery, which use far less invasive techniques, may represent the greatest challenge to traditional hospital inpatient services. Other new modalities of care, ranging from telemedicine to mobile imaging facilities, imply a future that is increasingly focused on the role of ambulatory rather than inpatient services. These innovations, combined with financial pressures from more stringent managed-care arrangements and government entitlement programs, suggest that these trends will accelerate in the future.

THE MANAGEMENT ROLE IN ORGANIZING AND OPERATING THE SYSTEM

The ambulatory care/group practice administrator is principally responsible for running the "system." The challenge of this responsibility is reflected by the immense array of duties reviewed in the remainder of this chapter and discussed in detail throughout the rest of this book.

Management of the operations of a practice has now moved toward a greater focus on productivity and efficiency; the utilization of information systems for management control and financial planning; and the development of strategic alliances, contracting, and managed-care arrangements. At the same time, managers face a continuation of traditional managerial functions, such as personnel administration, facilities planning and operation, and the like. All of these topics are covered extensively in other chapters of this book.

The external context within which the practice now operates is changing rapidly. This is exemplified by increased practice participation in various managed-care arrangements. Systems for enhancing accountability, such as management information systems for financial control and planning, are mandated by payers. A number of chapters of this book focus on these larger issues and their implications for ambulatory care and group practice management.

More than ever, the practice administrator must monitor the internal operations of the practice. At the same time, the manager must adapt to, and aggressively pursue, opportunities and challenges created by the evolution of the health care marketplace. As health services move increasingly toward a corporate model, with enhanced competitiveness, accountability, and market responsiveness, the manager must be more oriented toward producing the product, as in manufacturing and service industries. It is hoped that the pendulum will not swing so far in this direction that the human side of health care, the quality of care, the realities of patients' lives, and fundamental questions of survival are lost in the equation. As accountability to all constituencies has increased, the manager faces a starker and in many ways more threatening reality (Blair & Fottler, 1990).

Characteristics of Client-Oriented and Well-Managed Practices

There are a number of established, generally accepted principles for determining whether ambulatory care services are well organized and effective in meeting the needs of patients (Benson & Townes, 1990). Services can be assessed from the perspective of the payer community, the client or patient, or the provider. The extent to which an individual institution or organization views its own health care services from the community or client perspective varies considerably, in part depending on its degree of accountability to the population served, governing structure, and responsiveness to the marketplace.

Accountability to clients can be effected through ownership, governance, or economic, political, social, or ethical pressures. In the increasingly competitive health care arena in which services are now provided, it is important for most ambulatory care organizations to consider both community and client perspectives in the design of optimal health care systems.

The ability to attract and keep patients is dependent in part on the administrator's success in recognizing the client's perspective. Even in managed-care systems, patient satisfaction and retention are important. Among the desirable features of ambulatory care organizations,

from the client's perspective, is the assurance of accessible care and pleasant physical surroundings. The ambience of a practice correlates to a remarkable degree with patient satisfaction.

Access to services includes more than physical access. The availability of services must be assured in terms of hours of operation, after-hours coverage, and availability of consultation and referrals. Accepted criteria for designing ambulatory care systems suggest that practices should assume organizational responsibility for the well-being of their patients 24 hours a day, seven days a week. More tightly controlled managed-care environments enhance this attribute to decrease out-of-plan use (Shouldice, 1991).

Efficient scheduling of patients also contributes to a higher degree of client satisfaction and more efficient facility operations. Scheduling is often a difficult and imprecise activity. The development of scheduling and appointment systems that minimize patient waiting times and maximize the efficient use of personnel and other resources is essential. This subject is discussed further in a later chapter.

Access to care requires, in addition, that patients have adequate financial resources to purchase care. These resources can be obtained from the patient's own finances, government entitlement programs, or third-party insurance coverage and employers. In managed care, budgeting dollars for patient care demands a rationalization of the care process. Incentives for providers and patients must assure that resources are well managed. Indeed, efficient use of resources is a key objective of managed care.

Any ambulatory care practice must balance the realities of the financial operations of the practice with the needs of patients and their ability to pay for care. Philosophies and practical approaches to meet the health care requirements of poor patients are needed in every practice. Otherwise, attempts to control costs through managed care, coupled with funding reductions, may place poorer patients and local governments at increasing peril (Kongstvedt, 1989).

The quality of medical care involves far more than the level of technical services provided. Patient perceptions of ambulatory care services are frequently linked to the ambience of the physical facilities, as mentioned above, and to the success of one-to-one patient-provider interactions. Clients consider services of high quality when they are associated with a caring, concerned staff that is courteous and aware of patient needs and sensitivities.

High-quality services also require continuity and coordination of care. Continuity and coordination of care, in turn, require the development of referral systems, various forms of gatekeepers and primary care providers, scheduling and triage, timely access to needed care, and patient follow-up (Smith, 1995). Continuity and coordination are also supported by medical records that link patients with their own personal practitioners and by the organization's assumption of overall responsibility for patients.

Obviously not all ambulatory care organizations achieve the same level of continuity, coordination, and comprehensiveness of services, but the tenets of good medical practice now dictate an awareness of these issues and a conscientious attempt to address them wherever possible. Managed-care providers probably have the greatest degree of competitive advantage in these respects.

Services must also be assured with respect to the technical quality of care provided, which can be measured in three ways. First, the quality of care can be measured by the structure of the provider organization, such as controls over medical staff hiring. Second, quality can be measured by the process of care, through such indicators as the number and appropriateness of tests and procedures performed and the extent to which patients are followed up or referred to appropriate specialty care. Third, quality can be measured by the outcome of care, through such indicators as reductions in morbidity and mortality. The quality of care provided is also a function of the coordination, continuity, and comprehensiveness of care; the ambience of the practice; availability of multilingual staff, if appropriate; physical access for the handicapped; pleasant interpersonal relationships; and many other factors.

From the perspective of operating an efficient and profitable practice, there are many additional criteria that must be recognized. The work environment engendered by the practice and its management should represent a pleasant and humane surrounding that contributes to employee morale and enthusiasm. Each practitioner and staff member should have a well-defined and appropriate role in the practice, should be evaluated regularly and provided with incentives and encouragement, and should be treated fairly and with dignity and respect. Duties assigned to individuals should match their skills and training.

To maintain esprit de corps, all employees should be compensated adequately, and incentives should be available to encourage productivity, efficiency, good patient relations, and efficient internal operations. These incentives should be available to physician and non-physician employees alike. Balancing these incentives with the delivery of care is a challenge in many managed-care environments.

The use of equipment and facilities should also maximize productivity and efficiency. Technological resources should be used to improve the quality of care, increase productivity, and contribute to the economic well-being of the practice. Information systems are now vital to practice management, monitoring of care, and participation in managed care. Inappropriate use of personnel, capital, finances, and technological capabilities is symptomatic of poor management, lack of controls, and waste of health care resources.

Financial pressures from managed-care arrangements and restrictions in funding for government entitlement programs have also contributed to enhancement in productivity, coordination of care, rationing, and integration of health services. Quality-of-care issues remain an important concern, but bottom-line trade-offs have increasingly moved to the forefront of decision making and public policy. As a result, increasing rationalization of services, application of critical guidelines and algorithms, integration of information systems to monitor and control the delivery of services, and other innovations and trends have assumed a more central role in the operation of the health care system. Each ambulatory care practice is affected by these trends, although the nature and extent of the impact varies greatly, depending on the prevalence of managed care and other arrangements as well as on the nature of the practice itself.

The proper management of an ambulatory care practice requires that all supporting systems, ranging from facility operations to patient medical records, be constantly monitored and updated to meet ever-changing needs. The management of the physical, financial, and human resources of the practice and the operation of the patient care services and management support systems are the responsibility of the ambulatory care administrator. Monitoring the constantly evolving health care scene, keeping up with competition, and moving the practice forward require competent leadership on the part of the administrator and the medical director, as well as an aggressive, ongoing process of strategic management (Hillestad & Berkowitz, 1991).

ALTERNATIVE CHALLENGES FOR THE FUTURE

It should be obvious that ambulatory care management is a highly complex job requiring a wide range of knowledge, skills, and experiences. The scope and diversity of the administrator's role, given his or her ultimate responsibility for the success of the practice, require a staggering array of talents. In addition, dealing with the community and other external organizations, while satisfying the demands of the medical staff, may strain the mental health of even the most capable and enthusiastic individual.

Specific operational considerations in ambulatory care management that are pertinent to the future development of the health care system and to the role of the administrator are discussed in the remaining chapters of this book. Strategic alliances, managed care, the changing financial landscape, new considerations in the legal and physical environments, changes in strategic planning approaches and concerns, and many other considerations provide a critical focus for these chapters (Burns & Thorpe, 1993; Coddington et al., 1993). Their purpose is to alert the ambulatory care administrator to the ever-changing and challenging role that he or she plays in the provision of health care services to our nation.

REFERENCES

Benson, D. S., & Townes, P. G. (1990). *Excellence in ambulatory care.* San Francisco: Jossey-Bass Publishers.

Blair, J. D., & Fottler, M. D. (1990). *Challenges in health care management: Strategic perspectives for managing key stockholders.* San Francisco: Jossey-Bass Publishers.

Burns, L. R., & Thorpe, D. P. (1993). Trends and models in physician-hospital organization. *Health Care Management Review, 18*(4), 7–20.

Coddington, D. C., Moore, D. D., & Fischer, E. A. (1993). Integrated health care systems: The key characteristics. *Medical Group Management Journal,* (Nov/Dec), 76–80.

Havlicek, P. L. (1996). *Medical groups in the U.S., 1996 Edition: A survey of practice characteristics.* Chicago: American Medical Association.

Hillestad, S. G., & Berkowitz, E. N. (1991). *Health care marketing plans* (2nd ed.). Gaithersburg, MD: Aspen Publishers.

Iglehart, J. K. (1992). The American health care system: Introduction. *New England Journal of Medicine, 326,* 962–67.

Kongstvedt, P. R. (1989). *The managed health care handbook.* Gaithersburg, MD: Aspen Publishers.

National Center for Health Statistics (1996). *Health, United States, 1995.* Hyattsville, MD: Public Health Service.

Nelson, J. A. (1987). The history and spirit of the HMO movement. *HMO Practice, 1,* 75–82.

Roemer, M. I. (1981). *Ambulatory health services in America.* Rockville, MD: Aspen Systems Corporation.

Shouldice, R. G. (1991). *Introduction to managed care.* Arlington, VA: Information Resource Press.

Smith, S. (1995). The impact of an ambulatory care firm system on quality and continuity of care. *Medical Care, 33,* 221–26.

Starfield, B. (1992). *Primary care: Concept, evaluation and policy.* New York: Oxford University Press.

Stevens, R. (1989). *In sickness and in wealth: American hospitals in the 20th century.* New York: Basic Books.

Torrens, P. R. (1993). Historical evaluation and overview of health services in the United States. In S. J. Williams & P. R. Torrens (Eds.), *Introduction to health services,* (4th ed., pp. 3–28). New York: Delmar Publishers, Inc.

CHAPTER

Legal and Organizational Issues of Ambulatory Care Organizations

Mitchell J. Olejko

CHAPTER TOPICS

Overview of the Legal Issues
Legal Structures
Key Legal Characteristics
Organizational and Management Issues
Operational Issues
Challenges for the Future

LEARNING OBJECTIVES

Upon completing this chapter, the reader should be able to:

- Identify the different types of legal organizations commonly encountered in ambulatory care situations
- Outline the attributes of a variety of legal entities
- Describe and discuss the advantages and disadvantages of a number of different legal entities
- Identify and discuss other legal issues commonly encountered in the management of health care organizations

The legal and organizational context of health care entities is of increasing importance. The complex issues affecting the interaction of the laws that govern our economy and how they control, impact, and modify health care management in ambulatory care is the focus of this chapter.

OVERVIEW OF LEGAL ISSUES

For better or worse, all health care organizations, including ambulatory care organizations, are subject to increasing direct regulation by state and federal governments. Perhaps more important, the number and scope of legal issues that management must identify and take into account have grown at a seemingly exponential rate.

Legal concerns in health care range from basic issues regarding the legal organization of group practice to the legal implications of day-to-day management actions, such as billing, contracting, and special projects. One of the responsibilities of a manager is to identify, assess, and address these legal issues properly. The manager should know when to seek the counsel of lawyers and how to use lawyers in assisting management to achieve the goals of the practice.

The manner of addressing these legal concerns varies from organization to organization. Some organizations are large enough to justify employing lawyers as part of the management team. More typically, an organization has continuing relationships with independent lawyers who are called on by management when the need arises to provide general and specialty services to the organization.

LEGAL STRUCTURES

The choice of legal structure for an ambulatory care organization depends on a variety of factors, including the types of organizations permitted by state law, the nature of the organization's mission, the identify of the owners (in a proprietary organization), pension-planning requirements, and the perceived needs and goals of the organization. Some organizational structures result from historical accidents, others from the execution of plans developed after long study. In some cases, the management structure of the organization is driven by the legal structure; in other cases, it is organized without regard to, and perhaps in spite of, the specifics of the organization's legal structure.

Many commentators have stated that the legal structure of the large, modern corporation has resulted in alienating ownership from management, allowing management to ignore the needs or wishes of the owners (Conrad, 1981). This is not true of group practice organizations. The owners of a group practice are directly involved in providing services and, as such, can continually and closely evaluate management. Depending on the structure, owners are also able to direct the management of the organization.

The types of legal structures permissible for the organization of a group practice vary from state to state. The details of the rights and responsibilities of various types of legal entities are also a matter of state law, and these details may vary as well.

A Note Concerning Liability

Liability for an organization's debts and obligations is often one of the key factors considered in choosing the legal form of an organization. For present purposes, there are two principal types of liabilities and obligations. The first is the debts and obligations arising from the operation of a business (but excluding obligations for negligent acts). These business obligations include contractual undertakings, borrowing, and obligations for goods and services.

Claims of liability resulting from professional negligence, the second principal type of obligation, are typically treated differently from ordinary business claims. Responsibility for such claims is generally placed upon both the individual and the organization. Other individuals may also be liable for such acts, simply as a result of the form of the organization.

Types of Organizations

The typical types of organization for ambulatory care practice are:

- Sole proprietorships
- Sole proprietorships that share facilities and expenses
- Partnerships, joint ventures, and similar arrangements

- Limited liability companies
- Business corporations
- Professional corporations
- Nonprofit corporations
- Alphabet organizations, including IDs, PHOs, MCOs, Alliances, IPAs, and PPMs

In each of these legal structures, the owners have different rights and responsibilities in relation to one another and in relation to third parties.

Let us consider corporations first. Although corporations have existed for centuries, corporations organized to practice medicine are a relatively recent phenomenon. All states previously accepted the principle that a corporation could not practice a learned profession, including medicine, either directly or through its employees. The reason given for this prohibition was that professional licensing was specific to an individual and, for the protection of the public, a corporation—which could be controlled by unlicensed and therefore unqualified individuals—should not be permitted to engage in the practice of a profession (Fletcher et al., 1991–93; Eaton & Church, 1963–95).

From the 1950s until 1983, there were significant differences between the tax-deferred pension-planning opportunities for employees of a corporation and for employees of other types of organizations. Owners and employees of sole proprietorships and partnerships and the employees of nonprofit corporations were at a significant disadvantage when compared to the owners and employees of corporations, although these differences have become less dramatic over time (Cavitch, 1963–95).

As a result of these differences, a few states permitted professional service corporations to be created to allow professionals to take advantage of the pension-planning opportunities available under federal law (Fletcher et al., 1991–93; Eaton & Church, 1963–95). However, the Internal Revenue Service (IRS) took the position that a corporation in which a single professional was the sole shareholder, director, and employee providing professional services would not be recognized as a corporation entitled to these tax benefits, even if this type of corporation was permitted under state law (Fletcher et al., 1991–93; Eaton & Church, 1963–95). The IRS later extended this principle to corporations consisting of any number of professionals.

Eventually, the IRS, and later Congress, reversed this position and recognized as corporations for tax purposes various types of single-owner corporations (U.S. Department of the Treasury, 1995a). This change in position led many states to adopt statutes that permitted the organization of professional corporations to practice medicine. However, the statutes also protected the public by limiting stock ownership and board membership to persons who were licensed to practice the profession (O'Neal & Thompson, 1994). In addition, the statutes did not limit the liability of shareholders and directors for their own acts of malpractice to the assets of the corporation (Green et al., 1922–67).

Considering partnerships, there are many advantages to this form of organization for any small business owner. These include the elimination of double taxation, not only on current income but also on sale or merger. Partnerships, of course, do not have limited liability (except for limited partnerships, where limited liability is obtained only at the cost of the loss by each limited partner of any significant voice in management). A need was thus perceived for an entity taxed as a partnership but with the limited liability of a corporation or limited partnership.

As a result of this perceived need, a new form of organization with both of these characteristics was created: the limited liability company, or LLC. LLCs were proposed by a variety of interested persons and were based on types of companies common in Europe (Bagley & Whynott, 1995). The first legislation concerning LLCs was passed in Wyoming in 1977. The movement to LLCs accelerated in 1988 with the first IRS revenue ruling on these companies and, in 1992, with a model law prepared by the American Bar Association (Bagley & Whynott, 1995).

Alphabet organizations also respond to a perceived need, but they do so in a different manner than partnerships and other types of organizations. While these other types of organizations are legal organizations, alphabet organizations use contracts and one or more of the different types of legal organizations to respond to a need in health care. For example, a physician-hospital organization (PHO) can be created by using any one, or a combination, of the legal organizations described here. The same is true of managed-care organizations (MCOs), individual practice organizations or associations (IPOs or IPAs), and integrated delivery systems (IDSs). Use of the different types of organizations results in two key attributes of alphabet organizations: they are unique and flexible.

Another type of alphabet organization is the physician practice management company (PPM). PPMs are not only for-profit corporations; they are publicly traded companies whose stocks are traded on a national or regional stock exchange. These organizations are the medical complement to the hospital management organizations that emerged in the 1970s.

KEY LEGAL CHARACTERISTICS

The following section describes the key legal characteristics of these different types of organizations. Included are sole proprietorships, partnerships, corporations, and limited liability companies.

Sole Proprietorships

The most common form of organization for larger ambulatory care organizations is either a partnership or a corporation. However, sole proprietorships still account for a substantial number of smaller group practices. Legally, a sole proprietorship is a very simple organization. There is a single owner, or proprietor, who owns each asset and incurs each liability as an individual—even if the sole proprietorship is doing business under a trade name. The employees are also individually liable for their own acts of malpractice.

There is no legal limitation on the size of business that may be operated as a sole proprietorship or on the number of professionals who may be employed by the sole proprietor. Although a sole proprietorship can become quite large and the sole proprietor can delegate various aspects of management to employees, the control and reporting requirements are clear and simple: the sole proprietor is the ultimate and final authority.

A common variation on the sole proprietorship occurs when a number of sole proprietors band together in an office-sharing arrangement. The parties involved do not intend that this type of arrangement will create another legal entity, such as a partnership or corporation, but it may inadvertently have that result (Green et al., 1922–67).

This variety of sole proprietorship is also unlimited as to size, and each sole proprietor (separately or as a group) may employ an unlimited number of professionals or other employees. Such an arrangement involves an agreement among sole proprietors to share certain expenses, including, for example, rent, utilities, and the cost of employing persons to manage the practice or deliver health care services. However, the sole proprietors in this type of arrangement do not agree to share profits. Although revenues may be billed and collected through a single office, the revenues (and any related discounts or contractual allowances) are strictly allocated to the individual sole proprietor whose services generated the revenues. If profits were to be shared by the sole proprietors, then the arrangement would be a partnership, because the sharing of profits is a key attribute of a partnership. It is common in sole proprietor arrangement, however, to allocate an increased share of expenses to a sole proprietor who produces a higher proportion of the total revenue, on the assumption that the more productive sole proprietor incurs a larger proportion of the shared expenses.

Sole proprietors sharing office space often adopt a single practice name and present themselves to their patients and to other members of the public as if they constituted an integrated economic unit. Sole proprietors who share office space also often refer patients to one another and share patient coverage.

This type of arrangement is created by an agreement among the sole proprietors. Such agreements tend to be brief and incomplete if they are in writing and subject to rapid change or dispute over the precise terms if they are not. These arrangements can lead to other problems as well. For example, although the sole proprietors do not assume any risk for the malpractice liability of one another, such liability can be implied by law, resulting in a potentially devastating and unexpected liability

(Green et al., 1922–67). Each sole proprietor is also fully liable for all the debts incurred by the group of sole proprietors. In addition, unless the sole proprietors have agreed in writing to a particular management structure, management delegation in such an organization may be complex, difficult to document, and subject to serendipitous change.

Partnerships

Partnerships, coventures, and joint ventures are names used to describe different types of partnerships. The principal difference between a partnership and a group of sole proprietors sharing office space is that the partners have agreed (whether or not in writing) to share all profits from the partnership as well as all expenses and liabilities of the partnership (including malpractice liabilities). The sharing of profits need not be on an equal basis, but the key element of a partnership is the joining together to conduct a business for profit and to share those profits (Green et al., 1922–67). There is no limit to a partner's exposure to malpractice liability, for his or her own or another partner's acts of malpractice.

The partners in a partnership may themselves be various entities. A partnership for many purposes is a single legal entity. For some purposes a partnership is treated as a collection of individual partners.

A partnership may include as partners individuals or professional corporations or a combination of both. Each partner has an equal right to participate in the management of the partnership based on the partnership's state limited partnership act. However, the partners, in their partnership agreement, can delegate the right to manage the business to a particular partner (typically called the "managing" partner) or to a group of partners (either several managing partners or a management committee). The scope of delegation can range from complete delegation of authority, with the other partners retaining only the right to elect the managing partners or the management committee members, to very limited delegation, in which each act of the managing partner is subject to veto by a vote of the other partners.

The principal difference between a partnership and a corporation is that a corporation, as described in more detail below, provides a shareholder with protection from individual liability for corporate obligations and liabilities. However, a limited partnership can provide similar protection to limited partners in a partnership. The liability of a limited partner is limited to the capital that he or she has invested in the partnership and to the partnership's assets (Green et al., 1922–67). Limited partners, unlike general partners, are not permitted to participate in the management of the partnership. If a limited partner does become involved in management, that partner could become liable as a general partner (Green et al., 1922–67). A limited partnership is not commonly used as the legal structure for a group practice, more often being used as an investment vehicle to acquire land, buildings, or equipment used in the practice.

Corporations

A corporation is, for almost all purposes, an entity with an existence distinct from its shareholders, directors, officers, and employees. Although a corporation cannot take an action without an act by its human agents, a corporation is still treated as a separate entity.

Business Corporations

The most common form of corporation is the business, or for-profit, corporation. A corporation is a creation of state law. Thus, the specific rights and liabilities of shareholders, directors, and officers may vary depending upon state law. However, certain generalizations can be made. A corporation is liable for all of its obligations to the extent of its assets. Shareholders, directors, and officers are not ordinarily individually liable for the debts and obligations of a corporation, unless they take some action, such as executing a guarantee, to make themselves individually liable (Fletcher et al., 1991–93).

In certain circumstances, the existence of the corporation as a separate legal entity is ignored, and shareholders, directors, and officers (or any group of them) are treated as individually liable for a corporate obligation. Ignoring the separate existence of a corporation is uncommon, however, as long as the officers, directors, and shareholders have complied with the legal formalities necessary to maintain the separate existence of the corporation. These formalities include:

- Scrupulously treating the assets of the corporation as assets owned by the corporation
- Taking corporate actions through resolutions of the board of directors and its committees or pursuant to a delegation of authority from the board of directors
- Executing all corporate contracts and undertaking all corporate commitments in the name of the corporation

In a business corporation, a shareholder owns property rights that are represented by shares of stock. The property rights of a shareholder in a corporation may include the right to vote for the election of directors, the right to distribution of dividends from the corporation, and the right to assets remaining upon liquidation of the corporation after payment of the corporation's debts. The precise nature of the shareholder's property interest in a corporation's stock depends upon the type of stock issued by the corporation.

The board of directors elected by the shareholders is responsible for managing the corporation and its business. Typically, shareholders are entitled to one vote for each share they own. The board of directors may delegate some, all, or none of their management authority to particular officers, directors, or committees of the board of directors or to management.

Professional Corporations

Professional corporations (or professional service corporations) are business corporations whose shareholders must be licensed to practice the same profession as that practiced by the corporation (Fletcher et al., 1991–93). A shareholder is not legally required to practice as an employee of the professional corporation, although it is common for shareholders to do so.

Shareholders in a professional corporation have the same range of rights as do shareholders in an ordinary business corporation. They are not liable for debts and other obligations of the corporation. However, if they are employed by the corporation, they are individually liable for their own acts of malpractice.

Shares of stock in a professional corporation cannot be transferred to an unlicensed individual, except for certain brief periods in specifically limited circumstances. For example, stock in a professional corporation may be transferred to a shareholder's heirs upon the shareholder's death, subject to the requirement that the stock be redeemed by the corporation or transferred to a licensed professional within a particular period of time.

Nonprofit Corporations

Nonprofit corporations (known in some states as not-for-profit or public benefit corporations) are different from for-profit corporations. Although some types of nonprofit corporations may issue stock, the traditional nonprofit corporation does not give shareholders property rights in the corporation. In effect, there is no "owner" of a traditional nonprofit corporation. However, a nonprofit corporation may have members with the right to elect directors, the right to approve amendments to the corporation's organizational instruments, and other such rights, granted in the corporation's articles of incorporation and bylaws. A member of a nonprofit corporation that is itself a nonprofit corporation can become a holding company with ultimate control of the nonprofit corporation that it is a member of.

Not all states permit nonprofit corporations to employ licensed professionals or to deliver services through licensed professionals. States that permit nonprofit corporations to engage in this type of activity treat the corporations as professional corporations (Revised Code of Washington, 1995). For example, in some states, professional employees continue to be individually liable for their own acts of negligence.

With rare exceptions, a nonprofit corporation is the only type of organization described in this chapter that is exempt from federal income tax (U.S. Tax Court, 1981). The prerequisites for qualification as a tax-exempt organization are contained in the Internal Revenue Code

(U.S. Department of the Treasury, 1995b). To qualify as a tax-exempt, nonprofit corporation, a group practice is required, among other requirements, to demonstrate a charitable purpose (which may include the delivery of medical services on a free or part-pay basis) and an educational or a research purpose. The nonprofit corporation must also demonstrate that its net earnings do not benefit any shareholder or other individual. This provision requires that salaries paid to employees be limited to an amount reasonable to compensate for services actually rendered. This requirement is often met by having salaries and benefit packages planned, approved, or set by persons other than the employees receiving them.

Physician participation in the governance of nonprofit corporations that operate as integrated delivery systems may be limited (Arizon v. Maricopa County Medical Society, 1982). According to IRS policy, physician voting control in a nonprofit corporation should not exceed 20 percent of the membership of the governing body. However, this is policy, not law, and it is contrary to prior actions of the IRS (Jefferson Parish Hospital District #2 v. Hyde, 1984).

Limited Liability Companies

Limited liability companies combine the best aspects of partnerships and corporations. As in a limited partnership, the liability of members in a limited liability company is limited to the amount of capital they have contributed, unless the members guarantee or otherwise become liable for debts of the limited liability company. However, members who are also employees are individually liable for their own acts of malpractice. As in a partnership, most of the details of ownership and operation of a limited liability company may be set forth in a document separate from that filed with the state.

The principal difference between a limited liability company and a corporation is that any member or group of members of a limited liability company may be designated as managers, with an equal right to participate in the management of the company. The members can also delegate their right to manage the business

to a particular member or group of members, either completely or in part.

In a limited liability company, a member owns property rights, which may include the right to vote for the election of managers, the right to distribution of dividends from the company, and the right to assets remaining upon liquidation of the company after payment of the company's debts.

ORGANIZATIONAL AND MANAGEMENT ISSUES

This section of the chapter discusses the organizational aspects of business entities. Practical management issues, including contracting, are also addressed.

Organizational Issues

Any business organization is subject to filing and reporting requirements imposed by local, state, and federal licensing, taxing, and other authorities. There may be variations in the specific filings that must be made, depending on the type of business organization, but each organization is required to file a number of reports and returns.

More important for the present discussion are the legal requirements for establishing the organization and operating the organization once it has been established. The greatest number of legal formalities are required to establish a corporation. These requirements are described next.

In order to form a corporation, articles of incorporation must be prepared, signed, and then filed with the appropriate state office—typically the office of the state's secretary of state. The corporation does not exist until the articles of incorporation are filed. Operating as a corporation prior to this filing could make the shareholders, directors, and officers liable as individuals for any action taken on behalf of the "putative" corporation, simply because the corporation did not exist when the action was taken (American Bar Association, 1985–86).

A corporation's articles of incorporation contain a description of the basic structure of the corporation, including the type and number of shares that may be issued by the corporation, the rights attached to such shares, the names of the initial members of the board of directors, and certain other information, such as the purpose of the corporation and the method for amending the articles of incorporation.

After the articles of incorporation have been filed, the corporation's board of directors is required to hold an organizational meeting, at which the board adopts the bylaws of the corporation, elects officers, and takes other actions. The bylaws contain a detailed plan for operating the corporation. They address such issues as board meetings, election of directors, issuance of stock, and committees of the board of directors, which should include an executive committee.

In smaller proprietary corporations, the shareholders often enter into an agreement restricting transfers of stock so that stock is owned only by people who are part of the group practice (O'Neal & Thompson, 1994). Typically, a shareholder's stock is sold to the corporation upon the shareholder's retirement, death, or separation from service as an employee of the corporation.

Professional service corporations are subject to all of the foregoing requirements. In addition, the articles of incorporation of a professional corporation must refer specially to the profession that the corporation is organized to practice. It must also contain limitations on the transfer of shares to unlicensed persons.

Nonprofit corporations are similar to for-profit corporations with regard to the legal formalities required to establish them. The principal difference is that there is no reference to the issuance of stock in either the articles of incorporation or the bylaws of a nonprofit corporation unless the corporation issues shares. The qualifications and rights of members are set forth in the nonprofit corporation's articles of incorporation and bylaws.

Because a corporation is required by law to adopt certain organizational documents and take certain organizational actions, the corporate model is commonly used to evaluate organizational issues for other types of organizations, such as partnerships and sole proprietorships. However, because there are no legal requirements that the same issues need to be addressed in either the

partnership or the sole proprietorship agreement, these agreements may be incomplete.

In forming a partnership, the document that is similar to the articles of incorporation and bylaws of a corporation is the partnership agreement. This agreement is not required to be filed with any office of the state in order to be effective. Any partner can act for and obligate the partnership, unless this arrangement is changed by a partnership agreement. Thus, a partnership agreement should identify and delegate the rights and responsibilities of operating the partnership. Partnerships can replicate the structure of a corporation so that the owners may delegate to a smaller group—such as a management committee—the responsibility of managing the affairs of the partnership and the right to further delegate management authority. Partnerships can also provide for management by all of the owners, which may be appropriate for smaller organizations but may become quite cumbersome in larger partnerships.

The method for amending a partnership agreement is also normally found in the partnership agreement. Issues not addressed by the agreement may be decided as a matter of law, which may vary from state to state.

Limited partnerships, unlike other partnerships, normally require a filing with the secretary of state. In addition, certain provisions must be specifically set forth in the partnership agreement in order to form a limited partnership.

Limited liability companies are organized in a manner similar to limited partnerships: by filing a document, called the articles of organization, with the secretary of state. Unlike a partnership, a limited liability company may appoint a manager or managers. Only a manager can bind the limited liability company. The manager must be named in the articles of organization. If a manager is not named, then each member is deemed to be a manager. In that event, the management of a limited liability company becomes quite similar to the management of a general partnership. Additional details regarding management are set forth in the limited liability company's operating agreement.

Like partnerships, sole proprietorships, and sole proprietorships with office-sharing arrangements are not subject to any filing requirement with a state or federal office in order to be organized. All that is required for the organization and operation of a sole proprietorship is undertaking the business activity. All that is required for a sole proprietorship office-sharing arrangement is an agreement among proprietors, which need not be written.

Although not required by law, a written agreement among partners, members of a limited liability company, or sole proprietors can prevent significant problems. Such problems may range from simple management difficulties to disagreements among the owners as to their respective rights and responsibilities. The latter could result in dissolution of the organization in a way that was not contemplated by the parties involved.

Management Issues

In most cases, the legal requirements for the management structure of these types of organizations can be varied by agreement. Only the most common structures are reviewed here.

The classic management structure in a corporation provides for a representative form of corporate governance. Shareholders, as owners, have the right to elect directors who are legally responsible for the management of the corporation as the owners' representatives. The shareholders can enter into agreements among themselves concerning how they will vote in the future on particular issues. The board of directors of a corporation tends to set broad policy and to make major decision, but delegates to smaller groups (such as executive, finance, and strategic-planning committees) the supervision of actual operations. The board of directors and its committees may then delegate portions of the management responsibility to the chief executive officer and chief operating officers of the organization.

The manner of operating a partnership can mimic the management structure of a corporation. Unless otherwise agreed by the partners, however, a partnership, by law, operates as a committee of the whole. Unlike the traditional corporate structure, each partner in a partnership can act alone. A limited liability company's management structure is similar to that of a partnership, including the ability to mimic a corporation.

The management structures of nonprofit corporations vary widely. Although the most common structure for a nonprofit corporation is a self-perpetuating board, there are many variations. Members—whether corporations, groups of employees, or others—can be given the right to elect the board of directors. Members can also be given rights over the amendment of the articles of incorporation. In other ways, however, the organization of a nonprofit corporation follows the traditional corporate structure.

OPERATIONAL ISSUES

Most of the operations of an ambulatory care organization have legal implications. For example, determining who has final authority to make particular decisions is a legal question. Similarly, each relationship with a third party or an employee of the organization is a legal relationship. Happily, a lawyer need not be involved in each and every one of these decisions and operational issues. However, a manager must have a grounding in, and an awareness of, the legal implications of his or her activities in order to evaluate the attendant legal risks. Unfortunately, the complexity of organizational law makes it difficult to keep current in all areas.

Liability for acts of malpractice is the most common aspect of legal liability for group practices. The issue of patient relations is covered in more depth in a later chapter, but a few comments should be made in this context. Generally, a health care provider is liable for injury caused to patients as a result of the provider's acts of negligence. Negligence is defined simply as the failure to meet the standard of care in the community for services of the type performed (Speiser et al., 1983–93). The trend has been toward the establishment of a national standard of care. This has resulted, at least according to anecdotal evidence, in the practice of "defensive" medicine: performing extra tests and analyses that increase costs, in order to avoid malpractice claims.

Malpractice claims usually are managed by a program of risk management to identify practice risks and to maintain quality and help prevent injuries that could result in malpractice claims. Insurance is purchased or programs of self-insurance are established to provide a source for payment of attorneys' fees and other costs incurred in defending malpractice claims and to pay settlements or malpractice judgments.

There are new sources of potential liability for group practice that are not typically covered by insurance and can result in potential damages equal to or exceeding malpractice claims. The most important of these is the recent application of antitrust laws to the medical profession.

Prior to 1982, economic activities of the medical profession were exempt from antitrust laws, due to the "learned profession" exception to antitrust laws. The basis for this exception was that the practice of medicine and certain other activities were professions, not businesses, and thus should not be subject to the same economic regulations as businesses. In 1982, the United States Supreme Court effectively overruled the learned profession exception (Arizona v. Maricopa County Medical Society, 1982). As a result of this ruling, the activities of group practices are now subject to potential liability under antitrust laws. These laws provide for criminal and civil sanctions, and private parties who successfully claim that they are subject to injury as a result of anticompetitive activities may recover up to three times their actual damages and also attorney's fees.

Generally, antitrust laws prohibit attempts to monopolize a market in restraint of trade. Subjected to intense scrutiny are combinations with competitors, exclusive contracts and other agreements that have the effect of monopolizing the market, or the use of monopoly power to obtain a particular benefit. Antitrust laws may be enforced by federal and state authorities as well as by private parties.

There are three principal areas in which antitrust laws may apply to health care providers and group practices. First, hospital medical staff decisions—if they appear to be made to eliminate competition—can be the subject of antitrust claims. For example, in a recent case, which involved many years of litigation, the allegation was made that members of a clinic, who also served on a medical staff peer review committee, took their actions to eliminate a competitor. Second, exclusive contracts with third parties are permitted only if they achieve a substantial purpose other than the elimi-

nation of competition (Jefferson Parish Hospital District #2 v. Hyde, 1984). Third, mergers and acquisitions of health care providers that result in substantial increases in market share may be subject to antitrust scrutiny.

Another major area of developing regulation involves reimbursement programs. It has always been a crime to overbill or present false bills, but the difficulty of prosecuting such crimes has led to legislation designed to prohibit fraud and abuse. Congressional frustration with perceived physician referral abuses, for example, has led to regulation of financial relationships between physicians, and between physicians and other health care providers, whenever a referral for Medicare or Medicaid services is involved. This legislation is referred to as Stark I and II. Originally applying only to laboratory services, it was expanded as of January 1, 1995, to apply to virtually all health care services, including physician practices. The law also applies without regard to intent and specifies the elements of a permissible relationship between physicians and others. For example, it requires most leases or other arrangements between a physician and hospital to have a one-year term.

Of increasing importance to group practices and other health care providers in this country is the growing regulation of the disposition of medical waste. Important changes relevant to group practices have occurred, and more changes are likely to occur in the future.

Aside from these specialized regulations and laws, group practices are also subject to the same regulations and laws as other businesses. For example, construction projects are subject to land use and building permit requirements.

CHALLENGES FOR THE FUTURE

Ambulatory care administrators face important legal issues every day. Thus, their role requires an understanding of the complex legal environment in health care and intelligent use of legal advice. The rapid pace of change in tax, organization, liability, and other areas of law in recent years is likely to accelerate in the future, making legal knowledge and advice even more crucial for the administration of ambulatory care.

REFERENCES

American Bar Association Committee on Corporate Law. (1986). Model professional corporation supplement. In author, ed. *Model business corporation act* (3rd ed., pp.). Clifton, NJ: Law and Business.

Arizona v. Maricopa County Medical Society, 457 U.S. 332, 349–50, 73 L. Ed 2nd 48, 61–63 (1982).

Bagley, J., & Whynott, P. (1995). *The limited liability company.* Costa Mesa, CA: James Publishing.

Cavitch, Z. (1995). *Business organizations with tax planning.* New York: Matthew Bender & Co.

Conrad, A. (1981). Business corporations in American society. In *Commentaries on corporate structure and governance.* Philadelphia: American Law Institute.

Eaton, B. C., & Church, D. H. (1963–1995). *Professional corporations and associations.* New York: Matthew Bender & Co.

Fletcher, W. M., Bjur, T. P., & Elkins, K. (1991–1993). *Fletcher cyclopedia of corporations.* (perm. ed.). Wilmette, IL: Callaghan & Company.

National Conference of Commissioners on Uniform State Laws (1994). Uniform Partnership Act. In *Uniform Laws Ann* Vol. 6. St. Paul, MN: West Publishing Company.

Jefferson Parish Hospital District #2 v. Hyde, 466 U.S. 2, 80 L. Ed 2nd (1984).

O'Neal, F. H., & Thompson, R. (1994). *O'Neal's close corporation* (3rd ed.). Deerfield, MI: Clark Boardman Callaghen.

Revised Code of Washington, § 18.100.050 (1995).

Speiser, S., Krause, C. F., & Gans, A. W. (1983–1993). *The American law of torts.* Deerfield, IL: Clark Boardman Callaghan.

U.S. Department of the Treasury. (1995a). Treasury regulations, § 301.7701-2.

U.S. Department of the Treasury. (1995b). Internal revenue code, section 501(c)(3).

U.S. Tax Court. (1981). University of Maryland Physicians, P. A. V. Commissioner, Dec. 1981–23; 41 Tax Court Memorandum Decisions (CCH) 732.

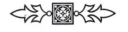

PART TWO

FINANCIAL MANAGEMENT IN AMBULATORY CARE

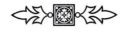

CHAPTER

3

The Fundamentals of Financial Management

Ernest J. Pavlock

CHAPTER TOPICS

Financial Information Needs

Basic Accounting Process

Reporting the Results and Status of Operations

Responsibility Accounting

Basic Concepts of Cost Accounting

Cost Allocation

Determining the Cost of Patient Services

Cost Accounting Systems

Financial Systems in Review

LEARNING OBJECTIVES

Upon completing this chapter, the reader should be able to:

- Describe the nature of the accounting process, its underlying assumptions, and the application of generally accepted accounting principles to medical practices
- Explain the content and significance of the basic financial statements and the messages they convey
- Apply the tenets of responsibility accounting in designing an accounting system and how it can be used
- Identify the various ways to classify costs, explain why costs behave in a certain fashion, and explain how to allocate costs to determine the cost of medical services
- Summarize the approaches to assigning and accumulating costs in developing the cost of patient services
- Distinguish between an actual cost system and a standard cost system

Financial management is a key process for assuring successful operations in any business organization. Typically, financial management is defined as planning for, providing, and controlling a business's capital to achieve its overall goals and objectives. Financial planning includes all the activities that support the forecasting or planning of the business's future flows of cash receipts and payments. Financial control includes all the policies and activities that help monitor financial operations and assure that cash flows are proceeding according to plan. Financial control also entails identifying deviations from plan and addressing them in a manner that assures financial health and the attainment of the organization's financial objectives. The following are some specific financial management functions:

- Designing the financial information system
- Financial planning
- Financial reporting and control
- Managing short-term resources (cash and receivables)
- Making long-range decisions and capital acquisitions
- Working closely with top management in strategic planning
- Analyzing and reporting data for decision-making
- Evaluating and training all personnel with financial responsibilities

The above definition of financial management applies without reservation to medical group practices. The fundamentals of financial management within the medical group setting are the focus of this chapter.

FINANCIAL INFORMATION NEEDS

Financial information is the lifeblood for managing the operations of medical practices. The heart of this information comes from the financial segment of the management information system established by the medical group. Commonly referred to as the accounting system, the financial information system records

and processes data that summarize business transactions affecting the practice. These data are used to provide a picture of the financial condition and operating results of the practice and to assist in planning and controlling its operations.

Financial data are usually called accounting information. An entire discipline, the field of accounting, has evolved over centuries to provide a conceptual framework for gathering financial data. It serves as the language for communicating these data to an organization's management, as well as to individuals and institutions outside the organization. Through evolution and technological advancement, a number of specialized fields of accounting have emerged. Two of the most important are financial accounting and management accounting.

Financial and Management Accounting

Financial accounting deals with the measurement and recording of transactions of a business entity and the periodic preparation of various reports from such records. The reports provide a reckoning of the financial affairs of the organization. A set of underlying concepts, assumptions, and standards, called *generally accepted accounting principles* (GAAP), guide the choice of information that is recorded and the manner in which it is reported. Application of these principles assures the consistency and comparability of financial statements issued by different business organizations.

Conventional financial statements typically derived from financial accounting are the following:

- The operating statement, or income statement
- The balance sheet, or statement of financial position
- The cash flow statement, which summarizes cash movements for a time period.

Examples of each of these statements are presented later in the chapter.

Management accounting relates to the use of accounting information for the planning and control of an entity's business and for making various kinds of business decisions. It makes use of historical data as well as financial estimates of future events. Management accounting overlaps financial accounting in that it uses

Some of the information in this chapter has been adapted from *Financial Management for Medical Groups* by Ernest J. Pavlock, PhD, CPA with permission of the Center for Research in Ambulatory Health Care Administration, 104 Inverness Terrace East, Englewood, CO, 80112-5306; (303) 799-1111. Copyright 1994.

financial statements to manage operations and plan future operations. In addition, management accounting employs market values and nonfinancial information. The criterion for adopting management accounting principles is whether the data are useful for management purposes.

Both financial and management accounting are used in medical practices. In the discussion that follows, however, both types of accounting will be referred to simply as "accounting."

Medical Group Needs for Financial Information

A medical practice has at least five different needs for financial information:

1. Information for financial planning and control
2. Information for decision making
3. Information for income distribution
4. Information required by law (the income tax return)
5. Information required by contract

Information for Financial Planning and Control

Planning for the future is a necessity for all practices. Managers must estimate the group's future directions and how to control its activities. Financial planning may entail no more than an evaluation of the past year's activities to assess which actions must be taken to avoid the difficulties of the past year and which to repeat or improve the favorable aspects of the past year. Or financial planning may include a much more formal process, such as the following:

• State goals and objectives
• Develop estimates of revenues and expenses for the next year, based on past data and forecasts of what conditions are likely to be in the future
• Integrate these estimates into a profit plan, cash budget, and projected set of financial statements
• If appropriate, break the profit plan into separate budgets for each identifiable part of the practice in

which fees are generated or expenses are incurred (such as each specialty or ancillary department)

For most practices, the financial planning and control activities fall somewhere between these two extremes. Presently, most groups tend toward the limited or informal end of the continuum; however, as activities become more complex and group size increases, planning and control systems must become more formalized. This evolution is especially likely when the practice acquires a larger share of the prepaid care market. Because of the increased risk inherent with prepaid contracts, good financial planning and control information become imperative.

Information for Decision Making

Most decisions center around choosing an alternative that provides the greatest benefits for the costs involved. Thus, practices must be able to identify, measure, and compare the benefits and costs attributable to different alternatives.

Generally, there are two classes of decisions: long-range decisions and short-range decisions. Long-range decisions involve the addition or replacement of service capacity, such as facilities or equipment. Short-range decisions involve the use of existing service capacity over a short time period, addressing such questions as what fees should be charged and what volume of services should be provided.

Measuring the benefits and costs of long-range decision alternatives depends on more than data obtained from the traditional accounting system. Because long-range decisions relate to the future, estimated future conditions also must be taken into account. Because facilities and equipment usually last a long time, the measurement of benefits and costs should be based on cash flows, not on accounting measurements of income.

In contrast, short-range decisions involve activities that recur each month and typically require knowledge of the volumes and mix of services and how costs change with activity level. The information needed for these decisions relates to a shorter time frame and is of a different nature than the information required for long-range decisions.

Information for Income Distribution

Medical groups conduct their practices using a variety of legal structures. In many cases, a particular structure is selected so that physician income can be distributed in a certain way. Three major organizational structures found in practices are the sole owner, the cost-sharing group, and the "true" group.

A sole owner is a single physician who owns a practice and employs associates on a salary basis. Salaries or bonuses may reflect the physician's production, but all of the net income of the practice goes to the sole owner. Since there is only one entity, there is only one set of accounting records.

In a cost-sharing group, several physicians practice as a group and remain as separate entities while sharing in the costs of common services for the group. Each physician receives his or her own receipts and pays the expenses directly related to his or her own practice, plus a share of the common expenses. There are separate sets of accounting records for each practice, each identifying the charges, collections, and expenses of a different, individual physician. Another set of records reflects the common expenses shared by all of the physicians and how the expenses are to be shared among the members.

In a "true" group, all of the physicians practice in a single business entity. There is one set of accounting records for the whole group. The income of each physician is determined by the income distribution formula of the group. The formula may provide for an equal distribution of income or some type of proration that may be contingent upon production.

Information Required by Law

The income tax code, which requires that an income tax return be filed for each business entity, is the most pertinent law affecting organizations. The code also requires that taxpayers' accounting records reflect the data used in the income tax return. Thus, most accounting systems are initially developed primarily to satisfy income tax–reporting requirements. As other needs for financial data evolve, the accounting system is modified or else supplemental information is generated from outside the accounting system.

There is considerable latitude in the way revenue and expense transactions are measured for tax purposes, and they do not necessarily use the same accounting principles as those used for external financial reporting. For example, there are two bases of accounting that can be employed in filing tax returns: the cash basis and the accrual basis. Under the cash basis, revenue is measured when cash is received and expenses are measured as cash is paid. Under the accrual basis, revenue is recognized when the service is provided to the patient (regardless of when cash is collected), and expenses are recognized when the resources are consumed in providing the service (regardless of when the cash is paid).

For medical practices that do not have capitation contracts, the cash-basis method is more advantageous than the accrual basis for tax purposes, because taxes are not paid until after the cash is collected from patients. Also, the timing of the payment of expenses may be advanced or postponed to gain further tax advantages. Although the cash basis provides tax advantages, it can also cause distortions in measuring results and reduce the comparability of accounting reports when evaluating the performance of different practices.

Unfortunately, many medical practices choose to adopt the cash basis of accounting, which is used in the practice's tax return, and for all financial reporting needs. The use of tax accounting for financial statements may not present a fair picture of a practice's operations nor provide the most useful kinds of information for appraising results and for financial planning, control, and decision making. Because the accrual basis of accounting allows a fuller and more complete portrayal of operations, it should be followed for internal and external financial reporting.

Information Required By Contract

Banks and long-term creditors generally require group financial statements before they grant and service loans. Other information may also be required, depending upon the nature and amount of the loan. If the loan is small or fully secured, the creditor generally accepts the financial statements prepared for the group's income tax return or for members of the group. However, if the loan is large and security is limited, the creditor may require additional financial statements that are based on accrual accounting and that conform with GAAP. In most cases, the statements must be audited by a CPA.

Prepaid contracts that are entered into under managed care also require the inclusion of certain accounting and financial information relating to the medical group's operations. In fact, this information is an integral part of the determination of capitation rates to be paid to the medical group.

BASIC ACCOUNTING PROCESS

This section covers the framework for structuring the recording of transactions, basic financial statements, and their underlying principles and assumptions. These areas constitute the essence of financial accounting.

Accounting Measurements

Business events that are represented by transactions form the basis for recording accounting information. Most small businesses and many small medical practices use the cash basis of accounting, as mentioned above. However, accrual accounting is being adopted by an increasing number of medical groups, and it is used by most businesses. The following descriptions and comparison of these two accounting methods explain the increasing use of accrual-basis accounting.

Cash-Basis Accounting

Under cash-basis accounting, revenues are recorded when cash is received, and expenses are recorded when cash is paid. In other words, cash must be involved in a transaction in order for it to be recorded. Thus, financial statements prepared using this basis exclude accounts receivable, accounts payable, accrued expenses, and deferred costs and deferred revenues related to the current period's operations. If a "pure" cash basis of accounting is adopted, all expenditures, including those for long-lived assets, supplies, and liability insurance premiums, are expensed only when the cash outlays are

made. A pure cash-basis balance sheet has only two elements—cash as the asset and the owner's equity. In practice, however, the pure cash basis is usually modified to record long-lived assets, as well as payables and receivables relating to the borrowing or investing of cash.

Accrual-Basis Accounting

The movement of cash as a receipt or payment does not affect the recognition of revenues and expenses under the accrual basis of accounting. Under this basis, revenue is recorded when services are performed or when the organization's products are delivered. For a medical practice, accrual accounting provides an accurate measurement of revenue for efforts expended, because revenue is recorded when patient services are rendered rather than when payment for them is received. Similarly, expenses are recorded when resources (assets) have been used up or consumed in the generation of revenue, regardless of when cash was expended to acquire those resources. In other words, cash receipts and payments do not govern the time period when revenue and expenses are recorded.

Comparing Cash and Accrual Basis of Accounting

The cash basis of accounting mismatches revenues and expenses among one or more accounting periods. No such mismatching occurs under accrual accounting because revenues recognized for any time period are matched with the best estimates of expenses used up in producing those revenues. Thus, accrual accounting allows for better monthly comparisons of achievements (revenues) and resource utilization (expenses) as operating results. Although a medical group may use the cash basis for income tax reporting, the accrual basis should be followed for internal reporting purposes because it provides a sounder basis for evaluating the performance of the practice.

Accrual-Basis Transactions

The occurrence of a recordable event or condition represents a business transaction under the accrual basis. All business transactions are recorded in terms of money, which serves as the uniform unit of measurement. Examples of transactions include:

- Receipt of $25,000 in capitation payments from an HMO
- Payment of a telephone bill of $120
- Purchase of a new X-ray machine for $10,000

A cardinal rule of accounting is that:

$$\text{Assets} = \text{Equities}$$

Assets are resources owned and used by a business. Equities are rights or claims to these resources. There are two main types of equities: creditors' rights and owners' rights. Creditors' rights, also called liabilities, are those represented by debts or obligations of the business. The rights of the owners are the owners' equity. Thus, the first equation can be expanded to:

$$\text{Assets} = \text{Liabilities} + \text{Owners' Equity}$$

This expanded equation is known as the basic accounting equation. It can be restated as:

$$\text{Assets} - \text{Liabilities} = \text{Owners' Equity}$$

The basic accounting equation is used in analyzing business transactions. Transactions are recorded as assets, liabilities, or equity. Each transaction is analyzed to determine which of the three elements it has increased or decreased. The new values for the elements must maintain equality in the equation.

For example, assume a medical group is formed by several physicians investing a total of $100,000 cash from their personal savings and obtaining a bank loan of $300,000. This transaction would be recorded as follows:

Assets	= Liabilities	+ Owners' Equity
Cash	= Notes Payable	+ Capital
increase	increase	increase
$400,000	= $300,000	+ $100,000

Entries like the above would be recorded for each transaction, with the monetary balance of the equa-

tion's three elements maintained. Every entry on one side of the equation would be offset by an equal entry on the same or other side of the equation to maintain equality. This system of accounting is called a double entry system for this reason, and it is followed by all businesses in this fashion.

A more detailed example of this system of recording is given in Table 3–1, which shows a series of transactions for the first three months of operation of the medical practice of Wills, Aust and Pall, PC. For a more detailed description of the accounting recording process, accounting textbooks may be consulted.

Basic Financial Statements

Three basic financial statements are the balance sheet, income statement, and statement of cash flows. Examples of each of these statements are shown in Table 3–1d–f for the Wills, Aust and Pall, PC medical group. Note that the two bases of accounting described earlier—accrual and modified cash—have been followed in recording transactions and in the preparation of the statements (Table 3–1b and c).

Balance Sheet

The construct of a typical balance sheet, such as the one in Table 3–1d, embodies the basic accounting equation give above. Assets (resources) owned and used in the practice are balanced against liabilities (debts or obligations owed to outsiders) and stockholders' equity, which represents the ownership interests if the practice is a corporation. Because many small groups still follow the modified cash basis of accounting, several important differences between this basis and the accrual basis should be pointed out.

A more inclusive picture of group assets is portrayed with the accrual basis because accounts receivable, supplies, and prepaid insurance are included. These items are excluded from the modified cash basis. The accrual basis also shows more liabilities, such as accounts payable, interest payable, and deferred revenue from prepaid services.

TABLE 3–1a   Summary of Wills, Aust and Pall, PC Transactions for First Three Months of Operation

(1) Three physicians—Wills, Aust, and Pall—formed a professional corporation and started a family practice medical group. Each invested equal amounts of cash totaling $200,000, and capital stock was issued to the new owners.

(2) Equipment was purchased for $250,000 and was paid for by $50,000 cash and a five-year, 12 percent note payable for $200,000.

(3) A one-year malpractice liability insurance policy was purchased for $24,000 cash.

(4) Supplies were purchased on credit for $36,000.

(5) During the three months, the delivery of patient services on a fee-for-service basis totaled $180,000; $40,000 was received in cash, leaving $140,000 in accounts receivable.

(6) During the three months, $50,000 of the above accounts receivable were collected.

(7) Shortly after the group was formed, a prepaid contract was entered into with a local HMO. Capitated payments received totaled $60,000.

(8) Rent was paid for three months at $24,000.

(9) Bills for laboratory, utilities, and telephone services were received and totaled $38,000.

(10) Payments on items procured on credit (above) were made as follows: supplies, $17,000; laboratory, utilities, and telephone services, $30,000.

(11) Nursing and support staff salaries were paid: gross wages were $18,000, withheld taxes were $6,000, net pay was $12,000.

(12) Physician salaries were paid: gross wages were $68,000, withheld taxes were $20,000, net pay was $48,000.

(13) Withheld taxes paid to the taxing authorities totaled $14,000.

(14) Payment on principal amount of note was made ($10,000), and interest was paid for two months ($4,000).

(15) Adjustments: depreciation expense, $12,000
(16)   amortization of prepaid insurance, $6,000
(17)   supplies consumed, $20,000
(18)   accrual of interest, $2,000
(19)   capitated revenue earned, $45,000
(20) Closing: net income to retained earnings

Both cash and accrual statements have the same elements of stockholders' equity—capital stock and retained earnings—but with different amounts. There is a positive balance of retained earnings reflected under accrual accounting. This indicates that physician cash withdrawals are less than the difference between revenues and expenses. The modified cash basis, on the other hand, reflects a deficit. This indicates that physician cash withdrawals are greater than the difference between cash receipts and cash expenses.

Income Statement

An income statement, such as the one shown in Table 3–1e, depicts revenues for the time period indicated, matched with expenses incurred to generate those

TABLE 3–1b Wills, Aust and Pall, PC: First Three Months of Operations

Accrual Transactions ($1,000s)

Accounts	Acct. Type	1	2	3	4	5	6	7	8	9	10	11	12	13	14	15	16	17	18	19	20	Balance
Cash	Asset	200	-50	-24		40	50	60	-24		-47	-12	-48	-14	-14							117
Accounts Receivable	Asset					140	-50															90
Supplies Inventory	Asset				36													-20				16
Prepaid Insurance	Asset			24													-6					18
Equipment	Asset		250													-12						238
Accounts Payable	Liabilities					36				38	-47											27
Payroll Tax Withholdings	Liabilities											6	20	-14								12
Interest Payable	Liabilities																		2			2
Deferred Revenue	Liabilities							60												-45		15
Notes Payable	Liabilities		200												-10							190
Capital Stock	St. EQ.	200																				200
Retained Earnings	St. EQ.																				33	33
Fee-For-Serv. Revenue	Revenue					180																180
Contract Serv. Revenue	Revenue																			45		45
Lab, Util.&Teleph. Expense	Expense									38												38
Rent Expense	Expense								24													24
Supplies Expense	Expense																	20				20
Non-Physician Salaries	Expense											18										18
Depreciation Expense	Expense															12						12
Insurance Expense	Expense																6					6
Interest Expense	Expense														4				2			6
Physician Salaries	Expense												68									68
Net Income																					33	33

TABLE 3–1c Wills, Aust and Pall, PC: First Three Months of Operations

Cash Transactions ($1,000s)

Accounts	Acct. Type	1	2	3	4	5	6	7	8	9	10	11	12	13	14	15	16	17	18	19	20	Balance
Cash	Asset	200	-50	-24		40	50	60	-24		-47	-12	-48	-14	-14							117
Accounts Receivable	Asset																					
Supplies Inventory	Asset																					
Prepaid Insurance	Asset				N					N							N	N	N	N		
Equipment	Asset		250		O					O						-12	O	O	O	O		238
Accounts Payable	Liability																					
Payroll Tax Withholdings	Liability											6	20	-14								12
Interest Payable	Liability				E					E							E	E	E	E		
Deferred Revenue	Liability				N					N							N	N	N	N		
Notes Payable	Liability		200		T					T					-10		T	T	T	T		190
Capital Stock	St. Eq.	200			R					R							R	R	R	R		200
Retained Earnings	St. Eq.				Y					Y							Y	Y	Y	Y	-47	-47
Fee-for-Service Revenue	Revenue					40	50															90
Contract Service Revenue	Revenue							60														60
Lab, Util. & Teleph. Expense	Expense										30											30
Rent Expense	Expense								24													24
Supplies Expense	Expense											17										17
Non-physician Salaries	Expense												18									18
Depreciation Expense	Expense															12						12
Insurance Expense	Expense				24																	24
Interest Expense	Expense														4							4
Physicians' Salaries	Expense												68									68
Net Income																					-47	-47

revenues. In the figure, modified cash-basis and accrual-basis income statements are compared. Because of differences in recognizing the timing of revenue, the accrual-basis total revenue is greater than the modified cash-basis total. Whereas the fee-for-service accrual portion is greater than the modified cash portion, the reverse is true for the prepaid service segment of the practice. Because of timing differences in expense recognition, expenses under the modified cash basis are somewhat greater than under accrual accounting. The significant difference in income before physician salaries results from these timing differences.

There seems to be a conscious decision not to distribute most of the income before physician salaries to the physicians for the quarter, because there is a sizable amount of net income after recognizing physician salaries under the accrual basis. The net loss for the quarter under the modified cash basis occurs because physician salaries exceed the amount of cash income.

Statement of Cash Flows

As indicated by its name, this statement presents a summary of all cash flows experienced by the group for

TABLE 3–1d Wills, Aust and Pall, PC
Balance Sheet

At the End of the First Three Months of Operations
($ 1,000s)

	Accrual	Modified Cash
Assets		
Cash	$ 117	$ 117
Accounts receivable	90	– –
Supplies	16	– –
Prepaid insurance	18	– –
Equipment (net)	238	238
Total	$ 479	$ 355
Liabilities and Stockholders' Equity		
Accounts payable	$ 27	$ – –
Payroll tax withholdings	12	12
Interest payable	2	– –
Deferred revenue	15	– –
Notes payable	190	190
Capital stock	200	200
Retained earnings	33	(47)
Total	$ 479	$ 355

TABLE 3–1e Wills, Aust and Pall, PC
Income Statement

For the First Three Months of Operations
($ 1,000s)

	Accrual	Modified Cash
Revenue:		
Fee-for-service	$ 180	$ 90
Prepaid service	45	60
Total	$ 225	$ 150
Expenses:		
Laboratory, utilities, and telephone	$ 38	$ 30
Rent	24	24
Supplies	20	17
Non-physician salaries	18	18
Depreciation	12	12
Insurance	6	24
Interest	6	4
Total	$ 124	$ 129
Income before physician salaries	$ 101	$21
Physician salaries	68	68
Net Income	$ 33	$ (47)

a specified time period. It is organized to reflect cash flows along three dimensions:

1. Cash provided (used) by operations
2. Cash provided (used) by investing
3. Cash provided (used) by financing

Along each of these dimensions, both inflows and outflows of cash are included.

Table 3–1f shows statements of cash flow for the Wills, Aust and Pall, PC medical group under the two bases of accounting. Because both statements summarize cash movements, they are identical. Both statements also reflect that cash is being used by operations (as opposed to being provided by operations, which is more desirable), largely due to physician withdrawals of cash (as salaries) in amounts greater than the difference between cash receipts and cash payments for expense items. A practice must generate positive cash flows from operations in the long run to remain a viable economic practice. Continued decrease in the cash balance necessitates

new infusions of cash through borrowing or additional investment by the physician-owners. The only other cash flows occurring during the quarter in the Wills, Aust and Pall, PC group were the initial investment of $200,000 in the practice, the purchase of equipment for $250,000, the borrowing of $200,000, and the payment of $10,000 on the note payable.

Generally Accepted Accounting Principles

As mentioned earlier, accrual accounting is based on a set of standards called *generally accepted accounting principles* (GAAP). These principles, which have been developed by individuals and professional groups over a long period of time, serve as the best guidelines for recording and reporting on business transactions. The principles are continually updated to keep pace with the changing economic environment. Responsibility for this updating rests with practicing accountants, accounting educators, business financial executives, and

TABLE 3–1f Wills, Aust and Pall,
PC Cash Flow Statement

For the First Three Months of Operations
($ 1,000s)

	Accrual	Modified Cash
Operating Activities:		
Collection for services	$ 150	$ 150
Pay various expenses	(111)	(111)
Pay interest	(4)	(4)
Salary distributions to physicians	(58)	(58)
Cash Used by Operations	$ (23)	$ (23)
Investing Activities:		
Purchasing equipment	$ (250)	$ (250)
Cash Used by Investing	$ (250)	$ (250)
Financing Activities:		
Investment in practice	$ 200	$ 200
Increase in long-term debt	200	200
Reduce long-term debt	(10)	(10)
Cash provided by financing	$ 390	$ 390
Increase (decrease) in cash	$ 117	$ 117
Beginning balance (cash)	0	0
Ending balance (cash)	$ 117	$ 117

others, through a private body called the Financial Accounting Standards Board (FASB). The board identifies problems in financial reporting, conducts research into the issues, and, after due deliberations, pronounces new or revised standards that add to the set of generally accepted accounting principles.

Some of the important GAAP used by all businesses, including medical practices, include the historical cost principle, revenue recognition rule, and expense recognition rule.

Historical Cost Principle

According to this principle, assets and liabilities are recorded at their initial cost or the value of consideration given at acquisition. This is the basic rule for recording the acquisition of assets and liabilities. Cost is used because it is a reliable measurement more easily subject to objective verification than other valuation methods, such as market values.

Revenue Recognition Rule

This rule prescribes that revenue be recorded when services are performed or products delivered. The receipt of cash for these transactions is of secondary importance and is treated as a second transaction. However, if there is a great deal of uncertainty about cash being collected, then revenue recognition may be delayed until the cash is collected. If some of the revenues are not likely to be collected, an estimate of the uncollectible amount may be made to reduce the revenue to the amount expected to be collected.

Expense Recognition Rule

This rule applies when assets or costs are used to provide a service. For costs directly related to a specific revenue, such as the sale of a prosthesis to a patient, the rule dictates that costs of the item should be carried as an asset (inventory) until revenue is recognized for the sale of the item. Then the cost of the sold item is treated as an expense (cost of goods sold). When there is no direct relationship between the cost of the asset and the revenue generated from its sale, such as for long-lived assets (equipment), the cost of the asset is allocated as an expense in a systematic and rational way over its useful life. This process is called *depreciation* for tangible, long-lived assets and *amortization* for other long-lived assets, such as prepaid insurance and goodwill.

Costs that do not relate directly to particular revenues or are not representative of long-lived assets are considered as expenses during the accounting period in which they are incurred. Many of these costs pertain to the passage of time, such as interest expense and practice promotional expenses. In applying all of the above rules, the objective is to use the matching principle, that is, to match appropriate expenses expiring in a period to revenues recorded in the same period.

Assumptions and Concepts Underlying GAAP

There is a set of fundamental assumptions and concepts with which users should be familiar in order to fully comprehend the significance of GAAP. These are the business entity, going concern, accounting period, objectivity, monetary unit, relevance, reliability, full disclosure, conservatism, consistency, and comparability.

The Business Entity

The business entity assumption separates the activity of a business from the personal affairs of the owners. Accounting records kept for the business are separate from business transactions involving the personal financial affairs of the owners or managers. For some medical practices, there may be more than one entity. One entity may be the legal organization owning and operating the practice. Another entity may be an affiliated legal entity, such as a realty corporation. Financial statements may be prepared individually for each entity, or the entities may be combined for the preparation of one consolidated statement, depending upon the purpose and use of the financial statement.

Going Concern

Unless there is information to the contrary, under this assumption a practice is perceived to have an indefinite life. Thus, the historical cost principle can be applied, because temporary fluctuations in market values and liquidation values of assets can be ignored. However, periodic evaluations over shorter time frames (months, quarters, or years) are necessary. The matching principle is used to match expenses with revenues to measure net income for whatever time period is prescribed. To do so requires systematic estimates of expenses, such as depreciation expenses, that represent allocations of assets' costs over periods of their useful life.

Accounting Period

Because entities are assumed to have an indefinite life, it is necessary to establish an arbitrary time period for taking periodic reckonings of the results of a business's operation and of its financial status. The periods set for most businesses are years, but, internally, shorter time periods are typically used, such as quarters or months. One should view periodic financial statements as products of exercising judgments about revenue and expense amounts for the time periods indicated.

Objectivity

Normal business activity involves an exchange of goods or services at an agreed-upon price by the parties in the exchange. The transaction is recorded at cost, which is measured by the value of resources given up in the exchange. The measurement of the exchange should be by objective and verifiable evidence, such as an invoice or contract. Subjective bases should be avoided.

Monetary Unit

The monetary unit is used to quantify business transactions. Thus, financial statements contain money measures. Financial statements of businesses in other countries are expressed in their own country's currency unit. In interpreting financial statement information, it is important to remember that the value of a country's currency fluctuates through time and that no adjustments are made in the statements for these fluctuations.

Relevance

Relevance refers to the ability of accounting information to make a difference in decision making. Users of financial statements have different decision-making needs. For example, a lender may be interested in assessing a potential borrower's ability to repay a loan. An owner or manager may be interested in the practice's ability to generate sufficient income. In addition to financial statement data, internal reports and nonfinancial data may be required for effective decision making. Relevancy also refers to the timely distribution of the proper type of information to users.

Reliability

Reliability refers to the assurance that the information is reasonably free from bias and error and that users can depend on it to represent the economic conditions or events in question. To be reliable, accounting information must be able to elicit a high degree of consensus among independent measurers who use the same measurement methods.

Full Disclosure

Users of financial statements must be able to obtain a complete picture of the organization's financial position, operations, and cash flows. As general-purpose documents, financial statements are intended to fulfill the needs of all external users who do not have access to the organization's internal records. Footnotes may be added to amplify information presented in the main body of the statements.

Conservatism

This accounting guideline means choosing the accounting approach that will be least likely to overstate assets and earnings. This is why the cash basis of accounting is used in medical practices. A conservative practice in accrual accounting is postponing revenue recognition until the collection of cash is relatively certain, if not already in hand. Another conservative practice is recording losses at the first sign that they are likely to occur. The convention does not mean, however, that accountants should deliberately understate assets or earnings.

Consistency

Consistency requires that entities apply the same accounting methods to similar transactions from period to period. Comparability of accounting data is assured through consistent application of methods over time. Consistency does not mean that a business cannot switch from one acceptable method of accounting to another. When it can be demonstrated that another method is preferable to the current one, it is permissible to adopt the new one, with full disclosure of the impact of the change.

Comparability

Many of the above assumptions allow comparisons of accounting data between periods. Since organizations have long lives and it is necessary to measure short-term results to assess progress, the capacity to compare one period's results with the results of other periods is critical to a continuing evaluation of the operations of any business. Accrual accounting practices assure comparability and are the basis generally recommended for use.

REPORTING THE RESULTS AND STATUS OF OPERATIONS

In this section, two of the basic financial statements—the income statement and the balance sheet—are expanded upon. These two statements are the major communication vehicles used to inform managers and others how the operations of a medical practice or other business are faring.

The Income Statement

The income statement provides information to answer the question: How well is the medical practice doing? It presents information on the accomplishments of the practice, measured by revenues, and matches them with the costs incurred to produce those revenues, that is, expenses. By comparing income statements for several consecutive periods, significant trends in the elements of the statement can be identified and projections can be made of the practice's future earning power.

Table 3–2 illustrates a typical income statement for the Ideal Medical Group, a medium-sized group practice. The following sections examine in detail three parts of the statement: revenue, expenses, and net income.

Revenue

Revenue during a period is the inflow of assets, usually cash or receivables, from performing a service (treating patients), delivering a product, or performing other activities that comprise the ongoing operations of a business entity. Under accrual accounting, revenue is created when service is performed if the following two conditions are met:

1. The earnings process is substantially complete by accomplishing the activities that comprise professional services
2. Objective evidence exists to show that the asset (receivable) will be collected

Two sources of revenue are reported by the Ideal Medical Group: $4,779,000 as its predominant source

TABLE 3–2   Illustration of an Income Statement (Accrual Basis)

Ideal Medical Group
Income Statement
for the Year Ended December 31, 19X1
($ 1,000s)

	Amount	Percent	Percent
Revenue			
Gross charges—fee-for-service	$ 5,140	100.0%	
Less: adjustments	257	5.0	
Adjusted gross charges	$ 4,883	95.0%	
Less: allowances	104	2.0	
Net revenue—fee-for-service	$ 4,779	93.0%	83.8%
Capitated revenue	922		16.2
Net revenue	$ 5,701		100.0%
Operating expenses			
Human resources (except physicians)			
Ancillary department salaries	$ 290		5.1%
Medical support salaries	584		10.2
Administrative salaries	165		2.9
Housekeeping and security salaries	47		.8
Total salaries	$ 1,086		19.0%
Employee benefits	219		3.9
Total human resources	$ 1,305		22.9%
Purchased services (medical/professional)			
Outside laboratory and radiology	$ 174		3.1%
Physical resources			
Supplies and cost of goods sold	$ 283		5.0%
Occupancy and use (building/utilities)	391		6.8
Occupancy and use (furniture/equipment)	62		1.1
Total physical resources	$ 736		12.9%
General and administrative			
Purchased data processing services	$ 69		1.2%
Professional liability insurance	218		3.8
Other general and administrative	277		4.9
Total general and administrative	$ 564		9.9%
Interest expense	23		.4%
Total operating expenses	$ 2,802		49.2%
Income before physician distributions and benefits	$ 2,899		50.8%
Distributions to physicians	2,615		45.8
Net income to retained earnings	$ 284		5.0%

(fee-for-service) and $922,000 as its secondary source (prepaid contracts). A comprehensive method of reporting the fee-for-service portion and arriving at net revenue is shown in the table. Gross charges for services ($5,140,000) is a standard measure of services provided to a group's patients. Gross charge data are important because the amount of resources consumed as expenses should have a direct relationship to gross charges. There may be supporting schedules disclosing different types of gross charges, such as charges for surgery, office treatments, specialty area, or laboratory services, among others. Reductions (adjustments and allowances, totaling $361,000) are made to gross charges for allowances and discounts to standard charge rates and for estimates of uncollectible accounts receivable. This produces the fee-for-service net revenue ($4,779,000).

Revenues earned by providing services to prepaid patients on a capitation basis should be realized in the time period services are made available to plan enrollees. Expenses related to these patients that are incurred internally or contracted outside the group should be accrued as expenses and recognized in the same period that the prepaid patients' revenues are recognized. Key provisions of prepaid plans should be included in the notes to the financial statement.

Any nonoperating revenues, such as interest, rental income, or gain on the sale of excess equipment, should be shown separately from patient service revenue on the income statement.

Expenses

Expenses are resources (assets) consumed or used up in the process of producing revenue. Operating expenses, in a medical practice, are expenses incurred in the process of treating patients. These expenses, matched with patient revenue, determine net operating income. Nonoperating expenses are expenses related to activities not associated with the rendering of patient services. Examples include research expenditures and interest on borrowed funds.

Medical groups organize their operating expenses according to the nature of the expenditures made in operating their practices. A standardized system of account structure is provided by the Center for Re-

search in Ambulatory Health Care Administration (CRAHCA) in their *Medical Group Practice Chart of Accounts.* The CRAHCA Chart of Accounts system is flexible and designed to accommodate a broad range of financial information needs for practices of all sizes, including both fee-for-service and prepaid-service types of practice.

The income statement of the Ideal Medical Group follows the CRAHCA major categories of operating expenses. Amounts for each category are as follows:

	Total Amount
Human resource expenses	$1,305,000
Purchased services	174,000
Physical resource expenses	736,000
General and administrative expenses	564,000

Within each of these categories, there are individual accounts of various expenses, with the larger ones detailed in the body of the statement, as illustrated by the Ideal example. Note that interest expense is shown separately so that the cost of financing a practice might be compared to the cost for other groups.

For incorporated medical groups, all salaries, including those of physicians, are deemed operating expenses of the corporate entity. In partnerships, partners' (physicians') salaries may be shown as operating expenses or treated as distribution of net income. Ideal Medical Group shows physician salaries as a separate item below operating expenses ($2,615,000) even though the group is a corporation.

Human resource expenses usually comprise the major operating expense for medical groups ($1,305,000 out of $2,802,000 in Ideal's case). Along with purchased services, human resource expenses should be analyzed to assess their impact on the cost of services rendered to patients and on gross charges.

Physical resource expenses include amounts for depreciation and amortization. Even though they are expenses that do not reduce cash or working capital when recognized, they reduce the book value of noncurrent assets, such as buildings, equipment, and goodwill. GAAP requires a general description in the notes to financial statements of the method of depreciation used by major classes of assets, the balances of the major classes, and the accumulated depreciation taken to date by class and in total.

Other physical resources expenses include rent, supplies, utilities, insurance, property taxes, maintenance, repairs, and cost of goods sold to patients. The main items under general and administrative expenses are professional liability insurance and purchased data processing services. Other expenses in this category relate to office supplies, legal expenses, and accounting and various administrative expenses.

It should be noted that no amount for income taxes has been shown on Ideal's income statement. It is assumed that the corporation is able to follow tax accounting rules (different from GAAP, which is used in preparing the income statement) so that little or no income tax is payable by the corporation. If the amount of taxes payable by the corporate entity was significant, there would be a separate line item on the income statement showing the amount of income taxes.

Net Income

The final item on the income statement is called *net income.* It represents the residual amount after all expenses—operating and nonoperating—have been deducted from net revenue and nonoperating revenue. If physician compensation is considered as an operating expense, then net income is the remainder after all expenses are covered (as in Ideal's case). If distributions to physicians equal or almost equal net income before physician salaries, net income will be zero or a small amount. In the case of Ideal, management chose to retain five percent of net income in the practice to help finance new acquisitions of long-lived assets and add to working-capital needs as a result of growth.

The Balance Sheet

The balance sheet, such as the one for Ideal Medical Group shown in Table 3–3, answers the question: What is the financial position of the medical practice at the end of the year? In fact, this statement is often called the *statement of financial position* or the *statement of assets and liabilities.* Generally, assets and liabilities are placed in two broad classes—current, or short-term, and noncurrent, or long-term. As mentioned earlier, the balance

TABLE 3–3 Illustration of a Balance Sheet (Accrual Basis)

Ideal Medical Group
Balance Sheet
as of December 31, 19X1

Assets	
Current assets	
Cash (unrestricted)	$ 67,683
Marketable securities	6,400
Accounts receivable	610,250
Less: Allowances	(48,100)
Supplies	93,800
Prepaid expenses	29,735
Total current assets	$ 759,768
Investments	
Investment in securities	$ 85,500
Property held for future use	150,000
Total investments	$ 235,500
Noncurrent tangible assets	
Furniture, fixtures, and equipment	$ 481,655
Less: Accumulated depreciation	(160,420)
Total noncurrent tangible assets	$ 321,235
Total assets	$1,316,503

Liabilities and Stockholders' Equity	
Current liabilities	
Accounts payable	$ 79,875
Notes and loans payable	35,500
Payroll withholdings and related liabilities	28,110
Accrued payroll liabilities	44,365
Deferred revenue	218,000
Total current liabilities	$ 405,850
Long-term liabilities (Notes Payable)	$ 200,000
Stockholders' equity	
Common stock	$ 250,000
Capital contributed in excess of par	100,000
Retained earnings	360,653
Total stockholders' equity	$ 710,653
Total Liabilities and Stockholders' Equity	$1,316,503

sheet shows resources, or assets, in balance with liabilities and owners' equity. For Ideal Medical Group (see Table 3–3), this balance is shown by the equation:

$$\text{Assets} = \text{Liabilities} + \text{Owners' Equity}$$
$$\$1,316,503 = \$605,850 + \$710,653$$

Assets

Assets are generally divided into four categories:

1. Current assets
2. Long-term investments
3. Noncurrent tangible assets (fixed assets such as buildings, equipment, and furniture)
4. Intangibles and other assets

The balance sheet for the Ideal Medical Group shows the following types of assets:

- Current assets, $759,768
- Investments, $235,500
- Noncurrent tangible assets, $321,235

Current assets include cash and other assets that will be converted into cash within one year through the normal operations of the practice. The Ideal balance sheet illustrates the typical types of current assets that most practices present in their balance sheets. Marketable securities are short-term investments, such as certificates of deposit, United States treasury bills, and money market accounts. Note that accounts receivable are reduced by an estimated amount that is not expected to be collected, called *Allowances for Uncollectible Accounts*. These allowances include adjustments to gross charges billed, discounts for contractual agreements, and estimated uncollectible amounts.

Investments are not used in group operations and are held for purposes other than conversion into cash to finance current operations. Items typically included in this category are investments in securities, long-term receivables, investments in affiliates, and property held for future use. Investments in securities include long-term bonds, certificates of deposit, and preferred and common stock. These securities may be kept in a separate fund for a special purpose, such as for expanding facilities or repaying long-term debt. When a group wants to exercise control or significantly influence the direction of a closely related entity, it may hold that entity's securities as an investment.

Noncurrent tangible assets include long-lived assets used in group operations. Examples are land, land improvements, buildings, equipment and furniture, and fixtures. Except for land, all assets in this classification are subject to periodic write-off of their cost as an expense, a process described previously as depreciation. As each asset is depreciated, annual depreciation amounts are entered into a separate account, called *accumulated depreciation.* Thus, Ideal's balance sheet shows the cost of furniture, fixtures, and equipment ($481,655) followed by a deduction for the accumulated depreciation as of December 31, 19X1 ($160,420), to arrive at the net value of noncurrent tangible assets ($321,235).

Intangibles and other assets include organization costs, goodwill, relocation costs, and any other assets not classifiable in the above categories. Organization costs pertain to legal, accounting, and state-imposed fees incident to incorporation. These costs are generally written off in a short time period, say 60 months. Goodwill is an intangible asset that is recognized only when another medical practice is purchased and the purchase price is greater than the value of the tangible assets acquired. This excess is called goodwill. According to generally accepted accounting principles, recognized goodwill is written off or amortized over its useful life, or 40 years, whichever is less. Relocation costs arise from moving the location of the group's operations, all or in part. These costs are capitalized and written off over a short time period, such as three to five years.

There are no intangible assets for the Ideal Medical Group. Indeed, few practices use the intangible assets category.

Liabilities

Liabilities are comprised of two types of obligations—short-term and long-term. Current liabilities are obligations arising from past transactions that must be paid within one year from the balance sheet date, either by using current assets or by incurring other current liabilities. Accounts in this category include accounts payable, claims payable, notes and loans payable, current portion due of long-term debt, payroll withholdings, accrued payroll liabilities, other accrued liabilities, patient deposits, accrued contract claims payable, and deferred revenue from prepaid plans or capitation contracts.

Most of these items are self-explanatory. Other accrued liabilities relate to amounts due for services that have been received and used by the group in operations prior to the supplier's billing date, which falls in the next accounting period. An adjustment is necessary to recognize the amount of services received as an expense in the income statement and to show a liability on the balance sheet. Called incurred but not received claims (IBNR), these expense estimates will be transferred to claims payable when bills have been received from the service suppliers. Deferred revenue from prepaid plans or capitation contracts represents payments received in advance of the period when the group is to provide services.

In Ideal's balance sheet, total current liabilities aggregate $405,850 and include many of the above items.

Long-term liabilities embrace obligations that will not mature nor require the use of current assets within one year of the balance sheet date. The current portion of this debt is carried as a current liability, as indicated above. In a note to the statement, disclosures for the major types of borrowings should include the interest rate, repayment schedule, security covenants, and other material information. The types of long-term liabilities are long-term notes payable, mortgages payable, construction loans payable, and capital lease obligations.

The first three types are self-explanatory. Capital lease obligations arise from lease agreements between two parties for the rental of a facility or equipment. Under generally accepted accounting principles, certain noncancellable leases that meet specified criteria must be recorded as capital lease obligations by the lessee. That is, the amount of future payments must be recorded as a long-term asset and a long-term liability on the balance sheet of the lessee. Once capitalized, the asset and lease liability are accounted for separately. The asset is depreciated over its useful life, and the lease liability is treated as a form of installment debt.

Leases that do not meet the capitalization criteria are called *operating leases*. In this case, lease payments are expensed as rent when payments are made, and there is no capital asset or liability on the balance sheet of the lessee.

A $200,000 long-term note payable appears on Ideal's balance sheet in this category.

Stockholders' Equity

When the medical group operates as a corporation, owners' equity is called stockholders' equity. Terms used on balance sheets for this category can be confusing because they include legal and accounting terms that are not fully standardized. Accounts appearing under stockholders' equity include preferred stock, common stock, capital contributed in excess of par, donated capital, retained earnings, and treasury stock.

Stockholders' investments in a corporation results in increases in both assets and stockholders' equity. Shares of stock are issued to the investors to represent ownership. If the amount invested exceeds the par, or stated value indicated on the shares issued, the excess is recorded in a separate account, called *capital contributed in excess of par*. The par value is a nominal amount representing the legal, or stated, capital that provides creditors a financial cushion. It is simply the legal capital per share. It is the minimum consideration the corporation must receive to issue shares as fully paid. Once issued, any shareholder's liability is limited to the amount invested.

Preferred stock has certain preferences and limitations written into the contract between the issuing corporation and the holder. Typical preferences are dividends up to some specified percent, if declared, and accumulations of dividends in arrears for years in which they were not distributed. Dividends must be declared by the board of directors of the corporation before they are carried as a liability. Preferred dividends usually must be paid before any dividend on common stock is declared.

The number of shares authorized, issued, and outstanding for both common and preferred stock must be disclosed in financial statements, along with the number of shares reacquired but not cancelled. The latter is called treasury stock and, if it exists, it is subtracted from total stockholders' equity when displayed on the balance sheet.

Retained earnings, a major component of stockholders' equity, shows the accumulation of net income and losses net of dividends declared and paid. At the end of each accounting period, net income appears as an increase to the retained earnings account (a net loss decreases retained earnings). When the entity declares a dividend or distribution of earnings, the dividend amount reduces retained earnings. Thus, at any balance sheet date, retained earnings are the accumulation of lifetime net earnings, offset by net losses and reduced by the amount of dividends declared and paid to stockholders to date.

The stockholders' equity category on the Ideal Medical Group balance sheet shows three types of equity, totaling $710,653.

Partners' Equity

If a medical group organizes as a partnership, the owners' equity is called partners' equity. The partners' equity, or capital, is comprised of two parts: contributed capital and undistributed earnings. Sometimes these two elements are combined. Recall that a partnership agreement, rather than a state incorporation statute, governs owner distributions in a partnership. Since general partners have unlimited liability for partnership debts, the record of contributed capital is not so important to creditors as it is in a corporation.

RESPONSIBILITY ACCOUNTING

The focus next shifts to management accounting and a framework for organizing financial information so that internal reports reflect the detailed operations of the medical group. This framework is called responsibility accounting.

What Is Responsibility Accounting?

Responsibility accounting is a system of accounting in which accounts are aligned with the organizational structure of the practice. This facilitates the collection and reporting of relevant information to managers who are responsible for various segments of the practice's operations. Responsibility accounting is most useful for large groups in which different individuals are given responsibility for specific areas of the practice. However, the structuring of accounting data in this way is also useful for smaller groups, even those in which one or a few individuals are responsible for all phases of operations.

A premise underlying responsibility accounting is that the accounting system should support the planning and control efforts of the organization. Indeed, this premise is at the heart of management control, which is defined as the process or system by which managers assure that resources are obtained and employed efficiently and effectively to achieve organizational goals and objectives.

In this context, *efficiency* refers to the relationship of inputs (costs) to outputs (revenues and quality care). A group is efficient when it delivers its services at the least possible cost for a given level of output, in terms of revenue dollars, and provides the best quality of care. *Effectiveness* refers to the achievement of an organization's goals and objectives. A medical practice is effective when it achieves all its stated goals and objectives. Failure to meet its goals and objectives implies that the practice is ineffective. A practice may be effective but inefficient if it achieves its goals and objectives but does so at a financial loss to its owners.

Responsibility Centers

Responsibility accounting in organizations is implemented by the designation and use of responsibility centers. A responsibility center is an identifiable organizational unit, headed by a designated individual, established to conduct certain assigned activities of the medical group. Usually the manager has decision-making authority and exercises some measure of control over a segment of the group's practice. The responsibility center consumes some resources and provides some benefit, either directly or indirectly, to patients. How responsibility centers are constituted may vary. A responsibility center may be an activity, a department, a function, or a specific geographic location.

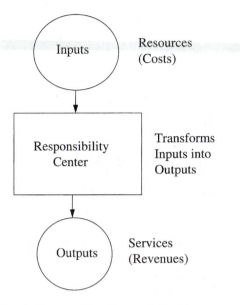

FIGURE 3–1 Resource Flows Responsibility Center

It may consist of the activities of a single employee or an entire department.

Figure 3–1 summarizes the basic operation of a responsibility center. The responsibility center transforms inputs, or costs of resources, into outputs, or services. Some responsibility centers' outputs are patient treatments that are represented by revenue dollars. Other re-

sponsibility centers' outputs include such items as accounting reports or human resource department services, which are difficult to measure in quantitative terms. These latter centers are called *indirect responsibility centers.*

Responsibility accounting provides information about inputs (costs) and outputs (revenues) for two purposes. One purpose is to supply information to control revenues and costs. The other is to provide information for decision making. For these purposes, three types of responsibility centers can be identified: expense, or cost, centers; profit, or contribution, centers; and investment centers. Table 3–4 summarizes each type of responsibility center. The centers differ in the types of financial information they generate and in the relative emphasis they place on flows of expenses, profits, and investments.

Expense, or Cost, Centers

The primary orientation of expense, or cost, centers is the measurement and reporting of expenses, or costs, incurred. Generally, these centers do not serve patients directly, but costs incurred are collected and traced to patient care through a process called *cost allocation.* Managers of these centers are evaluated on their ability to minimize the costs incurred to deliver their particular service, either in total dollars or in cost per unit of service. Some examples of cost centers in medical

TABLE 3–4 Types of Responsibility Centers

Characteristics	Expense, or Cost, Center	Profit, or Contribution, Center	Investment Center
Traceability of financial data	Expenses: total expenses, expenses per unit of output	Revenues: total revenues, total expenses, profit or contribution	Revenues, expenses, assets employed
Financial measures of performance	Amount of expenses; actual vs. previous period, actual vs. planned, actual vs. other comparable groups	Amount contributed by responsibility center to cover common costs and generate income for physicians	Return on assets employed (also measures cited for other types of centers)
Nonfinancial measures of performance	Time spent and quantity of resources consumed per unit of output	Number of patients served, time spent and quantity of resources consumed per unit of output	Number of patients served, time spent and quantity of resources consumed per unit of output
Evaluation criterion	Minimize expenses: minimize dollars of expense per unit of activity	Maximize profit or contribution	Maximize return on assets

groups are medical records, reception and appointments, accounting, and occupancy.

Profit, or Contribution, Centers

Profit, or contribution, centers perform services for patients. Services are measured by revenue, and the costs incurred in service delivery are tracked and matched against revenue to develop a profit, or contribution, measure for the center. Managers in these centers are evaluated on their ability to control costs in relation to the revenue generated and to produce a satisfactory contribution that covers common costs and provides the physicians with desired income levels. Contribution is defined as revenue less direct costs traceable to the contribution center. Examples of profit, or contribution, centers are the medical group's clinical and ancillary departments, such as family practice, pediatrics, and laboratory.

Investment Centers

Investment centers are responsibility centers within which the amount of assets employed can be determined, as can the revenues and costs generated by the center. Resulting profits or contributions produced by these centers can then be related to the amount of assets used, to compute a rate of return on investment. This type of center is used by large corporations with diversified operations and multiple products and services. However, in large medical groups, with independent satellite clinics scattered throughout several markets, this approach may be applicable, particularly if the clinics are self-supporting. Another area in which a return on assets is appropriate is in evaluating an ancillary department that has a large investment in equipment. In this case, the ancillary department could establish fees to generate a desired rate of return on assets employed.

Other Centers

In every organization, there are other responsibility centers to which financial data can be traced. Although it may not be feasible to trace revenues and costs, some types of nonfinancial data are available for all responsibility centers. These nonfinancial data may include time spent, hours of operation, quantity of resources consumed, and some physical measure of output.

BASIC CONCEPTS OF COST ACCOUNTING

An essential component of proactive management reporting is cost accounting. Accurate cost identification at all levels, but especially at the procedure and treatment levels, provides an effective basis for practice management, flexible budgeting, cost control, and contract analysis.

Cost accounting systems are part of management information systems, with data bases that provide medical groups with the so-called "true cost" of services and products. Before managed care, medical groups relied mostly on cost information broadly gleaned from billing data. The prices charged to patients for service were often based on optimizing reimbursement rather than on detailed cost analysis. Groups based their costs on the ratio of costs to charges and, as a result, may have made incorrect calculations. For example, managers may have assumed they were losing money on a certain diagnosis-related group (DRG) when they were actually making money, or vice versa. More accurate knowledge of costs enables group management to negotiate competitive health care contracts, market their services, and focus efforts on the review of unprofitable areas.

Use of Cost Data in Medical Group Practices

The importance of cost information for medical group managers parallels the general financial information needs cited earlier in this chapter. Specifically, groups benefit from having accurate and complete cost data in five distinct areas:

1. Measuring income
2. Distributing income to physicians
3. Controlling costs
4. Overall planning
5. Decision making of various types

Income Measurement

As stated previously, costs of services rendered must be determined for discrete time periods, such as years or quarters, and matched with revenues in order to calculate periodic net income. Fortunately, medical groups do not have the complex cost-measurement problems found in manufacturing or other businesses with myriad types of inventories. The basic issue for medical groups is whether a cash or accrual basis of accounting should be used. The position taken here is that accrual accounting provides the best measure of income for medical groups today, especially now that the prepaid component of health care services is increasing.

Distributing Income to Physicians

How a practice is organized and how income is distributed govern the practice's cost information needs. In the past, physician productivity generally was not a component of distribution schemes. The billing system, coupled with the convenient cash basis income system, provided the needed information for distributing income. The fee-for-service delivery mode rewarded physicians who saw more patients and had more patient visits. Cost data were not important as long as the practice received full, or almost full, reimbursement for the cost of services rendered.

Production-oriented income distribution systems are not consistent with prepaid medical care. Rather than treating sicker patients—or treating them more often—the motivation in the new environment is to keep patients well. Assuming maintenance of quality of care, there are now financial incentives for preventive rather than curative care. In groups with significant prepaid revenue components, income distribution methods are moving toward salary arrangements, together with incentives that include care utilization and referral control. Costs are now more important, and information needs center on cost per unit of activity and cost per member per month.

Cost Control

The control of costs is deemed by many to be the dominant purpose of cost data. The emphasis is now on determining cost per treatment, per procedure, and per patient. These determinations are effected largely through the tracing of costs and activities by the responsibility centers involved in the direct and indirect delivery of services to patients.

The control of costs depends on management's ability to clearly define responsibility center activities. In many businesses, managers of responsibility centers are held accountable for costs incurred by their centers. In many medical practices, however, the physician-manager of a responsibility center—particularly a specialty area—is expected to carry out the clinical activities of the center and leave cost control to the administrator or financial manager. As a result, the administrator or financial manager has responsibility for costs incurred through the decisions made by someone else in the organization. This sharing of responsibility leads to ineffective or no cost control. Clearly, there needs to be a shift in attitude among physicians who are *responsibility heads,* so that cost controls as well as clinical concerns are addressed.

Managers of centers must know what costs should be before activities are carried out. Such foreknowledge leads to decisions about patient protocols and procedures that are cost effective and cost efficient. This orientation requires involvement by physicians in budgeting costs and in developing standard costs, when feasible.

Overall Planning

Increasingly, medical groups are adopting formal budgeting approaches when planning the next year's operations. The growth of prepaid services as a larger proportion of total services is one factor driving the need to budget costs and expenses. Planning and controlling operations require two types of information: knowledge of what happens to revenues and costs as activity levels change; and knowledge of when cash is collected and when cash must be disbursed. Projections of cost must be based on the amount of resources used for various kinds of services performed.

Decision Making

Making decisions involves visualizing the future and the conditions that are likely to prevail in different situations. Some decisions, such as setting fees, are made routinely and are based on data from the financial information system. Other decisions, such as whether to perform a laboratory test in-house or to use an outside service, are made less often and require additional sources of information. In all decisions, special attention must be devoted to selecting the appropriate kind of cost information to assess the desirability of a particular course of action. Chapter 6 includes several examples that illustrate the use of cost data.

Classification of Costs

The term *cost* can be defined as the amount of resources consumed or used for a particular purpose. That purpose is labeled the *cost object* or *cost objective.* To understand the meaning of the term *cost* there must be a specific object or designated relationship toward which cost is directed. For example, one can speak of the cost of a service, cost of a product, cost of running a department, cost of a piece of equipment, or cost of treating a patient. Without a cost object, the meaning of the term *cost* cannot be determined. Furthermore, there are different kinds of cost—historical cost, replacement cost, joint cost, common cost, future cost. To be useful, the specific meaning of *cost* must be identified. The next several sections describe a number of key classes of costs.

Direct and Indirect Costs

In health care, this classification is widely used. It is an important categorization to follow in determining the cost of providing patient care. A direct cost is a cost that can be traced to, or is caused by, a particular cost object, such as a service, product, activity, or segment of the practice. In patient treatments, direct costs are the salaries of the physician and other medical personnel involved in care delivery, the supplies used, and, in some cases, the outside referral costs.

An indirect cost is a cost that cannot be traced to a particular cost object—a service, product, activity, or segment of the practice—but that is necessary to support the total practice. An indirect cost is generated by two or more cost objects jointly, but it is not traceable directly to any one cost object individually. The nature of indirect costs is such that it is not possible, or at least not feasible, to measure directly how much of an indirect cost is attributable to a single cost object. Thus, these costs must be allocated to all the cost objects on some equitable, but arbitrary, basis. Examples of indirect costs are the salaries of employees in the business office, malpractice insurance premiums, and occupancy costs. Frequently, indirect costs are referred to as "overhead."

The designation of a particular cost as direct or indirect depends upon the cost object, and the same cost may be construed as direct indirect in different contexts. For example, the financial manager's salary is a direct cost when the cost object is the cost of managing the practice. But the manager's salary is an indirect cost when the cost object is the cost of treating patients.

Full Costs and Differential Costs

Full costs represent the cost of all resources used for a specific cost object, such as treating a patient or running a specialty department. The full cost is determined by combining the total direct costs of that activity with a fair share of indirect costs. For example, the full cost of treating a patient would include the direct costs (share of physician and other delivery personnel salaries, and supplies) plus an allocation of applicable indirect costs (occupancy, business office expenses, malpractice insurance, and so on that support the activity.

Differential costs, sometimes referred to as incremental costs, are the difference in cost of alternative courses of action in specific situations. For example, if a physician has a choice of treating a patient with procedure A ($300 cost) or procedure B ($500 cost), the differential cost between procedures A and B would be $200. The term *differential* can also be employed in the context of revenue. Differential revenue is the difference between alternatives in the revenues they produce.

Controllable Costs and Noncontrollable Costs

Like direct and indirect costs, classifying costs as controllable and noncontrollable depends upon the context. At some level in any business, all costs are controllable, but not all costs are controllable at the same level of management. Costs are considered controllable at a particular level if the manager at that level has the power to authorize or influence the amount of costs incurred.

For example, a manager of a specialty department is responsible for controlling the use of supplies within that department. But the manager has no control over the amount of occupancy costs allocated to the department. The manager has little influence over the amount of rent, maintenance costs, and depreciation charged to the department, except, perhaps, for the percentage allocation of the total occupancy costs. In this case, occupancy costs are deemed noncontrollable by the specialty manager. However, at another level in the organization, someone else—perhaps the administrator or governing body that makes decisions on rented facilities and maintenance—assumes control for those occupancy costs.

Costs are classified as controllable and noncontrollable at various levels of management. Internal reports that are prepared for each manager should break down costs into those that are controllable by that manager and those that are not.

Sunk Costs

A sunk cost is a cost that has already been incurred and, thus, cannot be changed. The historical cost and the book value (historical cost less accumulated depreciation) of a long-lived asset are examples of sunk costs.

The concept of sunk costs is useful in certain short-run decision-making situations. For example, assume a medical group purchased an expensive piece of equipment (with an estimated life of five years) for $50,000 two years ago. Its book value is now $30,000 ($50,000 less two years' depreciation of $20,000). A technologically improved model is now available. It performs more efficiently than the old equipment and would save $150,000 per year in operating costs. The $30,000 book value of the old equipment, which is still productive and usable, is a sunk cost that should not figure in the decision to replace the equipment with the new model. The only relevant factors to consider are the cost

savings plus other gains from higher performance levels and the cost of the new model.

Discretionary Costs

When certain costs are not considered absolutely essential to the short-term operations of a practice, they are classified as discretionary costs. For example, the costs of continuing education for office employees are classified as discretionary—they could be foregone without great harm in the short-run, except perhaps for the ill feelings and disappointment felt by the employees. Other examples of discretionary costs are promotion expenses, management consulting fees, and charitable contributions to local community organizations. In tight budgetary situations, these costs are usually the first to be reduced or eliminated, because their discontinuance does not affect short-term results to any large degree. However, these costs should be examined periodically to ascertain their long-run impact.

Opportunity Costs

Opportunity costs measure the potential benefits that are lost when an alternative is *not* chosen. Assume a financial manager has excess cash of $75,000 in the practice for the next six months. At the end of this period, these funds will be needed to run the practice. Two choices are available for short-term investment of the funds—a money market account that pays 5 percent or the purchase of a six-month United States treasury bill, currently yielding 6.5 percent. If the manager decides to invest in the money market account, the opportunity cost of *not* investing in the Treasury bill is $2,438 ($75,000 × 6.5 percent × 1/2 year). Based on this calculation, the manager might consider switching investments to maximize the return to the practice and to minimize the opportunity cost.

Opportunity costs differ fundamentally from other types of costs because they do not represent a transaction involving a cash outlay. Nevertheless, they should be considered in all decisions involving the commitment of resources because generally there is at least one alternative to any expenditure of funds, even if it is only to not spend the money. If a medical group is contemplating opening up in a new location, for example, management should consider the opportunity cost of investing the resources in other activities or alternatives before committing funds to the new location.

Cost Behavior

Cost behavior relates to changes in cost as activity levels go up or down. Some costs rise or fall in synchronization with activity changes; other costs tend to remain constant. When managers understand the relationships between cost behavior and activity level changes, they are able to use cost data meaningfully to predict how costs will fluctuate under different operating conditions. Without this ability, serious mistakes in decision making can occur. For example, in contracting for the delivery of medical services under an HMO contract, the group must know which costs will change and by how much in order to negotiate a favorable rate for their services. In these situations and many others, this knowledge is crucial to reaching decisions that are advantageous to the medical group.

In every organization there are literally hundreds of unique relationships of cost and activity levels. However, cost data can be generalized to just four different configurations for ease in using cost data in decision-making. These four configurations are variable costs, fixed costs, semivariable or mixed costs, and step-fixed costs. They are illustrated in Figure 3–2. The cost structure of organizations varies, depending upon the relative importance of each type of cost. Some organizations, such as steel or aluminum manufacturing companies, have many fixed costs but relatively few variable or mixed costs. Most medical practices have this same structure. Other organizations, such as management consulting firms, have more variable costs than fixed costs. Each of these four types of cost configuration is discussed further below.

Variable Costs

Costs are variable when the total cost of an item varies both directly and proportionately with changes

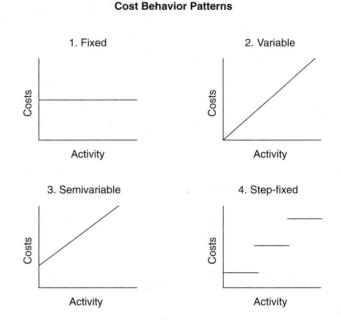

Cost Behavior Patterns

FIGURE 3–2 Illustration of Four Cost Behavior Patterns

in volume or level of activity. If activity rises 15 percent, then the total variable cost also increases by 15 percent; similarly, if volume goes down 5 percent, the total variable cost also falls by the same percentage.

For example, a medical group specializing in obstetrics/gynecology provides each patient with a videotape summarizing the typical experiences of pregnancy and outlining steps prospective mothers can take to relieve or cope with their condition. Each videotape costs the group $20.

Number of patients	Cost per videotape	Total variable cost
1	$20	$ 20
10	$20	$ 200
100	$20	$2,000

Although the unit cost of $20 per videotape remains constant, as the number of patients increases, the total variable cost rises proportionately. Thus, the activity measure, that is, the number of patients, drives the variable cost total.

In general, a *cost driver* is an activity that seems to "cause" the amount of a variable cost to fluctuate with changes in the level of that activity. Other examples of variable costs in medical settings are the costs of medical supplies and laboratory testing costs. The cost driver for these examples, as well as for many other types of costs in medical practice, is the number of patients. In hospitals, the cost driver may be the number of patients or the number of occupied beds. Increasingly, other types of cost drivers are being used, such as the procedures undertaken in treating patients.

Fixed Costs

Fixed costs are costs that remain the same regardless of the level of activity experienced. Fixed costs seem to predominate in medical practices. They include physician and administrative salaries, rent for equipment and facilities, malpractice insurance premiums, and depreciation on equipment. It is important to note that it is the total amount of a fixed cost that stays the same as volume fluctuates. However, the average, or unit, fixed cost changes as volume fluctuates. As activity or usage increases, for example, the average fixed cost per unit decreases, because the constant fixed cost total is spread out over more units. Conversely, as activity or usage decreases, the average fixed cost per unit rises, because total fixed costs are spread out over fewer units. The example below, involving the rental of an X-ray machine for $5,000 per month, illustrates this point.

Monthly rental cost	No. of patients treated	Avg. cost per patient
$5,000	5	$1,000
$5,000	50	$ 100
$5,000	500	$ 10

Sometimes it is useful to distinguish between two different categories of fixed costs: committed fixed costs and discretionary fixed costs. Certain fixed costs are related to the basic organizational structure of the practice and to the cost of investments in the fixed assets. These costs are committed in the sense that they cannot be eliminated or reduced significantly in the short run without affecting the continuity and long-term objectives of the practice. Examples of committed costs are the salaries of top management and key personnel,

depreciation on the building and equipment, and taxes and insurance on real estate. Most practices maintain these investments because the costs of replacing them far outweigh the short-term benefits.

Discretionary fixed costs include the costs of such items as promotional activities and continuing education. The benefits flowing from such costs are long-term and difficult to correlate with specific expenditures. Management decides upon a stipulated sum to budget and spend each year, but the amount can be changed at management's discretion if dire circumstances necessitate a reduction of practice costs.

The major differences between variable and fixed costs are summarized in Figure 3–3.

Mixed, or Semivariable, Costs

Both variable and fixed cost components are included in mixed, or semivariable, costs. At some activity levels, mixed costs appear to be variable; at others, they appear to be fixed. Mixed cost totals change in the same general direction as the change in activity level, but the amount of change in the total cost is less than proportional to changes in volume. For example, when an activity goes up 10 percent, the total cost of a mixed item may go up less than 10 percent.

There are many examples of mixed costs. In fact, some experts argue that most costs are mixed over the long run. Typical examples are operating an automobile, renting a copying machine, or processing accounting data through a service bureau. In all these

	In Total	Per Unit
Variable Cost	increases/ decreases proportionately with changes in activity level	remains constant
Fixed Cost	remains constant with changes in activity level	changes (rises or falls) as activity level changes

FIGURE 3–3 Comparison of Behaviors of Variable and Fixed Costs

cases, there is a fixed, or flat, charge for the use of the asset, with the variable cost portion rising as usage increases. When cost behavior patterns are analyzed for the purpose of predicting future levels of cost, items showing a mixed pattern must be separated into their variable and fixed components.

Step-Fixed Costs

Step-fixed costs are fixed over a certain range of activity but increase in a stair-step fashion at higher levels of volume. Many medical practice cost items seem to follow this pattern of behavior. When a new physician is added to a medical group, for example, many costs increase in this way, such as costs for clinical staff, nonclinical staff, expenses, rent, and depreciation on equipment.

Relevant Range of Activity

The time frame is an important variable in classifying costs in the four behavior patterns described above. Over long time periods, more costs are variable. Conversely, as one shortens the time perspective, more costs become fixed. For example, most costs in a medical practice do not change over the course of an hour or a day, regardless of the number of patients seen or the specific procedures performed. As the time frame expands, however, more and more costs become variable as more activities occur—so much so, in fact, that the expression "all costs vary in the long run" is often used. In most cases, a time period of a year is used. This is because budgets and reports of operations are generally prepared on an annual cycle.

The step-fixed pattern of cost-activity levels pose the interesting question of when it is necessary to include a cost with this configuration among the total fixed costs of a practice. Consider the step-fixed costs in Figure 3–4. For a range of volume from 0 to 500 patients, there are three cost levels, one for each of three different ranges of volume. The question is: Which one should be chosen to depict the level of fixed cost for the forthcoming year? The answer is: the level that is most likely to occur. Thus, if the middle level is believed to be the level that is most likely to occur, the middle range

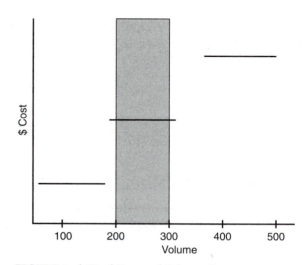

FIGURE 3–4 Fixed Costs and Relevant Range

is used as the "relevant range" for arriving at the amount of fixed cost.

Determining Cost Behavior Patterns

When information from cost behavior patterns is used, total costs must be broken down into variable and fixed costs. Two practical approaches are used to break down costs in this way: the inspection of accounts and the study of past cost behavior patterns. The two methods differ in the sources of data used in the analysis and in their accuracy.

The inspection of accounts involves simply examining the amounts of costs, incurred at various activity levels, that are accumulated in the group's accounting records. If the time period examined is sufficiently long, the cost patterns should be fairly evident. The basis for this method is largely intuitive and arbitrary; thus, it is likely to be less accurate than other methods. However, if only an approximation of cost patterns is needed, this approach may be cost effective.

An illustration of the inspection of accounts method is shown in Table 3–5, which presents a list of accounts and their probable cost behavior patterns. It should be noted that each medical group's situation is unique and that cost behavior patterns should be determined from the group's actual costs, operations, and style of practice.

The study of past cost behavior patterns is a more formal approach than the inspection of accounts. Past

TABLE 3–5   Illustration of Inspection of Accounts

	Determination of cost behavior patterns	
Account	**Account title**	**Cost behavior pattern**
5100	Physician salaries, distributions, and bonuses	Fixed—amount of distribution to doctors depends upon many factors other than activity level. A salary based upon production should be segregated and classified as a variable.
5200	Physician benefits	Fixed—see explanation for account 5100.
5400	Ancillary department salaries	Step-fixed—most medical practice personnel are hired in steps, resulting in a stair-step pattern.
5500	Medical support salaries	Step-fixed—see explanation for account 5400.
5600	Administrative salaries	Fixed—most medical practice administrative personnel costs will not depend upon activity levels.
5700	Housekeeping, maintenance, and security salaries	Fixed—see explanation for account 5600.
5800	Other salaries	Fixed—these salaries depend more on style of practice than activity level.
5900	Nonphysician employee benefits	Fixed—benefits are largely fixed by contract. To the extent that some of the salaries are variable, a portion of the benefits may also be variable.
6100	Supplies expense	Variable—with minor exceptions supplies relate to patient visits.
6200	Ancillary department supplies expense	Variable—see explanation for account 6100.
6400	Occupancy and use—buildings and grounds	Fixed—these costs relate to the provision of capacity rather than to various levels of activity in the use of capacity.
6500	Occupancy and use—building depreciation	Fixed—see explanation for account 6400.
6600	Occupancy and use—furniture, fixtures, and equipment	Fixed—see explanation for account 6400.
6700	Occupancy and use—furniture, fixtures, and equipment depreciation	Fixed—see explanation for account 6400.
6800	Occupancy and use—furniture, fixtures, and equipment expenses	Fixed—see explanation for account 6400.
7100	Purchased supplies—nonprepaid professional and medical	Variable—amount will depend upon the style of practice.
7200	Purchased services—nonprepaid professional and medical	Variable—amount will depend upon the amount of care the group must refer outside.
7300	General and administrative—purchased services	Fixed—amount will depend upon factors other than level of activity.
7400	General and administrative—employee-related	Fixed—most expenses in this category are discretionary and do not relate to volume of service.
7500	General and administrative—liability insurance	Fixed—this expense relates to the number of doctors and the types of specialities.
7600–7700	Other general and administrative expenses	Fixed—these expenses relate to the style of practice and discretion of management.
7800	Interest expense	Fixed—these expenses have no direct relationship to level of activity.
8200	Nonoperating expense	Fixed—these expenses have no relationship to operations.

SOURCE: Center for Research in Ambulatory Health Care Administration, 1990.

data are studied graphically or mathematically to discern relationships between cost amounts and activity levels. This method is used when greater accuracy is required, because empirical evidence is used to determine the cost patterns. To avoid distorting the patterns, accrual accounting measures of resource use must be used rather than cash accounting measures. This is because cash measures indicate only when a resource was paid, not necessarily when it was consumed.

In practice, three general methods are used to determine cost behavior patterns from past data:

1. Scatter-graph approach, which relies upon a visual fit of a number of observations using a graph
2. High-low method, which fits a line to two representative points of data using simple mathematics
3. Linear regression method, which fits a line to several observations using statistical methods

Readers who are interested in learning more about these approaches are encouraged to consult a cost accounting textbook.

In Figure 3–5, the analyst has "fit" a straight line to cost-activity data, under the assumption that cost and activity vary linearly, that is, in a straight line. The point where the fitted line meets the x-axis, FC, denotes the level of fixed costs. The slope of the fitted line provides VC, the variable cost per unit of activity. Thus, at any activity level, the fixed cost would be the same amount and the variable cost would be the number of units of activ-

ity times VC. Mathematically, a straight line can be fitted to any set of two or more points. However, evaluating the quality of the fit and the reliability of the resulting cost-activity formula requires sound judgment.

COST ALLOCATION

Calculating the cost of medical services requires knowledge of the way in which costs are allocated among the various types of activities, departments, and segments of a medical practice. This section examines how costs are accumulated into various pools and segments of the practice and then reassembled to determine the cost of treating patients.

What Is Cost Allocation?

Cost allocation is a process of taking costs from one cost objective and reassigning them to others. Although there are many types of cost allocation, only two are examined in detail here:

1. Allocating indirect costs within a department to specific individual patients (for example, allocating the medical director's salary to each patient)
2. Allocating one department's or cost center's costs to another center (for example, allocating the accounting department's costs to the patient-treating center)

All departments have direct and indirect costs. The salary of a technician performing a test for a specific patient and the cost of reagents used to perform the test are examples of direct costs. The salary of the lab manager, who performs many management activities but no testing, and the cost of clerical supplies used in the lab are examples of indirect costs. To determine the full costs of providing care to a specific patient, one must aggregate the direct costs and assign or allocate to the patient an appropriate share of the indirect costs.

Costs that are indirect and not easily associated with individual patients are referred to as overhead costs. Overhead costs require some form of aggregation and allocation to patients. One goal of cost allocation is to associate overhead costs as closely as possible with the patients who cause the costs to be incurred. In some cases, overhead costs can be assigned directly to

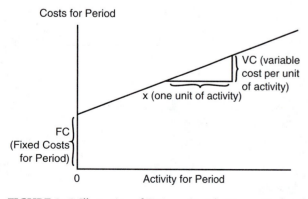

FIGURE 3–5 Illustration of Fitting a Straight Line to Cost and Activity Data

patients. In other cases, departments must assign their overhead costs to other departments first before they are assigned to patients. In all cases, the benefits of more accurate cost assignments must be weighed against the costs of collecting such data.

Consider the following example. A clinic's patients directly and indirectly receive the benefits of the housekeeping department. Housekeeping may clean patient consulting rooms and offices and perform other chores that enable the clinic to operate efficiently. It might be possible to measure the direct benefit as a direct cost. However, the amount of direct housekeeping cost for any one patient is low relative to the cost of measuring it and assigning it directly to the patient. Therefore, all housekeeping costs are usually considered as indirect to patient care. These costs are assigned to the various departments that consume housekeeping service, such as patient-treating centers. Each patient-treating center, in turn, allocates the housekeeping costs (along with other costs) to the various patients cared for by that department. Another example of cost allocation is given in Case Study 3–1.

Overhead Application Rates

In order to assign costs from one area or cost center to another, there must be a cost pool and a base. A cost pool is any grouping of costs to be allocated. A base is the criterion upon which the allocation is to be made. For example, costs might be allocated on the basis of patient-days or hours of services provided.

Consider the following example. To obtain an allocation rate, we divide the cost pool by the base. Assume the base is the total number of housekeeping hours of service. If housekeeping costs total $200,000 and housekeeping services total 20,000 hours, the allocation rate is:

$$\frac{\$200,000}{20,000 \text{ hours}} = \$10 \text{ per hour}$$

Each department using housekeeping services would be allocated a housekeeping charge equal to its number of hours of housekeeping services consumed, multiplied by the $10 per hour rate.

If total costs of the department were based on patient-days instead of hours of service, the $200,000 housekeeping costs would be divided by the number of patient-days to get a cost per patient-day. Thus, if the patient-days volume was 50,000 patient-days, the rate would be:

$$\frac{\$200,000}{50,000 \text{ patient-days}} = \$4 \text{ per patient-day}$$

When rates calculated in this manner are used to determine "product" costs, they are called *overhead application rates*. Each time a patient-day is incurred, the rate is applied to that patient. For example, assume housekeeping costs are allocated on the base of patient-days in a large clinic, and the ambulatory surgery department has accumulated 700 patient-days in a given month. Multiplying the overhead rate of $4 by the 700 patient-days in the center results in a housekeeping cost allocation to surgery of $2,800.

Overhead application rates are usually determined at the beginning of each year. The base for the allocation is determined (e.g., patient-days or direct labor hours) and then divided into a budgeted cost. The result is a budgeted cost per unit of the overhead base, or a budgeted overhead application rate. For example, assume that annual fixed costs for housekeeping are $240,000, and variable costs are $20 per hour of service provided. If 15,000 hours of service are expected for the year, the budgeted overhead application rate would be calculated as:

$$\frac{\text{Budgeted fixed costs} + \text{Budgeted variable costs}}{\text{Budgeted base volume}} = \text{Overhead rate}$$

$$\frac{\$240,000 + (\$20 \times 15,000 \text{ hours})}{15,000 \text{ hours}} = \frac{\$540,000}{15,000} = \$36/\text{hour}$$

This rate would be charged to each department consuming housekeeping services throughout the year. In this manner, the total cost of housekeeping would be spread out at an even rate over units of service each month.

Using an overhead rate based on budgeted data is referred to as *normal costing*. If the application rate is based instead on actual costs and actual usage, the process is called *actual costing*. To calculate an actual

CASE STUDY 3–1

ALLOCATING SERVICE DEPARTMENT COSTS

The Western Clinic had an ambulatory surgery department housed in a separate building. The department head, Dr. Greg Burns, wanted to know the full costs of its two major services, the operating room and other outpatient services. Dr. Burns wished to compare these costs with the revenues produced by the two services in order to evaluate their relative profitability.

To obtain full costs, it was necessary to allocate the costs of two service departments (Occupancy and Support Services) to the two profit centers (Operating Room and Outpatient Services). To perform the analysis, the following data for a recent quarter were compiled for Dr. Burns:

Responsibility Centers	Revenue	Direct Costs
Operating Room	$ 800,000	$ 300,000
Outpatient	2,400,000	900,000
Occupancy	0	240,000
Support Services	0	120,000

Allocation Basis and Percentages:

	Total	Profit Centers		Service Departments	
		Operating	Outpatient	Occupancy	Support
Square feet	100%	40%	45%	—	15%
Square feet (revised—after first allocation)	100%	47%	53%	—	—
Number staff	100%	15%	80%	5%	—
Number staff (revised—after first allocation)	100%	16%	84%	—	—

Case Discussion Questions

1. Allocate the direct costs of the two service departments to the two profit centers using the direct method.
2. Allocate the direct costs of the two service departments to the two profit centers using the step-down method, selecting occupancy as the first department to allocate.
3. Using the direct method of allocation, develop a profitability analysis, showing the relative contributions to profit for each profit center.

rate requires waiting until the accounting period has ended and patient care has been rendered. Normal costing, in contrast, provides a predetermined rate that can be used to determine each patient's cost on an ongoing basis. Normal costing also can provide management with the information needed for negotiating prices, evaluating the profitability of specific types of patients, and other important activities.

Allocation Bases

Selecting an appropriate base for cost allocations is an important and difficult issue. The base should make sense and cause the minimum amount of distortion in the accuracy of product costing. For example, for an admitting department, assignments of costs to patients should be based on the amount of time spent admitting the patient. This reflects a cause-and-effect relationship, the ideal basis. However, for other overhead areas, such as administration, supervision, depreciation, the basis of allocation is less obvious. The objective is to allocate overhead in a way that matches as closely as possible the changes in overhead costs incurred.

In health care, commonly used bases include patient-days or patient visits, hours spent on various activities, square feet of space occupied, quantity of units used, personnel count, total direct costs, gross payroll costs, and revenue. Table 3–6 shows some examples of allocation bases for several cost centers.

Use of Multiple Bases

Some medical practices use more than one basis of allocation. Each department may have its own unique rate. Also, within a department there may be different rates for allocating different types of costs.

TABLE 3–6 Common Allocation Bases for Medical Groups

Cost center or cost pool	Allocation bases
Occupancy (rent, depreciation, property taxes, maintenance)	Square footage Utilization
Data processing (rent, depreciation, maintenance)	Utilization Combination (square footage plus utilization)
Administration	Personnel count Equal to all departments
Central supplies and purchasing	Specific identification
Reception and appointments	Physician count (provider count) Patient visits
Medical records	Patient visits
Accounting	Personnel count Revenue production

Each rate should be based on a distinct cost driver. As defined above, cost drivers are activities that are responsible for fluctuations in costs. In the case of admitting, above, the cost driver is the hours of personnel time. Thus, costs from the admissions department are allocated on the basis of the amount of staff time consumed.

Consider a more complex example. For a radiology department, there might be one application rate for radiology supervision, based on the number of technicians, and another application rate for supplies, based on the number of X-rays developed. In cases such as this, indirect costs are segregated into several cost pools and a different application rate is determined for each pool. This approach is the basis for activity-based costing (ABC), which is being adopted widely by businesses.

Allocation Criteria

Responsibility center managers should agree on the technique, order, and basis of allocation before any numerical data are used. These issues should be decided on the basis of fairness, equity, understandability, and cost to implement. This approach is important, because managers are accountable for costs assigned to their departments.

There are three broad criteria for selecting allocation bases: cause-and-effect, facilities provided, ability to bear. Each is discussed briefly below.

Cause and Effect

The cause-and-effect criterion is a logical framework for ascertaining allocation bases. It normally results in fair and equitable cost allocations that are mutually acceptable to both the provider and the user of the service. Cause-and-effect is best measured through usage records. For example, using a vehicle owned by the practice may be charged to users directly. Ideally, to employ this criterion, the relationship between the cost to be allocated and the responsibility center receiving the allocation must be clear. Unfortunately, in most cases this relationship is casual or indeterminate.

For some responsibility centers, such as administration, there is no adequate measure of cause and effect. Attempts to measure cause and effect based on the time the administrator devotes to each responsibility center usually cause more problems than they solve and are very costly.

Facilities Provided

The logic underlying this criterion is that facilities are provided for all users and it is up to each responsibility center manager whether or not to use them. As a result, each manager should share responsibility in the possible, not the actual, use of facilities. Occupancy costs fit this criterion.

Ability to Bear

This criterion is arbitrary, because costs are allocated on the basis of those centers most able to cover additional costs. The fairness of this approach is questionable, especially in view of the fact that costs of services are often independent of their results. Any allocation scheme that uses revenues, gross charges, contributions, or a similar allocation base, without consideration of services provided in roughly the same proportion, is based on the ability to bear.

Cost Allocation Techniques

The approach followed by most health care organizations for internal cost determinations is that required for Medicare cost reports, often called *institutional cost reports* (ICRs). This approach specifies that all resource consumption first be associated with either a support center or a revenue center. For instance, housekeeping and finance are examples of support centers, and cardiology or other specialty and laboratory are examples of revenue centers. Each center accumulates its direct costs, such as labor and supplies. Then, all costs of the nonrevenue or support centers are allocated to the revenue centers that treat patients directly. Three techniques for allocating these costs to revenue centers are presently in use: direct allocation, step-down allocation, and simultaneous equations, or matrix algebra, allocation. Figure 3–6 shows a flow chart of data for the direct and step-down allocation methods. Table 3–7a

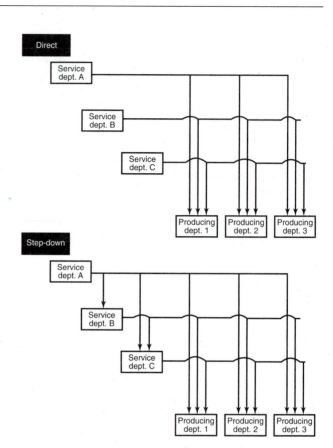

FIGURE 3–6 Service Department Allocation Methods

and b shows an example of the application of the direct and step-down allocation methods.

Direct Allocation

In this technique, costs of each service department are allocated directly and only to revenue centers. No costs of services are allocated to other service departments. When there are few service centers in a group, this technique produces equitable allocations at a reasonable cost. This is also the simplest technique, requiring a minimum of clerical effort.

In a complex organization with many shared services, the direct allocation method has a major disadvantage. It fails to recognize that services performed by one service department may benefit another and, consequently, does not develop the full cost of

TABLE 3–7a   Illustration of Direct and Step-Down Allocation

Allocation Bases Cost Centers	Direct Costs	Allocation Statistics	
		Maintenance Sq. Feet	Administration No. Personnel
Support:			
Maintenance	$ 80,000	—	10%
Administration	$ 120,000	30%	—
Revenue:			
Orthopedics	$ 800,000	40%	60%
Internal Medicine	$ 300,000	30%	30%
	$ 1,300,000	100%	100%

TABLE 3–7b   Illustration of Direct and Step-Down Allocation

Direct Distribution Cost Centers	Direct Costs	Allocation				Total Costs
		Maintenance Sq. Feet		Administration No Personnel		
Support:						
Maintenance	$ 80,000	$ (80,000)		—		—
Administrative	$ 120,000	—		$ (120,000)		—
Revenue:						
Orthopedics	$ 800,000	$ 45,715	[4/7]	$ 80,000	[2/3]	$ 925,715
Internal Medicine	$ 300,000	$ 34,285	[3/7]	$ 40,000	[1/3]	$ 374,285
	$ 1,300,000	$ 0		$ 0		$ 1,300,000

Step-Down Distribution Cost Centers	Direct Costs	Allocation						Total Costs
		Maintenance Sq. Feet		Subtotal	Administration No. Personnel			
Support:								
Maintenance	$ 80,000	$ (80,000)						
Administrative	$ 120,000	$ 24,000	[30%]	$ 144,000	$ (144,000)			
Revenue:								
Orthopedics	$ 800,000	$ 32,000	[40%]	$ 832,000	$ 96,000	[2/3]	$	928,000
Internal Medicine	$ 300,000	$ 24,000	[30%]	$ 324,000	$ 48,000	[1/3]	$	372,000
	$ 1,300,000	0		$ 1,300,000	0		$	1,300,000

operations in service departments. Thus, unfair allocations may result.

Step-Down Allocation

The step-down technique is also relatively simple. The fairest result seems to arise from the manner of identifying responsibility centers that provide the most support and the order in which these service department costs are allocated. In this technique, costs of service departments providing the most services to all departments—revenue-producing and service—are allocated first. All remaining service departments' costs are then allocated in descending order of their services-rendering experience. Thus, as the costs of a service department are allocated to revenue centers and remaining service departments, there is a step-down or continuation to the next service department. Once the costs of a service department are allocated, that service department is considered closed and no subsequent allocations are made to it from other service departments. Because no subsequent allocations are made to a closed service department, the step-down technique does not produce the full cost of each service department.

This technique is the most widely used method of cost allocation and is reasonably accurate for most purposes. It is also a systematic approach that involves only moderate clerical effort, especially with the use of a computer.

Simultaneous Equations

Also known as matrix algebra allocation, this technique provides the most precise information and develops full costs for each responsibility center through the use of simultaneous algebraic equations. The technique can be used effectively by a large organization with highly sensitive data, if the benefits exceed the costs of using the method. Because of the complex mathematical calculations required, a computer is necessary. Although most medical groups do not need the degree of accuracy the technique yields, the increasing use of computer software programs has led more and more groups to adopt this technique.

DETERMINING THE COST OF PATIENT SERVICES

Determination of the cost of providing patient health care services has evolved steadily, starting with fairly simple calculations and progressing to increasingly more refined approaches. In this section, the current method of determining these costs is presented. Future refinements will lead to greater accuracy and better understanding of what constitutes the cost of these services.

Assigning Costs to Units of Service

In the previous section, all costs of the organization were allocated into cost centers and then into the rev-

enue centers where patients are treated. The next step is to assign each revenue center's costs to the units of service that the group provides to its patients. For example, a patient-treating center assigns its costs to the surgical procedures that take place within it; a laboratory assigns its costs to the various laboratory tests it performs. Finally, costs are assigned to individual patients or to groups of patients, such as DRG.

To allocate costs to units of service requires the use of an allocation base. Bases used by practices include the number of procedures, tests, treatments, patients, or cases. These bases are sometimes referred to as *macro bases.* In some instances, groups or departments within groups can assign costs to patients more accurately using *micro bases,* such as person-minutes. Use of micro bases results in a more direct association of resource consumption with individual patients. Table 3–8 presents examples of macro and micro allocation bases.

The choice of which basis to use—macro or micro—depends on the accuracy of cost determinations and the cost/benefit relationships desired. Macro bases are broader and more global, and they require larger aggregations of cost and supporting data. Micro bases are narrower in scope and require more detailed data and calculations; thus, they are more costly to develop and apply.

Job-Order and Process Costing

The assignment of costs to patients can be accomplished using the principles of job-order or process costing. These methods have been in use for many years in the manufacturing industries, and medical group financial managers have borrowed many of their techniques to develop patient costing systems in health care. In process costing, all units produced or serviced within a given time period are assigned the same cost. In job-order costing, the cost of producing the units for each job (patient) are measured separately. An example of job-order costing is given in Case Study 3–2.

Job-order costing is used in product or service industries in which the products or services consume different amounts of inputs. For instance, a custom furniture manufacturer might use different amounts of labor,

TABLE 3–8   Macro and Micro Allocation Bases

Department	Macro (Gross) Production Unit	Micro (Weighted) Production Unit
Surgery	Surgical case	Person–minutes
Anesthesiology	Anesthesia case	Anesthesiology–minutes
Radiology	Examinations	Relative value units
Laboratory	Tests	Relative value units
Physical therapy	Modalities	Person–minutes
Delivery room	Deliveries	Person–minutes
Emergency department	Visits	Person–minutes
Social service	Visits	Person–hours
Nursing	Patient-days	Hours of care

materials, and overhead for each job. A management consulting firm might employ different amounts of resources for each engagement. Process costing is widely used when all products or services consume about the same amount of inputs. For example, a soft drink producer uses up about the same amount of resources for each bottle of soft drink produced. In practice, many organizations employ a hybrid system that combines job-order and process costing in varying degrees.

Table 3–9 compares process and job-order costing for two patients treated by a dermatology group. In process costing, the total costs for treating both patients are aggregated and divided by two to reach an average cost per patient. Recall that process costing assumes that all units of service consume equal amounts of labor, supplies, and indirect costs. In job-order costing, it is necessary to determine the amount of labor and materials used by each service unit. Thus, costs are tracked individually for each patient. Note that Patient A consumed more hours of labor and that each hour of labor was more expensive than the labor used by Patient B. Also, Patient A consumed more clinical supplies. With job-order costing, a specific cost per patient is obtained, which is in sharp contrast to the average cost per patient provided by process costing.

In the job-order illustration, overhead is allocated equally between the two patients. A more accurate amount of overhead consumed by each patient would be based on the amount of time involved in performing the procedure or treatment. Another refinement in assigning costs to jobs is to consider differences in the rel-

ative values of the procedures used to treat each patient. This would require special studies to develop a relative value scale of procedures and to apply cost allocation to the units indicated in the relative value scale. Alternatively, the relative values included in the Resource-Based Relative Value System (RBRVS) used in Medicare reimbursement might be used in allocating costs to units.

Historically, health care organizations have used more elements of process costing than job-order costing. In an era when groups were reimbursed for all costs, there was little incentive to establish cost accounting systems that tracked costs more precisely than by broad averages for each patient. Since the advent of the Medicare prospective payment system using DRGs, and with the increasing movement toward managed-care contracts, job-order costing is gaining favor among medical practices. Job-order costing recognizes the unique needs and resource consumption of each patient and provides cost information that is more useful in profitability analysis and contracting.

Table 3–10 summarizes the essential differences between the two methods of product or service costing. A major decision that any health care organization must make is the level of detail desired in its cost determinations. When greater specificity is chosen to enhance cost accuracy, there is more complexity and cost in record keeping. Where to draw the line between specific costs and average costs is a decision each organization must reach in designing its own product costing system. No matter what approach is chosen, there will invariably be some averaging of costs. Process

CASE STUDY 3-2

DETERMINING THE COST OF A PROCEDURE

The financial manager of the Western Clinic, Erin Figures, is concerned about the profit margin of sigmoidoscopies performed at the clinic for Medicare and nonMedicare patients. She completed a special study of activities undertaken to perform the sigmoidoscopic procedure and compiled the following cost information:

Physician salary	$200,000 desired annual income
	Works 40 hours per week with four weeks vacation and professional development
Technician salary	$24,000 per year
	Works an average of 1,800 hours/year
Direct material	Per sigmoidoscopy, $5.75 (Cidex, gauze, gloves, table paper, gown, etc.)
Indirect overhead	Annual fixed costs:

Office salaries	$ 56,800
Benefits	22,600
Rent	48,000
Malpractice and other insurance	10,000
Office equipment depreciation	8,600
Total	$146,000

Total procedures administered for all treatments to all patients during the year—9,000

Direct overhead	Sigmoidoscope depreciation ($12,000 cost divided by 4-year life = $3,000 per year divided by 600 budgeted procedures/year)
Physician time	15 minutes
Technician time	60 minutes

Case Discussion Questions

1. Calculate the full cost of a sigmoidoscopic procedure, using a job-order costing approach.
2. Calculate the per-patient profit for each sigmoidoscopy patient, assuming the clinic receives $81.25 per procedure for a Medicare patient and $110.00 per procedure for a nonMedicare patient.

costing does its averaging over a larger number of units (patients), whereas job-order costing uses a much smaller number.

Assigning Costs to Patients

The discussion thus far of how costs are accumulated, assigned, and allocated to determine the total cost of treating a patient is summarized in Figure 3–7. The figure shows the flow of costs through the various stages

of accumulation. It also shows the major processes that are carried out to arrive at the cost of patient care.

The first flow illustrates the allocation of service center costs to revenue centers, using the direct, step-down, or multiple-equation allocation methods. After all costs have been accumulated in the revenue centers, they are assigned to service units. If the service unit is the individual patient or a group of patients, such as a designated DRG, the entity decides what type of cost accounting system it wants to use—job-order or process.

TABLE 3–9   Process Costing for Surgical Patients

Cost Elements	Amount
Total labor (nursing and technicians):	
20 hours @ $28	$ 560
Surgical supplies	3,440
Overhead costs (depreciation, administration, etc.)	1,000
Total costs	$5,000
Divided by number of patients	÷2
Cost per patient	$2,500

Job-Order Costing for Surgical Patients

	Amounts	
Cost Elements	Patient A	Patient B
Total labor (nursing and technicians):		
16 hours @ $30	$ 480	
4 hours @ $20		$ 80
Surgical supplies	640	2,800
Overhead costs (depreciation, admin., etc.)	500	500
Total costs	$1,620	$3,380

TABLE 3–10   Advantages of Process and Job-Order Costing

Advantage	Process Costing	Job-Order Costing
More detailed information		x
Less expensive system	x	
More accurate information		x
Less burdensome to maintain	x	
Better for decision making		x
Less potential employee resistance	x	
Usefulness for responsibility accounting	x	x

Comparison of Costing Process and Job-Order

	Process Costing	Job-Order Costing
Labor	Averaged	Specific
Materials	Averaged	Specific
Overhead	Averaged	Averaged

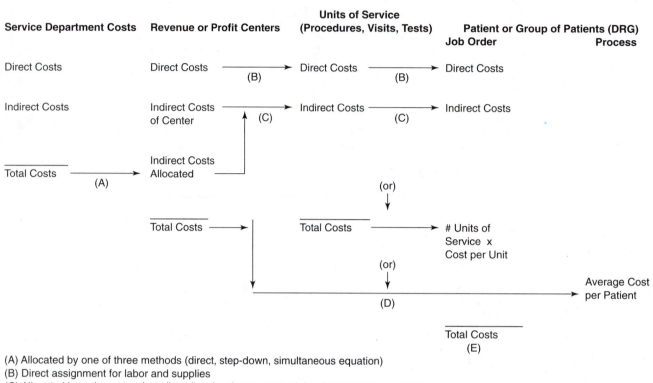

(A) Allocated by one of three methods (direct, step-down, simultaneous equation)
(B) Direct assignment for labor and supplies
(C) Allocated based on rates (per diem, hourly-minute rate, weighted procedures, or RVUs)
(D) Total cost per center divided by the number of patients
(E) For a group of patients, total costs are averaged to obtain cost per patient.

FIGURE 3–7 Cost Flows: Determining Patient Costs

If process costing is used, the total cost of each revenue center that treats a patient is allocated to the patient(s) by some averaging method. The allocation bases might be the number of patients, visits, procedures, tests, or days of treatment, or an hourly or per-minute rate. If job-order costing is used, the direct costs of labor and materials are traced directly to each patient's record. The indirect costs are allocated to the patient(s) through a similar averaging method by using allocation bases, as described above for process costing. If a more sophisticated allocation base for indirect costs is deemed necessary, a weighted procedure or relative value-units method might be developed and used. There might be an intermediary step between the assignment of revenue

center costs to the patient(s) in a job-order system, if specific procedures or treatments are the service unit cost object. That is, total direct and indirect revenue center costs might be assigned to specific procedures using a scale of relative value units to obtain a cost per procedure. Then, the final assignment of procedure costs would be made to the patient(s) depending upon the type and quantity of each procedure administered to each patient.

No detailed examples of these cost flows are provided in this chapter. Interested readers should consult a cost accounting text that covers health care costing for a fuller understanding of the more elaborate cost determinations that are now being adopted by medical practices.

COST ACCOUNTING SYSTEMS

Cost accounting systems can be based on either past or future costs. An actual cost system keeps track of past costs, while a standard cost system uses future costs in conjunction with past costs. In practice, some combination of the two systems is used by most medical groups.

Actual Cost System

An actual cost system deals only with historical or past costs that have been incurred. These costs appear in the accounting records and are shaped by the application of generally accepted accounting principles. As a reflection of past events, management can do nothing to change the amounts of actual costs once incurred. For the same reason, the utility of actual cost data is somewhat limited for current decision-making or planning purposes. Planning in particular requires management to look forward and estimate what costs are likely to be in the next few years.

Even though actual costs may not represent future costs, managers can use actual cost data as the starting point to predict future costs. Also, actual cost data can be analyzed to identify problem areas where inefficiencies are occurring and where investigations may be undertaken to correct or improve certain activities. Most cost accounting systems in medical practices today are based on actual costs.

Standard Cost System

A standard cost system employs standard costs of services rendered as the basis of costing data. Standard costs are predetermined estimates of what it should cost to produce a unit of a product or deliver a unit of service. A standard cost for a health care organization would be the expected cost to treat a specific type of patient. Standards for activities performed in providing services are developed by studying past results, doing time-and-motion studies, and making theoretical calculations tempered by past experiences.

The development of standard costs can assist managers by telling them how much it will cost to treat pa-

tients before services are rendered. This knowledge is useful in making decisions concerning negotiations with other health care organizations for contract services or in deciding whether to offer a particular program or service. Also, actual costs of procedures and treatments can be tracked and compared with the standard costs of these items to identify variances or departures from the expected levels of costs. These variances can then be investigated to determine their causes. Unfavorable variances usually indicate some form of inefficiency, which, once detected, can be altered for more efficient delivery of the group's services.

Practices that use standard costs develop a standard cost profile for their products. Products may be patients or intermediate products, such as tests, treatments, or procedures. Generally, standards are set by making technical estimates of the types and quantities of resources expected to be used in delivering the services. Costs are broken down into direct and indirect. A standard cost is calculated by adding together the direct labor, direct material, and indirect costs for each service unit. An example of a standard cost profile for a chest X-ray is shown in Table 3–11.

Standard cost systems are more detailed and accurate than actual cost systems. However, the development of a standard cost system takes a significant effort. Standards must be developed for the myriad procedures undertaken in patient services, and they must be

TABLE 3–11 Standard Cost Summary Chest X Ray

Cost Element	Amount
Direct labor Technician: 15 minutes @ $32/hour	$ 8.00
Direct materials Film	35.00
Department indirect costs Variable costs per X ray	6.00
Fixed costs: $80,000 divided by 20,000 expected X rays	4.00
Allocated overhead costs from other departments $120,000 divided by 20,000 expected X rays	6.00
Total	$ 59.00

integrated into an existing cost system. Groups must evaluate their needs for a sophisticated, standard costs accounting system before they decide on adopting one, including whether its benefits exceed its costs. A more extensive treatment of standard costs can be found in cost accounting textbooks.

FINANCIAL SYSTEMS IN REVIEW

Medical practices need financial information to plan and control their operations, decide on various alternatives, distribute income, and satisfy certain legal requirements and contractual provisions. The accounting process provides an effective way to collect, arrange, and report financial information about the practice. Through a time-tested model, with specifically espoused assumptions, the accounting process produces financial statements that show the results of operations and the status of the practice. Commonly used financial statements include the income statement, balance sheet, and statement of cash flows. A system of accounting to link financial statements with internal analysis and reporting is responsibility accounting, which employs cost and management accounting concepts.

Costs can be classified in many ways and terms, including direct-indirect, full-differential, controllable-noncontrollable, sunk, and opportunity. Knowing how costs behave in relation to changes in activity levels—whether they will be variable, fixed, or mixed—is helpful in planning and controlling costs. Cost allocation is a necessary and important process in arriving at the full cost of medical services and in determining the cost of patient care. Medical entities usually establish and use a system of actual costs, but the use of standard costs is becoming more common.

REFERENCES

Feuerstein, Thomas M., & Anderson, Craig A. (1990). *Budgeting and cost management for medical groups.* Englewood, CO: Center for Research in Ambulatory Health Care Administration.

Medical group practice chart of accounts, 1st ed. (1996). Englewood, CO: Center for Research in Ambulatory Health Care Administration.

Pavlock, E.J. (1994). *Financial management for medical groups.* Englewood, CO: Center for Research in Ambulatory Health Care Administration.

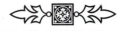

CHAPTER

4

Financial Planning for Operations

Ernest J. Pavlock

LEARNING OBJECTIVES

Upon completing this chapter, the reader should be able to:

- Describe the planning process and distinguish between strategic and operational planning
- Elaborate on the benefits and uses of budgeting
- Identify the components of a comprehensive operational budget, and explain how to prepare the major elements of revenue and expense estimation, cash budgeting, and pro forma financial statements
- Recognize the nature of flexible budgeting and state how it can be used to adjust for activity volume levels
- Explain the uses and elements of the cash flow statement and how it can be used to appraise the adequacy of present cash flows and to estimate future cash flows
- Summarize various approaches medical practices can follow in managing accounts receivable, collections, and claims outstanding

Planning is a process by which management visualizes the future and develops specific courses of action to achieve organizational goals. Planning embraces all aspects of a business, such as deciding on what kinds of services to offer and how much to charge for them; how to recruit, train, and manage the appropriate type of staff; how much financing is needed and where to get it; and so on. Managers approach planning in two ways: strategically and operationally.

PLANNING STRATEGICALLY AND OPERATIONALLY

Strategic planning focuses on developing long-range plans to attain goals. Strategic plans usually range from five to ten years. This type of planning sets the group's approach to acquiring the resources it needs to carry out its goals and objectives. It also provides the parameters for committing the group's resources in the long run. Strategic planners rely on broad frames of reference and set directions and frame policies that are deemed the best in light of present conditions. Because conditions change, strategic planning must be an ongoing process that entails periodic review of plans and revision of them when changing times make this appropriate.

Operational planning focuses on developing short-term plans to achieve specific objectives identified in the strategic plan. Operational plans complement the strategic plan and are usually set for time periods ranging from one week or month to several years. Examples of operational plans are a plan for determining the staffing levels for the next six months and a plan for forecasting the cash needs of the practice over the next year.

The need for formalized planning is greater than ever today because of rapid changes in the health care industry. Providing health care services on a prepaid basis will become a larger component of all practices in the

future, creating new stresses and challenges for the management of groups. Thus, it is crucial that medical groups establish more formalized approaches to planning, both short- and long-range. Strategic planning is especially important when conditions are uncertain. It is covered in more depth in Chapter 16. Contingency planning is also wise, preparing group management for whatever unfolds in the future.

The Planning Process

Whether planning is done formally or informally and whether it relates to strategic or operational planning, there are several basic steps in any planning process. These steps are most apparent when planning

Some of the information in this chapter has been adapted from *Financial Management for Medical Groups* by Ernest J. Pavlock, PhD, CPA with permission of the Center for Research in Ambulatory Health Care Administration, 104 Inverness Terrace East, Englewood, CO 80112-5306; (303)799–1111. Copyright 1994.

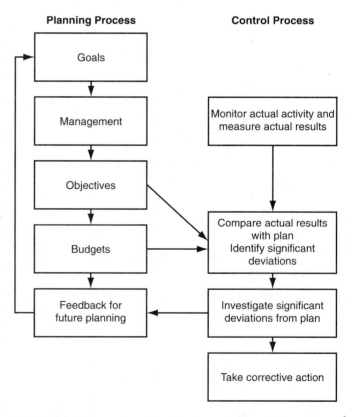

FIGURE 4–1 Illustration of the Planning and Control Process

is linked with control, as in Figure 4–1. The steps in the planning process are:

1. Obtain an understanding of the environment in which the practice operates by scanning its elements to detect trends and changes that are occurring
2. Develop and record the goals and objectives of the group, including specific targets and dates for accomplishing them
3. Design strategic plans that relate to the type of resources needed and the approaches to follow in reaching the specified goals and objectives
4. Establish short-term operating budgets consistent with the strategic plans and the goals and objectives
5. Compare actual results to budgets periodically and consider the need for corrective action or to alter the goals and objectives of the practice

Environmental scanning is largely an awareness process that organizations use to systematically examine the surrounding conditions and identify, quantify, and adopt environmental factors into the planning process. Areas scanned include all events, institutions, social policies, and governmental regulations and programs that have an impact on the delivery of health care services. As factors are identified, an assessment should follow of the degree of importance each has and what effect it will have on the group's operations. Those factors having a major import should become part of the strategic planning process.

Goals are broad, timeless statements that indicate, in general, what an organization wishes to achieve. Objectives are more specific. They identify certain ends that are to be attained within a limited time frame. Goals should emanate from beliefs shared by the group's governing body. Objectives should flow from goals and be stated in terms that are measurable.

Some of the areas in which medical groups should establish goals include:

- Professional services (What services will be offered?)
- Human resources (What kinds of personnel should be recruited and what methods should be used to train, develop, and retain them?)
- Physical resources (What facilities and equipment will be needed?)
- Financial resources (Which funding sources should be used to finance the plans? What are the financial information reporting needs?)
- Salary requirements (What levels should be set for physicians and for staff?)
- Productivity (What levels of output and input expectancies should be set?)
- Management information systems (What are the management information needs and how should they be satisfied?)
- Innovation (What new methods of practice should be used?)
- Social responsibility (What should be the role of the organization in meeting health care needs in the community?)
- Accountability (What types of identification and what forms of reporting should be established to instill accountability among all members of the group?)

Short-term operating budgets are covered in detail next. The comparison of actual results with budgets is covered in the next chapter.

OPERATIONAL BUDGETING

Operational budgets express short-term plans in terms of dollars. Frequently, these budgets are called *profit plans* because they show the activities that segments of a business plan to undertake in order to reach their profit goal. The time period of an operational budget is generally one year; there may another year or two added on, but the budgets for these added years would be less detailed.

Benefits of Budgeting

Budgeting the forthcoming operations of a medical practice requires managers to think about the future and to plan for operating the practice in an organized and coordinated fashion. The budgeting process also aids in integrating the input of managers at all levels. Communicating the agreed-upon budget plan to every manager allows everyone to carry out his or her activities under the same set of guidelines. In addition, the budget serves as a means to motivate managers to achieve their individual and organizational goals by providing target indicators. It also establishes benchmarks to control ongoing activities and to set criteria for evaluating managers' performances. A budget provides authorization for staff personnel to acquire and use resources during the budget period and to expand existing activities where so indicated. Finally, budgeting enables managers to anticipate conditions in order to capitalize on favorable ones and take steps to minimize unfavorable ones.

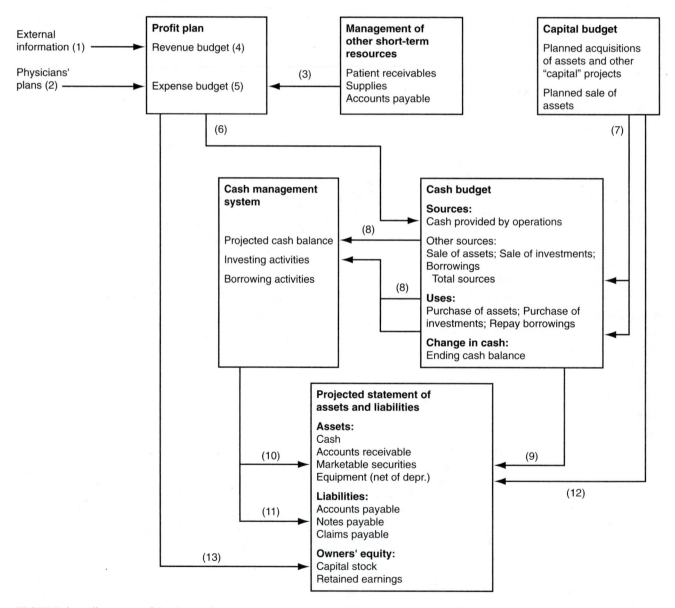

FIGURE 4–2 Illustration of the Comprehensive Budget

Components of the Comprehensive Budget

A comprehensive budget, sometimes called a *master budget,* consists of a series of informal projections and a number of formal statements. A medical practice may adopt all or part of the comprehensive budget framework, depending upon the group's size and scope of operations. A comprehensive budget is comprised of two major parts:

1. The formal comprehensive budget, which consists of a profit plan, a cash budget, a capital expenditures budget, and a projected balance sheet or position statement
2. Cash and other short-term resource management systems, which provide the means for managing these short-term resources.

These components are illustrated in Figure 4–2. The group in the figure is assumed to have both a fee-for-service and a prepaid component in its practice. Each number on the figure indicates a step in the budgeting process. These steps are described next.

Step 1: External Information

The medical group must develop a picture of the environment in which it is operating, including projections of the local economy, anticipated price increases, expected demands for medical services, competition, and any other external influences that are expected to affect the group. HMOs and others with which the group is contracting should provide projected enrollment and utilization data.

Step 2: Physician's Plans

The physicians/owners must examine both their personal goals and the goals of the group. Through this process the physicians indicate their expectations and desires concerning personal income levels; changes in hours of service; changes in the style of the practice; changes in productivity; planned addition or reduction of providers; and planned changes in the number of nurses and medical assistants. Many of these expectations should be expressed as objectives

(that is, as time-limited, quantified targets of planned accomplishments).

Step 3: Management of Other Short-Term Resources

A number of short-term resource control systems are used in any medical group. These systems provide planned levels for patient receivables, supplies, and short-term payables.

Step 4: Budgeted Revenues

The group's income from prepaid contracts (HMO payments, capitation payments, patient co-payments, risk-sharing payments, and so on) and the planned fee-for-service production of each provider may be projected, given changes in the environment, physicians' plans for changes in the style of the group, and the planned level of patient receivables.

Step 5: Budgeted Expenses

Projected expenses are made by three broad categories—variable or fixed, functional class, and responsibility center. Because variable expenses relate to the level of production, variable expense projections are based on the projected production volume, determined in Step 4. Fixed costs are determined by contracts, the level of capacity, and the physicians' plans.

Step 6: Cash Provided by Operations

Budgeted revenues and expenses use the accrual basis and include noncash items such as depreciation. These must be removed to arrive at cash provided or used by operations.

Step 7: Planned Acquisition or Sale of Assets

Planned acquisition or sale of assets will reflect the cash budget segment involving the expected sources and uses of cash from purchase and sale of assets. The cash budget should be accompanied by a capital expenditure budget to include all capital expenditures over a specified amount. The amount and timing of these out-flows can be critical and place significant demands on short-term resources.

Step 8: Projected Cash Balance

Planned sources and uses of cash are determined in the process of developing the cash budget. Investing and borrowing of cash may be necessary to manage the cash position and finance the capital acquisitions of the group. These activities must be reflected in the cash budget.

Steps 9 Through 13: Projected Balance Sheet

The interrelation of the steps in the planning process becomes clear when the projected balance sheet is prepared. The beginning balance sheet and the changes generated by the previous steps provide the information to determine the individual asset, liability, and owners' equity balances in the ending balance sheet. The ending cash balance is a product of the cash budget. Cash management activities project the amount of estimated collection of accounts receivable and the amount of investment in marketable securities. Cash management activities also project the amount of accounts payable for supplies, group credit cards, and outstanding bills; the amount of borrowing, repayment, and the resulting balance of notes payable; and the amount of outstanding medical claims payable. The capital expenditures budget determines changes in the long-lived assets and, with depreciation from the profit plan, the resulting balances of property, plant, and equipment. Finally, the profit or loss from the profit plan provides the change in retained earnings.

The Dilemma of Cash and Accrual Bases

In the previous chapter, the difference between cash and accrual methods of record keeping was explained, and the accrual basis was shown to produce a better picture of operating results. The issue of cash and accrual measurements often raises some problems in the budgeting process. The budget must be both a plan-ning tool (through the expression of management's plans) and a control tool (by providing a benchmark with which to compare actual results). The budget should reflect what is expected to happen as well as re-late to the actual measurements recorded in the ac-counting system.

Actual activities of the group involve the generation of assets, by providing medical services to patients, and the consumption of assets, in rendering these services. Recall that accrual accounting measures revenue in the period that service is performed and measures expenses in the period that resources are used. Thus, a profit plan prepared on the accrual basis does a better job of re-flecting the activities of the group and, therefore, pro-vides a better basis for evaluating performance. For a medical group with a significant prepaid component, the use of the accrual basis is the only way to get a proper measurement of activities and performance for a period of time.

In contrast, under the cash basis lags, in collection and payments, as well as purposeful manipulations of cash payments and collections to reduce the tax burden, distort the picture for short periods of time. As the mea-surement period is lengthened, to a year, for example, these cash-basis distortions are significantly reduced. Because of monthly distortions caused by cash-basis ac-counting, most medical groups on a cash basis use a quarterly planning period for their operating budgets. In this way, a balance is reached between the level of dis-tortion in the data and their usefulness. As a medical group becomes more mature in financial planning and control, the accrual basis may be used for financial planning, control, and other internal purposes, while cash-basis measurements are retained for the prepara-tion of income tax returns.

THE COMPREHENSIVE BUDGET

Accrual accounting principles are followed in this detailed narrative of the comprehensive budget. Three portions of the comprehensive budget are presented: the profit plan, cash budget, and balance sheet. The Western Clinic serves as an example to show how the budget for a medical group is developed.

Developmental Sequence

The goals and objectives of the group are the basis for developing the operational budget. Each responsibility center plans its activities and prepares its profit plan. Then, these individual profit plans are integrated into the overall profit plan for the group. To assure realistic profit plans and commitments, center managers should take an active role in planning their budgets and in follow-up control efforts. Good budgetary practices embrace a bottom-up approach.

When responsibility centers are involved, a typical sequence in the development of a comprehensive budget includes the following steps:

1. Group owners/stockholders of the practice corporation state goals and objectives, identify budgeting responsibilities, project overall activity levels, and determine resource availability
2. Administration further defines objectives and prepares working documents for responsibility center heads
3. Responsibility centers project activity levels, determine staffing, project direct costs of responsibility centers, and compile preliminary profit plans for responsibility centers
4. Administration combines preliminary profit plans into an overall plan, prepares a cash budget, and prepares a projected balance sheet
5. Group owners/stockholders of the practice corporation review, amend, and approve the comprehensive budget

Budgeting Revenues

The key element in any operating budget is the projection of operating revenues. This is key because expense projections, distributions to physicians, cash flow projections, and, to some extent, capital expenditure projections all depend upon the projection of operating revenues. Medical groups use various approaches in estimating future revenues. The following three approaches are explained in this section: projections based on estimate of demand, past activity, and estimate of the number of procedures or patient visits.

Projection Based on Estimate of Demand

Every medical group should periodically assess the future demand for its medical services in its geographic area. This information assists management in setting goals and objectives for the group's size and rate of growth. As in most other businesses, this assessment in a medical group amounts to determining its share of the local market. Also, projections might involve studies to determine the medical treatment needs of the populations to be served by the prepaid component of the practice.

The process of estimating demand for the group's services requires three types of data:

1. Demographic characteristics of the area
2. Patient usage rates for each department
3. Desired share of the market, that is, the share of potential patient visits that the medical group expects to have.

TABLE 4–1   Estimated Demand for the Western Clinic

Specialty	Potential Patient Visits	Physicians Total in Area	Physicians No. in Group	Percent of Total	Group's Share of Patient Visits	Group's Actual Patient Visits	Group's Percent of Potential Patient Visits
Family practice	101,136*	13	6	46%	46,523	39,600	39%
Pediatrics	39,232	3	2	67%	26,285	14,400	37%
Obstetrics/gynecology	8,030	2	2	100%	8,030	9,360	117%
Internal medicine	50,568	7	2	29%	14,665	10,080	20%
Total	198,966	25	12		95,503	73,440	37%

*Family practice visits assumed to be ⅔ and internal medicine ⅓.

TABLE 4–2   Projected Enrollment and Patient Visits, Prepaid Practice

Month	Projected Enrollment (Member-Months)	Projected Patient Visits		
		Care Provided In-house	Referred Outside	Total
1	130	40	10	50
2	216	66	17	83
3	328	100	25	125
4	1,165	356	89	445
5	1,721	526	131	657
6	1,875	573	143	716
7	1,976	604	151	755
8	2,426	742	185	927
9	2,590	791	198	989
10	3,290	1,006	251	1,257
11	3,778	1,154	289	1,443
12	3,850	1,177	294	1,471
24	10,245	3,131	783	3,914
36	19,061	5,825	1,456	7,281
48	27,734	8,475	2,119	10,594
60	34,942	10,678	2,670	13,348

To employ this approach, many assumptions are required. For example, the group must assume both the average patient usage rates and the group's estimated share of the total market, which together yield the total number of potential patient visits. Also, in estimating the group's share of the market, the extent of competition from other medical groups must be taken into account. Because several estimates are involved, this method may have a high degree of error.

Table 4–1 presents the results of estimating demand for the Western Clinic in the specialty areas they offer. With the exception of obstetrics/gynecology, actual patient visits are less than the estimated shares of the market. With more than 50 percent of the physicians in the area, the center is only serving approximately 37 percent of the estimated demand.

It was this kind of analysis that led the Western Clinic to consider prepaid practice. If the clinic considers providing physician services for Coastal HMO, enrollment and patient-visit projections for Coastal

would be required. Table 4–2 presents Coastal HMO's enrollment and patient-visit projections by month for year one and for the last month of years two through five. The projected prepaid patient visits to Western Clinic for the first year are 7,135, an addition of approximately 10 percent to the present year's patient visits. If the clinic maintains its present number of visits for fee-for-service patients (73,440 annual visits, or an average of 6,120 visits per month), the prepaid component will represent nearly one-sixth of the total patient activity by the end of the first year (1,177 prepaid and 6,120 fee-for-service visits in the twelfth month).

The Western Clinic's projected patient visits for the pediatrics department are presented in Table 4–3. Prepaid patients will generate an estimated 235 patient visits per month at the end of the first year. Note that prepaid patient visits are converted to a fee-for-service equivalent so that gross charges can be determined for the combined practice.

TABLE 4–3   Projected Patient Visits for Pediatrics

| | Fee-for-service | | Prepaid | | Total | |
Month	Patient Visits	Gross Charges[1]	Patient Visits	Fee-for-Service Equivalent[2]	Patient Visits	Gross Charges
1	1,150	$ 21,126	8	$ 129	1,158	$ 21,255
2	1,060	19,472	13	210	1,073	19,682
3	1,200	22,044	20	323	1,220	22,367
4	1,210	22,228	71	1,148	1,281	23,276
5	1,200	22,044	105	1,698	1,305	23,742
6	1,200	22,044	115	1,860	1,315	23,904
7	1,250	22,962	121	1,957	1,371	24,919
8	1,100	20,207	148	2,393	1,248	22,600
9	1,300	23,881	158	2,555	1,458	26,436
10	1,300	23,881	201	3,250	1,501	27,131
11	1,300	23,881	231	3,735	1,531	27,616
12	1,200	22,044	235	3,800	1,435	25,844
	14,470	$265,814	1,426	$23,058	15,896	$288,872

[1]Fee-for-service average fee = $18.37
[2]Discounted fee-for-service equivalent fee = $16.17 (88%)

Projection Based on Past Activity

Many groups believe that the best indicator of physicians' activity levels for the following year is their current patient load. This assumes that present conditions and productivity levels will not change significantly. The method generally is used for fee-for-service practices.

The projection starts with each physician's production for the past year, or year-to-date (annualized) if the budget is prepared before the end of the year. For example, if the budget for 19X1 is being prepared in November 19X0 and production of one physician for the first 10 months of 19X0 amounts to $364,878, then production for 19X0 is annualized as follows:

($364,878/10) × 12 months = $437,854 (annualized)

Annualizing in this manner assumes even production throughout the year. Any seasonal pattern in production must be considered in annualizing the data.

After the current year's data are annualized, expected changes are applied to the current year's production. Changes for a particular physician might include changes in hours of work (for example, a physician nearing retirement might wish to reduce his or her workload, or a physician might want to increase or decrease hours worked for personal reasons). There might also be changes in the mix of procedures (thereby changing the average fee charged) or in the fee schedule. By applying these changes to the current year's production, production for the next year can be projected. An example of projecting production by adjusting past activity in this way is shown in Table 4–4. Table 4–4 shows only one quarter. The analysis would have to be extended for an entire year. Note that this example does not consider the impact of prepaid patients. A separate forecast would be done for this element.

Projection Based on Number of Procedures or Patient Visits

A final method of projecting revenues is based on either the number of procedures or the number of patient visits each physician expects to handle per month during the budget year. Because of the large number of

TABLE 4–4 Projection of Production Based on Past Activity

	Actual Quarter 1 19X5	*Changes*	*Projected Quarter 1 19X6*
Physician A	$27,889	Increased production due to additional hours = $837 Increase in fee schedule during 19X5 (approx. 10%) = $2,789	$31,548
Physician B	24,122	No changes proposed in activity Increase in fee schedule during 19X5 (approx. 10%) = $2,412	26,534
Total production	$52,011		$58,082

possible procedures a medical group may perform, groups generally use the number of patient visits for this projection. Another alternative is the estimated number of days each physician will work per month. The disadvantage of projecting only days worked, and therefore production per day, is that seasonality in patient load is not considered. If good data are available by week or month for at least the last two years, it is possible to consider seasonality in patient load in a meaningful fashion. Because estimates of the number of procedures or patient visits are made by physicians, these estimates are likely to be fairly realistic, and, once set, they may provide an incentive for physicians to meet their targets.

To use this approach, the financial manager of the group must provide each physician with information on the number of days the group will be open during each month of the budget year and on the number of patients the physician saw in each month of the past year. Then, each physician must estimate the number of days he or she expects to work each month and the number of patient visits expected each month, for both old and new patients.

Budgeting Expenses

The importance of identifying cost behavior patterns for a medical group was emphasized in the previous chapter. As mentioned there, costs may be variable, fixed, mixed or semivariable, or step-fixed. Variable costs change in proportion to changes in activity, whereas fixed costs do not change as activity changes. Some costs exhibit both characteristics (mixed), and other costs increase in a step-like fashion as activity levels increase (step-fixed). In estimating specific expenses in the bud-

geting process, it is useful to identify the flexible budgeting formula for each type of cost or expense and to apply the formula in making expense projections.

The Flexible Budget Formula

The flexible budget formula is a mathematical statement of the relationship between activity and costs:

$$\text{Total costs} = \text{Fixed costs} +$$
$$(\text{variable costs per unit of activity} \times \text{activity level})$$

By expressing all costs as either fixed or variable, the flexible budget formula allows costs to be projected for any activity level. For the sake of simplicity, a linear, or straight-line, relationship between activity level and cost level is assumed. It is also assumed that all costs can be identified as fixed or variable. Mixed or semivariable costs thus must be separated into their fixed and variable components.

The following example illustrates the application of the formula. Assume that a laboratory has only four costs: rent at $3,000 per month, salaries at $3,600 per month, supplies at $3.00 per test, and equipment rental at $2,400 per month plus $6.00 per test. The flexible budget formula for each individual cost and for the total laboratory costs is:

Total Costs	=	Fixed Costs	+	Variable Costs
Facilities rental	=	$ 3,000	+	[$0 × (x)]
Salaries	=	$ 3,600	+	[$0 × (x)]
Supplies	=	$ 0	+	[$3 × (x)]
Equipment rental	=	$ 2,400	+	[$6 × (x)]
Total		$10,000	+	[$9 × (x)]

TABLE 4–5 Classification of Costs for Pediatrics Department

Costs	Cost Behavior Pattern	Flexible Budget 19X4 (Average Month)	Expected Changes in 19X5
Physician salaries	Programmed fixed	$11,500	Increase on Jan. 1 to $12,600
Physician benefits	Programmed fixed	a) 20% of salaries b) 2% of salaries meetings and professional development	a) No change b) Increase to 5% salaries
Staff salaries	Programmed fixed	$2,700	Increase at anniversary dates (approx. 10%)
Staff benefits	Programmed fixed	20% of salaries	No change
Supplies	Variable	$1.00 per patient visit	No change
Equipment rental	Committed fixed	$100 per month	No change
Professional liability insurance	Committed fixed	$300 per month per physician	No change

The total costs for any level of activity can be projected by substituting the number of tests in place of (x) in each formula. For example, if 2,000 tests were performed, the individual and total costs budgeted would be:

Facilities rental	$ 3,000	=	$3,000	+	[$0 × (2,000)]
Salaries	3,600	=	$3,600	+	[$0 × (2,000)]
Supplies	6,000	=	$ 0	+	[$3 × (2,000)]
Equipment rental	14,400	=	$2,400	+	[$6 × (2,000)]
Total cost	$27,000	=	$9,000	+	[$9 × (2,000)]

This budget is applicable only at the 2,000-test level. If 3,000 tests were performed, then a new budget would have to be calculated. The total cost would then be:

$$\$9,000 + [\$9 \times (3,000)], \text{ or } \$36,000$$

With these flexible budget formulas, costs can be projected at any level of activity when developing an operating budget and profit plan. Also, at the end of a period,

actual costs incurred can be compared to the flexible budgeted amount based on the actual activity level achieved.

Table 4–5 lists the costs of the pediatrics department of the Western Clinic, classifies them by behavior pattern, and indicates the flexible budget formula based on last year's (19X4) costs. For purposes of projecting fixed costs, these costs are identified in the figure as either committed or programmed. Committed fixed costs arise from long-range decisions and usually remain unchanged for long periods of time. Examples of committed fixed costs include depreciation of buildings and equipment, lease expense, insurance premiums, and property taxes. Programmed fixed costs arise from short-range decisions and may be changed by management. Programmed fixed costs are usually step-fixed in pattern. They include most of the staff salaries, employee benefits (particularly professional development), and repairs and marketing costs.

Seasonal expenses, such as utilities, and fixed expenses that vary from month to month, such as telephone, should be projected by applying expected

TABLE 4–6 Profit Plan for Pediatrics Department

	Jan.	Feb.	Mar.	Quarter 1 Total	Total Year
Fee-for-service gross charges	$21,126	$19,472	$22,044	$62,642	$265,814
Adjustments and allowances	(1,268)	(1,168)	(1,323)	(3,759)	(15,949)
Fee-for-service net revenues	$19,858	$18,304	$20,721	$58,883	$249,865
Prepaid gross charges (fee-for-service equivalent)	129	210	323	662	23,058
Total revenues	$19,987	$18,514	$21,044	$59,545	$272,923
Operating expenses:					
Physician salaries	$12,600	$12,600	$12,600	$37,800	$151,200
Physician benefits	3,150	3,150	3,150	9,450	37,800
Staff salaries	2,970	2,970	2,970	8,910	35,640
Staff benefits	594	594	594	1,782	7,200
Supplies	1,158	1,073	1,220	3,451	13,804
Equipment rental	100	100	100	300	1,200
Professional liability insurance	600	600	600	1,800	7,200
Total expenses	$21,172	$21,087	$21,234	$63,493	$254,044
Contribution to common costs and income	$(1,185)	$(2,573)	$ (190)	$(3,948)	$ 18,879

increases to the previous year's monthly amounts. In the example in Table 4–5, note that the flexible budget formula is provided for the average month in 19X4 and the expected changes to be incorporated into the formulas for 19X5.

Preparing the Profit Plan

The profit plan integrates budgeted revenues and budgeted expenses to show the net income, or contribution income, for the total practice or for segments of the practice. Planning, control, and decision making are most effective when the profit plan and subsequent performance reporting are related to responsibility centers. Most medical groups are organized along responsibility center lines, with each medical specialty a separate responsibility center.

Responsibility Center Profit Plan

A profit plan for each responsibility center that serves patients should be prepared. For the Western Clinic, a profit plan for the pediatrics department is shown in Table 4–6. This figure, as well as the two succeeding ones, includes amounts for each of the three months in quarter one and for the total year. (Quarters two, three, and four are omitted to simplify the figures). Only expenses directly traceable to the responsibility center are included in the responsibility center's profit plan. The bottom line shows the center's contribution to common costs and income.

Prepaid Practice Profit Plan

Every group entering prepaid practice must establish accountability for its prepaid contracts. Each medical and ancillary responsibility center providing service to prepaid patients should be given fee-for-service equivalent credit for patient visits or procedures performed in the responsibility center. This rewards each responsibility center with a satisfactory revenue measure. It does not, however, provide an evaluation of the prepaid practice. A separate responsibility center should be created for this purpose. Table 4–7 illustrates a profit plan for the prepaid practice segment of a group. It uses enrollment data from Table 4–2.

TABLE 4–7   Profit Plan for Prepaid Practice

	Jan.	Feb.	Mar.	Quarter 1 Total	Total Year
Enrollment (member-months)	130	216	328	674	23,345
Revenues:					
Capitation (inside services)	$1,446	$2,402	$3,647	$7,495	$259,596
Capitation (outside referrals)	1,008	1,674	2,542	5,224	180,924
Total revenues	$2,454	$4,076	$6,189	$12,719	$440,520
Expenses:					
Inside services to prepaid patients (fee-for-service equivalent)	$1,358	$2,238	$3,433	$7,029	$241,905
Outside referrals	1,008	1,674	2,542	5,224	180,924
Total expenses	$2,366	$3,912	$5,975	$12,253	$422,829
Contribution to common costs and income	$ 88	$ 164	$ 214	$ 466	$ 17,691

Capitation for inside services	$11.12
Capitation for outside referrals	7.75
Total capitation for services	$18.87
Projected cost per member per month for inside services	$ 9.95
Projected cost per member per month for outside referrals	7.75
Total projected cost per member per month	$17.70

Revenues in the prepaid practice responsibility center are the capitation payments from the HMO. Expenses include the cost of inside services provided to prepaid patients, expressed in fee-for-service equivalents, and the cost of outside referrals. If there are incremental costs traceable to the prepaid practice (for example, a nurse or clerk assigned to utilization review and control), these costs should be included in the profit plan of the prepaid practice and in subsequent reporting.

The real cost for inside services is the cost per member per month. The difference between the fee-for-service equivalent for service provided to prepaid patients and the real cost of serving the patients is included in the reports of the medical and ancillary responsibility centers. The cost per member per month should be included as a note to the profit plan of the prepaid practice.

In Table 4–7, the prepaid practice projects a contribution to income of $17,691 for the year. A further gain will be shown in the reports of the medical and ancillary responsibility centers for the difference between the cost per member per month for inside services of

$9.95 and the fee-for-service equivalent for service provided. This example does not consider the potential risk of hospital costs. If hospitalization is greater than expected, the center will experience a financial loss. Conversely, if hospital utilization is less than expected, the center will experience a gain.

Combining Department Profit Plans into a Group Profit Plan

The final budgeting effort culminates in the combination of individual department profit plans into a total profit plan for the group. Table 4–8 consolidates the separate responsibility centers' profit plans into an overall group plan. Production, adjustments and allowances, and net revenue are presented as single amounts for the entire group. Expenses, however, are presented by responsibility centers. An alternative presentation would list the contribution of each responsibility center and then deduct common costs from the total contribution for the group. Total production is

TABLE 4–8 Profit Plan for the Western Clinic

	Jan.	Feb.	Mar.	Quarter 1 Total	Total Year
Fee-for-service gross charges	$227,089	$209,115	$227,412	$663,616	$2,852,561
Adjustments and allowances	(13,625)	(12,547)	(13,645)	(39,817)	(171,153)
Fee-for-service net revenues	$213,464	$196,568	$213,767	$623,799	$2,681,408
Capitation (inside services)	$ 1,446	$2,402	$3,647	$7,495	$259,596
Capitation (outside referrals)	1,008	1,674	2,542	5,224	180,924
Total revenues	$215,918	$200,644	$219,956	$636,518	$3,121,928
Expenses by responsibility center:					
Family practice	$ 60,168	$ 59,930	$ 60,335	$180,433	$726,810
Internal medicine	22,499	22,435	22,553	67,487	272,006
Pediatrics	21,208	21,123	21,000	63,331	256,126
Obstetrics/gynecology	28,265	28,094	28,379	84,738	342,759
Laboratory	20,028	19,284	20,114	59,426	256,667
Radiology	14,090	13,787	14,125	42,002	175,743
Prepaid practice (outside referrals)	1,008	1,674	2,542	5,224	180,924
Reception and appointments	3,200	3,200	3,200	9,600	38,400
Medical records	5,598	5,554	5,603	16,755	68,150
Occupancy	22,200	22,200	22,200	66,600	166,400
Administration	20,290	20,068	20,316	60,674	248,348
Total expenses	$218,554	$217,349	$220,367	$656,270	$2,732,333
Net income (loss)	$ (2,636)	$(16,705)	$ (411)	$(19,752)	$ 389,595

shown in the table because most medical groups prefer to see total revenues for the group in the budget and income statement.

Preparation of the profit plan may go through several iterations using different projections of production and expenses if the physician-owners are not satisfied with the income level. The physician-owners may consider cost reductions, fee increases, or increases in the level of production of individual responsibility centers before a final profit plan is approved.

Preparing the Cash Budget

The second part of the comprehensive budget is the cash budget, which shows the anticipated sources and uses of cash for the coming year. The cash budget is developed after the profit plan is prepared and the capital expenditures are finalized. Ideally, both the profit plan and the cash budget should be structured as rollover budgets, meaning that they keep adding a new month at the end of each month (and a new quarter at the end of each quarter) and always show the next three months (and the next three quarters). In this way, the profit plan and cash budget are always current.

The cash budget represents the major instrument for planning the use of cash during the year. The final cash budget results from a series of trial estimates of cash forecasts. Each trial raises questions about whether the operating plans are too ambitious for the cash that will be generated in the next year. If so, revisions in the operating plans may be necessary. The cash budget also indicates whether capital expenditures are being financed in such a way as to create a chronic cash drain and thus a need for longer-term financing. In addition, the cash budget shows when and if a short-term loan is needed and when it can be repaid; the cash budget identifies the month that is best for scheduling discretionary or unusual payments, such as bonuses, once-a-year debt service, and annual

TABLE 4–9   Sample Cash Budget

High Desert Medical Group
Cash Budget
for the First Quarter of the Year, 19X1
($1000s)

	Jan.	Feb.	Mar.
Cash collected from patients	$148	$160	$185
Cash received from prepaid contracts	39	41	52
Total cash receipts	$187	$201	$237
Less: cash operating expenses	234	172	177
Cash increase (decrease) from operations	$(47)	$ 29	$ 60
Add: beginning cash balance	12	10	10
Cash subtotal	$(35)	$ 39	$ 70
Add: cash from sale of short-term investments	22	0	0
Cash available for investing and financing	$(13)	$ 39	$ 70
Less: cash payments for nonoperating items			
Payment on short-term debt	$ 2	$ 2	$ 2
Payment on long-term debt	0	30	0
Purchase of plant and equipment assets	0	0	24
Purchase of short-term investments	0	0	32
Subtotal	$ 2	$ 32	$ 58
Ending cash balance before borrowing	$(11)	$ 7	12
Add: borrowing to maintain minimum cash balance	21	3	0
Ending cash balance	$ 10	$ 10	$ 12

professional liability insurance premiums. It also anticipates the development of continuing cash excesses that call for a review of investment possibilities, a reduction of debt, or an additional distribution to the physician-owners. Once adopted, the cash budget may be used as a control benchmark, which, when compared with actual cash flows, indicates the accuracy of cash flow predictions and the need for revision of projections for future months. Finally, the cash budget can be used in negotiating loans or lines of credit from banks or other lending institutions.

Cash Budget Data and Sources

To prepare a cash budget the following data must be compiled and analyzed:

• Beginning cash balance

• Projected cash receipts from patients (also miscellaneous income)
• Projected cash operating expenses
• Projected cash expenditures for capital acquisitions and long-term investments
• Projected cash receipts from other sources (e.g., sale of investments)
• Required cash borrowing and debt repayment
• Ending cash balance

The data may be arranged in any format that is useful to the group's management. Table 4–9 highlights the importance of the end-of-the-month cash position. It also shows the impact of nonoperating sources of cash, nonoperating uses of cash, and cash borrowings. Supporting schedules for the components of the cash budget provide greater details for study and review.

CASE STUDY 4-1 [1]

DEVELOPING THE BUDGET

Assume you are the financial director of Catskill Clinic. The clinic serves a suburban community with a population of about 24,000, of which 25 percent are expected to become patients of the clinic. Each patient is expected to average five visits per year. Assume that visits occur evenly throughout the year. The average physician's salary is $11,000 per month. The current practice is all fee-for-service and includes Medicare and nonMedicare patients. The clinic has been approached by several HMOs to provide services to their enrollees, but the board of directors has decided to defer participation until 19X9.

After adjustments and allowances, average charges are $50 per visit. You believe that patient receivables are too high. You expect to improve collections, resulting in a balance of $220,000 patient receivables at the end of the year.

The flexible budget for operating costs for the clinic follows:

	Variable Expenses per Visit	Fixed Expenses per Month
Nurses' salaries	0	$18,000
Administrative and technical salaries	0	$19,000
Medical supplies	$6.00	0
Rent	0	$4,000
Service bureau for medical and financial records	$1.00	$2,000
Other operating expenses	$3.00	$6,000

Planned purchases of medical supplies are $16,000 per month. Supplies are paid in the month following purchase. Service bureau expenses are paid in the month following service. All other expenses are paid in the month of incurrence.

During 19X8, the clinic plans to purchase $80,000 worth of equipment, which will be depreciated on the straight-line basis over five years. A $75,000 line of credit has been arranged at the bank if needed. Assume a desired minimum cash balance of $10,000. You may assume that interest on any amounts borrowed is already considered in other operating expenses.

The statement of financial position at the end of 19X7 follows:

Catskill Clinic Statement of Fiscal Position, December 31, 19X7

Assets	
Cash	$ 20,000
Patient Receivables	240,000
Supplies	8,000
Total	$268,000

Equities	
Accounts Payable: Supplies	$ 6,000
Accounts Payable: Service Bureau	4,000
Total Liabilities	$ 10,000
Partners' Equity	258,000
Total Equities	$268,000

Case Discussion Question

1. Prepare a comprehensive budget for Catskill Clinic for 19X8.

[1]This case was adapted from a case appearing in Ross et al., 1991.

Cash Budgeting with Prepaid Contracts

Practices with large numbers of prepaid patients need to be aware of certain cash flow nuances arising from prepaid contracts. For example, payments for services in the form of capitations or prepayments are received before cash outlays are made for the cost of delivering the services. This flow is the reverse of the cash flow involved in a fee-for-service practice. Also, there is a lag in cash outflows resulting from incurred but unreported claims for outside referrals. The typical fee-for-service medical group does not have a liability for services provided outside the group. However, the medical group that has agreed to provide services to members of an HMO on a capitation basis typically has a liability for physician services performed outside the group. The need for estimating these outstanding claims and ways of measuring this liability are covered later in this chapter.

Preparing the Projected Balance Sheet

The third and final step in developing a comprehensive budget is preparation of a projected balance sheet. Figure 4–2 illustrated the flow of data through the profit plan and cash budget to the projected balance sheet. When the cash budget is developed, many of the ending balances of assets and liabilities for the balance sheet are produced. For example, projection of the cash payments lag for incurred but unreported claims also produces the balance of the liability for incurred but unreported claims.

The projected balance sheet has limited uses. Its major purpose is to link planning documents and show the estimated financial position at the end of the planning period. If the group has active cash management, a strong credit and collection function, and a good supply control system, the balances on the projected balance sheet should produce very few surprises.

THE FLEXIBLE BUDGET

The comprehensive budget described above can be prepared in either a static form, in which volume is as-sumed to be unchanging, or a flexible form, which adjusts for different levels of volume activity. With the exception of service volume, all of the assumptions are identical in both forms of the comprehensive budget. In practice, the flexible budget is prepared as a series of static budgets, each reflecting a different level of activity and incorporating appropriate details of revenues and expenses at that activity level.

It is difficult to estimate accurately the activity volume for any health care organization, and especially for a medical group practice. The volume of activity depends on a number of external and internal factors, many of which are not entirely within management's control. Fluctuations from planned activity volume causes variances from budgeted revenues and expenses. When it is difficult to estimate future activity volume and when costs vary in response to volume changes, use of a flexible budget provides an excellent approach to both planning and performance reporting.

The Nature of Flexible Budgeting

The flexible budget accommodates volume changes that can be specified by a variety of unit measures, such as the number and type of patient encounters or the number and type of procedures. For planning purposes, a flexible budget enables management to analyze costs based upon a series of individual volume forecasts, coupled with estimates of fixed and variable costs for each type of medical group activity. For performance reporting, a flexible budget allows responsibility center managers to evaluate periodically how budgeted resource consumption (costs) compares with actual production. This application is demonstrated in the next chapter. A flexible budget also provides a structured tool for addressing the two most common budget variance problems: inaccurate volume estimates and underestimates of needed services because of changes in patient mix and in severity of patients' illness. Both of these are common analytical problems with static budgeting. The advantages and disadvantages of static and flexible budgeting approaches are shown in Table 4–10.

TABLE 4–10   Static and Flexible Budgets

Static Budget

Advantages:
- Preparation is relatively easier and less time-consuming than a flexible budget.
- Can be a meaningful tool for performance measurement, if actual level of activity is reasonably near budgeted level.

Disadvantages:
- If actual activity level varies widely from budgeted activity level, it becomes very difficult to analyze variances caused by changes in volume, prices, and efficiency.
- Explanations for variances are often attributed to volume changes only rather than being segregated into more factors, some of which are controllable.

Flexible Budget

Advantages:
- Can be adjusted to reflect actual activity level that serve as more realistic norms for comparing actual results.
- Comparison of actual and budgeted amounts produce realistic variances that enable analysis of probable causes for differences between budgeted and actual performance.

Disadvantages:
- Requires more time and resources to develop and to analyze performance with budget.
- Generally a higher level of sophistication is required by the group's administrative, financial, and operating personnel to properly understand and utilize the budget.

Preparing a Flexible Budget

Selecting an appropriate unit of volume is one of the most complex requirements in preparing a flexible budget. Within each responsibility center that adopts flexible budgeting, an output measure (volume unit) must be identified for the center and for each activity within the center. Volume units may be defined with various degrees of specificity, depending on the needs and resources of the medical group. For example, volume units can be defined at the various service levels of the responsibility center, such as the procedure level. The degree of detail selected will affect the complexity of the data collection process and, consequently, the investment necessary to implement and maintain the data base. The greater the level of detail, however, the greater the opportunity for exercising management control.

The simplest measure of volume is the unit of service. Commonly used units of service are the number of patients and the number of patient encounters. These inexpensive indicators use readily available data, so they are used most extensively by medical practices. More detailed measures of volume include procedures or treatments. For other units of service, appropriate measures might be tests, hours, sessions, prescriptions, or transactions, among others. Table 4–11 presents a listing of these and other unit-of-service measures used in medical practices.

Procedures as Units of Service

If the procedure is used as the unit of service, each procedure performed equals one unit, and the number of procedures carried out in a responsibility center becomes the basis for establishing its flexible budget. Budget formulations are then derived by estimating the number of procedures to be administered for the budget period. These estimates are best developed by the

TABLE 4–11 Typical Unit of Service Measures

Responsibility Center	Unit of Service
All types of centers	Patient encounter
Physician's practice	Procedure or patient encounter
Surgery	Operating room hour or procedure
Emergency services	Procedure or patient encounter
Laboratory test	Laboratory test
Pharmacy	Prescription
Physical therapy	Workload measures or number of patients
Respiratory therapy	Procedure
Speech pathology	Session
EEK/EEG	Procedure
Radiology/imaging	Radiology/imaging procedure
Patient reception	Number of appointments or patients
Medical records	Number of appointments or patients
Building operations and maintenance	Square feet
Data processing	Number of transactions
Administration	Operating cost or number of staff

physicians, using past data and projections of the number of procedures to be performed in the next budget period. Revenues can be estimated by applying the expected fee amounts for each procedure to the estimated number of procedures to be performed. Similarly, budgeted cost of patient treatments can be developed by multiplying the estimated number of procedures to be administered by the average cost per procedure.

To illustrate budgeting the direct cost of patient treatments under this approach, consider a simplified organization for an obstetrics/gynecology practice. The steps to calculate an average direct cost per total procedures performed are as follows:

1. Determine total ambulatory care procedures performed in the practice (2,000)
2. Determine total direct costs of the practice ($300,000)
3. Divide direct costs by total procedures to obtain an average cost per procedure ($300,000/2,000 = $150 per procedure)

The result of this calculation is a single macro measure. It represents the average cost of resources consumed to produce a single unit of service, the procedure. In addition to the procedure, health care organizations commonly use other macro measures, such as the patient, case, test, or treatment. These measures are considered macro measures because they merely sum up the frequency of occurrence without regard to the relative mix or intensity of resource usage. If the mix and intensity of resource usage is taken into account, some form of a micro measure should be used. Micro measures in use include relative value units (RVUs), hours of care, and person-minutes. As stated earlier, micro measures require greater data-collection and cost-allocation efforts; thus, their use has been limited to those practices that have developed sophisticated approaches to budgeting and costing of patient services. The development of relative value units of service, combined with cost accounting, will be covered in the next chapter.

MEASURING CASH FLOWS

To forecast cash needs requires the history of cash flows during the last year or two of the operation of the practice. Having a sense of the sources and uses of cash during recent past periods serves as a basis for managers to estimate future cash flows and to prepare the cash budget. The financial statement that provides a picture of cash flows during the past year is the cash flow statement.

Uses of the Cash Flow Statement

The information on the cash flow statement can assist managers to assess several factors about the practice: the financial and operating risks, the financial flexibility of the practice, its liquidity position, and the likelihood of profitability. Each of these factors are covered next.

Financial Risk

This risk relates to the likelihood that the cash flow of a practice may be insufficient to cover its debt service requirements, which include periodic debt and principal payments. The degree of financial risk is a function of the practice's capital structure, that is, its relative proportions of debt and equity. The lower the proportion of debt to equity, the smaller the financial risk. Because debt interest and principal requirements are satisfied by cash payments, and cash is provided largely from operations, information about the group's cash flow from operations is useful in evaluating its ability to cover its debt service requirements. The greater the ability to cover these requirements, the lower the financial risk.

Operating Risk

This risk pertains to the probability of a practice experiencing unexpected reductions in the demand for its services. If this risk is high, cash flow from operations may become inadequate to provide funds to continue the practice at its normal level. Then funds may have to be obtained from outside the group, unless owners are able to provide them. The availability, amount, and timing of these needed funds may place a serious burden on the ability of the group to maintain its financial position and operating capability.

Financial Flexibility

Financial flexibility refers to the ability of a business to weather bad times and respond to new investment opportunities as they come along. Financial flexibility is related to operating risk. A high level of operating risk can sometimes be offset by the practice's ability to borrow funds or sell unneeded assets. Having this financial flexibility enables the group to continue operations at a desired level until cash flow from operations improve.

Liquidity

Liquidity refers to the composition of a practice's current assets and the proportion of those assets that are comprised of cash or near-term cash items such as marketable securities. The more liquid a group's financial assets, the less likely that the group will experience cash flow problems. The group will also survive downturns more easily and be able to take advantage of new investment opportunities if it has cash available.

Profitability

An important function of the cash flow statement is to show the relationship between accrual net income, reported on the income statement, and cash flows. Sometimes a practice shows a high level of net income but lacks sufficient funds to distribute cash to the physicians or invest in new options. Identifying the relationship between income and cash flow helps in projecting realistic forecasts of earnings and cash flows.

Summary

In summary, a cash flow statement provides management with information to assess a practice's future cash flow potential and predict its ability to pay debt service obligations and other liabilities and distribute cash to the physicians. A cash flow statement can reveal why a practice's earnings and net cash receipts and payments differ. It can also be used to assess investing and financing transactions. Thus, the cash flow statement can help to provide answers to such questions as:

- Why are cash distributions to physicians less than the net income of the practice?
- Is the group borrowing funds in order to continue the distribution of cash to physicians at a certain level?

- What other sources were used to raise cash besides operations?
- How are new acquisitions, such as equipment, being financed?

Elements of the Cash Flow Statement

On the cash flow statement, cash flows are categorized into three specific types: operating, investing, and financing. Both cash inflows and cash outflows are included in each category. This is because the statement shows related cash flows in the same category, such as cash proceeds from borrowing transactions and cash repayments of borrowings, both of which are shown under the financing category of the statement. The next sections describe each of the three categories of cash flows on the cash flow statement. Some of the items included under each of the three categories are shown in Table 4–12.

Operating Activities

These activities represent delivery of services or products to patients as part of the normal activity of the practice. Cash inflows are collections from patients and third-party payers, and cash outflows are payments for salaries, supplies and other expences. Generally, most of these items ap-pear on the income statement, although

when they appear on that statement may differ from when they appear on the cash flow statement because of the accrual-cash difference in timing.

Investing Activities

In this category, cash inflows and outflows relate to investments, such as the purchase or selling of equipment or the purchase or selling of investment securities.

Financing Activities

These activities pertain to various aspects of financing, such as obtaining and repaying loans from creditors, receiving additional contributions from physicians as further investments in the practice, and distributing cash to the physicians for their services and as a return on their capital investments.

Illustration of the Cash Flow Statement

The format of the cash flow statement is governed by generally accepted accounting principles. Table 4–13 illustrates the typical format that is followed by most businesses. The statement is broken down into the three basic segments: operating, investing, and financing. Combined changes in these three categories explain the net change in the cash balance ($63,000). The

TABLE 4–12 Statement of Cash Flows: Three Categories of Cash Inflows and Outflows

Cash Inflows	*Cash Outflows*
Operating Activities	
• Cash from patients	• Cash purchases of supplies
• Collections of accounts receivable	• Payment of accounts payable and other services
• Receipt of interest, rent, dividends, and other cash revenues	• Payment of interest, rent, and other cash and accrued expenses
Investing Activities	
• Sale of investment securities	• Purchase of investment securities
• Sale of property, plant and equipment, and intangible assets	• Purchase of property, plant and equipment, and intangible assets
• Collections of notes receivable and other loans	• Loans made or purchased
Financing Activities	
• Obtaining short-term loans	• Repayment of loans
• Issuance of capital stock, mortgages, notes, etc.	• Repurchase of capital stock, and retirement of bonds and other long-term debt
	• Payment of dividends

TABLE 4–13   Sample Cash Flow Statement

Ideal Medical Group
Cash Flow Statement
for the Year Ended December 31, 19X1
($1,000s)

Cash flows from operating activities:		
Net income		$284
Noncash expenses and other adjustments:		
Depreciation	$16	
Gain on sale of investments	(1)	
Increase in accounts receivable (net)	(56)	
Decrease in payroll withholdings	(3)	
Decrease in accrued payroll liabilities	(2)	
Decrease in supplies	12	
Decrease in prepaid expenses	2	
Increase in accounts payable	8	(24)
Net cash flow from operating activities		$260
Cash flows from investing activities:		
Sales of investments in securities	$12	
Purchase of investments in securities	(25)	
Purchase of equipment	(121)	
Net cash flow from investing activities		(134)
Cash flows from financing activities:		
Retirement of short-term notes payable	$(28)	
Retirement of long-term notes payable	(50)	
Proceeds of long-term notes payable	10	
Proceeds from issuance of common stock	5	
Net cash flow from financing activities		(63)
Net increase (decrease) in cash		$ 63
Cash balance at beginning of the year		5
Cash balance at end of the year		$ 68

beginning balance of cash ($5,000) is added to the net change in cash to produce the ending cash balance ($68,000). This is also the cash balance on the balance sheet.

Two options are available to the preparer of the statement when presenting operating activities: the direct method and the indirect method. The direct method shows the major types of operating cash receipts (from patients and third-party payers) and cash payments (for salaries and other services) to arrive at cash provided (used) by operating activities. The in-direct method arrives at the same net cash provided (used) by operating activities but uses a less direct route. It starts with the accrual-based net income from the income statement and adjusts it to determine the net cash provided (used). Table 4–13 summarizes these adjustments. Although the adjustments may seem confusing, they explain the differences between accrual net income and cash flows from operations that are included in the body of the cash flow statement under the direct method. Thus, most businesses use the indirect approach in presenting their cash flow statement.

MANAGING RECEIVABLES AND COLLECTIONS

Receivables for patient care constitute one of the most important assets of a practice. Consider the following scenario: the Burninger Medical Group has an average of $100,000 of billings per month that are outstanding an average of 90 days. This creates a non-interest-earning asset of $300,000. If the collection period can be reduced by three days, $10,000 will be freed for other uses. However, if collections are slowed even further, say by another three days, an additional investment of $10,000 will be required to maintain the same level of business. Thus, the control of receivables is a very important aspect of cash management.

Before self-pay patients are treated, it is helpful to determine their credit worthiness and to grant credit only to those who have responsible credit records and who fully accept the credit terms offered. Adding a prepaid component to the group should not change this fundamental consideration. The amount of receivables from prepayers should be nominal because the payment for prepaid services is usually received in advance of service delivery. These prepayments accelerate the collection of cash and reduce the administrative costs of billing and collecting. However, it is necessary to monitor or payers payments due from prepayers because these patients may be late in remitting monthly capitation amounts. Also, in these contracts co-payments may be required when patients visit the office. Staff members must be alert to this type of collection.

CASE STUDY 4–2[1]

CLINIC PERFORMANCE EVALUATION

During 19X8, the following actual events were recorded for the Catskill Clinic, for which a comprehensive budget for 19X8 was prepared in Case Study 4–1.

1. Patient visits amounted to 28,000 in 19X8, with an average billing rate of $48 per patient visit.

2. Expenses for 19X8 were as follows:

Physician's salaries	$552,000
Nurses' salaries	195,000
Administrative and technical salaries	198,000
Medical supplies	159,000
Rent	48,000
Service bureau (fixed portion, $24,000)	52,000
Other expenses (fixed portion, $70,000)	158,000
Depreciation	16,000

3. At the end of the year, payables for supplies were $10,000, payables for the service bureau was $2,500, inventory of supplies was $4,000, and patient receivables were $160,000; equipment was purchased as planned, but only $5,000 was borrowed in the line of credit (ignore interest on the borrowing).

Case Discussion Question

1. Evaluate the performance of Catskill Clinic for 19X8.

[1]This case was adapted from a case appearing in Ross et al., 1991.

| Net income | + | Depreciation expense
Increase in deferred taxes
Decrease in accounts receivable
Decrease in inventories
Decrease in prepaid expenses
Increase in payables[1]
Loss on disposal | − | Decrease in deferred taxes
Increase in accounts receivable
Increase in inventories
Increase in prepaid expenses
Decrease in payables[1]
Gain on disposal | = | Net cash flow from operating activities |

[1]Includes accounts payable, wages payable (accrued wages), interest payable (accrued interest expense), and taxes payable; does not include notes payable or current portion of long-term debt.

FIGURE 4–3 Calculating Operating Cash Flow from Net Income

Techniques of Receivable Management

A good management technique is to maintain a list of past-due accounts by payer. Follow-up actions should be specified and the results of these efforts documented. Write-offs should be supported by reasons for this action. Monitoring the status of third-party payers is crucial, and activities taken to speed up these collections should be noted. Care should be taken to exclude prepayments from any analysis efforts because these data can distort trends and ratios. Several specific techniques of receivable management that are used by medical practices have been found to be effective. These are presented next.

Payments-Pattern Approach

This approach helps managers plan and monitor the collection of patient receivables. It is based on the historical collection pattern of the group's receivables. Once established, the information can be used to plan and control receivables. For example, after an analysis, the Pack Medical Group discovered that its patients' payments pattern was 50-30-10-5-5 (50 percent collected in the month of service, 30 percent in the next month, and so on). These percentages can be multiplied by the forecasted billings for each of the next 12 months to estimate monthly receipts for the cash budget. Also, these percentages can be compared with recent collection experience to identify any control problems that have developed and may require corrective action.

Ratio Control Methods

Traditionally, various ratios have been used to monitor the collection experience of practices. When the trend in any one or in several ratios indicates a deteriorating condition, actions can be taken to improve collections. The ratios typically used are:

$$\text{Collection Ratio} = \frac{\text{Collections for the period}}{\text{Billings for the period}}$$

$$\text{Days Billing Outstanding} = \frac{\text{Accounts receivable balance}}{\text{Net billings for the period}/360}$$

$$\text{Accounts receivable turnover} = \frac{\text{Billings for the period}}{\text{Average accounts receivable}}$$

$$\text{Age of patient receivables} = \begin{array}{l}\text{Percentage of patient accounts} \\ \text{receivable in each age category} \\ \text{(30, 60, 90, over 90 days)}\end{array}$$

Patient Receivables Aging Schedules

This approach presents the amounts and percentages of receivables in different age classes. The schedules include the names of patients or payers with overdue amounts and the length of time they have been overdue. Table 4–14 presents a typical aging schedule of receivables.

TABLE 4–14   Patient Receivables Aging Schedule

	Age of Patient Receivables			
	0–30 days	31–60 days	61–90 days	91–120 days
January	60%	20%	13%	7%
February	64%	22%	9%	5%
March	65%	22%	9%	4%
April	58%	26%	11%	5%
May	56%	24%	14%	6%
June	59%	22%	12%	7%
July	64%	21%	10%	5%
August	64%	23%	9%	4%
September	57%	26%	12%	5%
October	55%	25%	14%	6%
November	54%	24%	14%	8%
December	52%	26%	14%	8%

An aging schedule is an excellent tool for managing receivables because it can be integrated with the best control concept—the management-by-exception principle. Improved cash collections can be accomplished by following up with payers having overdue balances.

Management Strategies

In this era of cost management and rapid change, efficient management of receivables and collections is most important. Efficient management improves cash flows and reduces the need for large amounts of working capital in the practice. Zimmerman (1992) proposes 12 practical strategies to improve cash flows in medical groups of all types:

1. Develop control prior to service (at previsit, get information from patients that is needed for credit decisions and billing, and get signatures of those financially responsible)
2. Safeguard control at the time of service (follow up on payment arrangements and old account balances, establish good collection procedures and record keeping, and handle patients responsibly)
3. Neutralize small-balance accounts (collect charges at the time of service, have a separate billing cycle for fast turnaround, and minimize time spent on these accounts)
4. Improve staff ability to collect (instruct staff in collection techniques, employ staff with good people skills, and identify possible payer problems)
5. Concentrate collection efforts on insurance (because most collections come from this source, focus on initial data collection procedures and use state-of-the-art billing and follow-up systems)
6. Reduce self-pay payment contracts (have financial institutions carry balances, and use credit cards)
7. Design form letters that work (keep letters short and to the point, use them for small-balance accounts, and use simple notices and statements)
8. Expand data processing payoff (rely on these systems more, use exception reporting to isolate problems, and design innovative communications to payers)
9. Analyze efforts to get the "biggest bang for the buck" (perform payment history analyses, issue prompt billings, address problem payers, develop third-party payer and debtor profiles, and emphasize point-of-service collection)
10. Build good public relations (be aware of group image, handle complaints fairly, and follow a code of ethics for collection)
11. Set goals for direction, motivation, and results (involve staff in focusing on better ways to achieve collection goals, and reward performers for effective results)
12. Maximize collection agency recovery (study feasibility of using an outside collection agency; if an agency is to be used, evaluate its fee structure, recovery track record, and tactics before deciding whether to use it)

MANAGING CLAIMS OUTSTANDING

When medical groups cannot, or choose not to, provide all services that patients need, they may enter into agreements to refer patients to outside providers as part of a prepaid plan. As mentioned previously, an important liability that must be budgeted is an estimate of financial liability of the medical group for these outside services. In many prepaid contracts, employers and enrollees pay premiums to the managed care contractor (HMO and others) for health care service coverage during the period of contract. The HMO, in turn, contracts with the medical group to deliver all, or a specified set of, services to the enrollees of the plan. Generally, payment for these services is incorporated into a capitated payment amount. The medical group has the responsibility of delivering the agreed-upon services, either by physicians of the group or by outside referral physicians and ancillary service providers. At the end of each month, it is very important for both the medical group and the HMO to make accurate estimates of all potential liabilities resulting from the provision of health care services.

The liability stemming from this arrangement is referred to as the *incurred-but-not-reported* (IBNR) *claims outstanding.* Hospitals, physicians, and other providers frequently take lengthy periods of time to submit bills to the medical group (or HMO) for the reimbursement for services rendered. Thus, there is a delay in the processing of these claims, which are expenses to be matched against the capitated revenue recognized each month. For a medical group to reflect all appropriate expenses for services provided patients, estimates of IBNR claims outstanding must be made each month. Otherwise, there will be an understatement of expenses for these unbilled and unprocessed claims.

Two approaches are used by practices to estimate this liability: the nonstatistical method and the statistical method.

Nonstatistical Method

When the volume of IBNR claims is low, this method is followed. Using manual accounting methods involving forms (referrals and hospital admissions) and activity logs (inpatient admissions, telephone confirmations) with key providers, the frequency and type of referrals are documented. The liability estimate is determined by multiplying the unrecorded units of services (provided by the referral provider) by an estimated charge per service, to arrive at the monetary amount.

Statistical Method

As the volume of IBNR claims grows (say, when capitation revenue becomes 40 percent or more of total revenue), the statistical method should be considered. To use this approach, it is necessary to determine the typical lag time experienced by the medical group (or HMO), between the month when claims from referral sources are received and the month in which services are provided. The lag time translates into a ratio of a to b, where a is the month the service is incurred and b is the month the claim

is received. Once this lag time is discerned, it can be used in estimating the IBNR claims-outstanding liability by determining the difference between the incurred claims estimate and the claims paid to date. An example employing this statistical method is beyond the scope of this chapter.

FINANCIAL PLANNING IN REVIEW

Planning is important for all medical practices and can be separated into strategic planning, which is oriented to the long-term time frame and achieving practice goals, and operational planning, which is oriented to the short-term time frame and achieving specific objectives as identified in the strategic plan. Operational budgets set forth short-term plans in a quantitative form and serve as planning and control tools for operations during the next year. Flexible budgets, which are actually a series of budgets, are better measures for comparing actual results with budgeted amounts. Profit plans integrate budgeted revenues and expenses and, when prepared for responsibility centers, constitute a mechanism for evaluating performance. Other elements of comprehensive budgets include cash budgets and projected financial statements. Statements of cash flows provide useful reports on cash flows for the past period, which is important in estimating these flows for future periods. Successful practices show effective management of collections, receivables, and claims outstanding.

REFERENCES

Pavlock, E.J. (1994). *Financial management for medical groups.* Englewood, CO: Center for Research in Ambulatory Health Care Administration.

Ross, A., Williams, S.J., & Schafer, E.L. (1991). *Ambulatory care management* (2nd ed.). Albany, NY: Delmar Publishers.

Zimmerman, D.H. (1992). *Twelve strategies to improve cash flows in medical groups* (2nd ed.). Englewood, CO: Center for Research in Ambulatory Health Care Administrators.

CHAPTER

Evaluating and Controlling Operations

Ernest J. Pavlock

CHAPTER TOPICS

Financial Performance Analysis

Key Operating Reports and Indicators

Resource-Based Relative Value Scale

Other Types of Performance Reporting

Activity-Based Costing

Improving Operations

Outcomes Management

Evaluating Performance in Review

LEARNING OBJECTIVES

Upon completing this chapter, the reader should be able to:

- Summarize the approaches to analyzing and evaluating the financial performance of medical practices, with a focus on internal norms and external sources
- Identify the various types of operating reports and indicators that depict results in significant areas of the practice
- Relate the nature and development of resource-based value scales, including the Medicare system and others developed internally, and explain how value scales can be used in planning and controlling operations
- Describe the types of reporting and variances that arise from the use of flexible budgets and standards and from the adoption of internal analytical software tools
- Explain the nature and purpose of activity-based costing and how it differs from the traditional costing-of-service approach

• Specify various ways to improve operations, including productivity enhancements, cost reductions, and the raising of income opportunities that incorporate recent developments in outcomes management

As a follow-up to financial planning, performance results must be measured and reported to the various operating levels in any organization (Pavlock, 1994). When medical practices are small, a single set of reports may satisfy the informational needs of management. As groups become larger, there may be one or more tiered types of reports, each addressed to a particular level of management. Ideally, actual performance should be compared with the goals and objectives of the practice to generate variances, or departures from expected results. Various normative criteria may be established to determine the validity of the deviations from planned results. Then management can take appropriate actions to close the gap between achieved performance and desired outcomes. This chapter explains how practices can summarize their operations in report form and learn how to achieve their goals.

FINANCIAL PERFORMANCE ANALYSIS

Under responsibility accounting, the responsibility center is the unit within an organization that controls performance and consumption of resources. The precepts of responsibility accounting prescribe that revenues and expenses be traced to profit and investment centers and that expenses be traced to cost or expense centers, so that managers of these respective centers can be held accountable for the results achieved. In this way, revenues, expenses, or profits become the indicators of performance for each type of responsibility center.

Evaluating Responsibility Center Performance

Each type of responsibility center is based on the level of responsibility assigned to it. For example, if a re-

Some of the information in this chapter has been adapted from *Financial Management for Medical Groups* by Ernest J. Pavlock, PhD, CPA with permission of the Center for Research in Ambulatory Health Care Administration, 104 Inverness Terrace East, Englewood, CO, 80112-5306; (303) 799-1111. Copyright 1994.

sponsibility center treats patients, it is labeled a profit or revenue center. If it does not treat patients, it is probably called a cost or expense center. If a testing laboratory or satellite office is largely free-standing and has a discrete quantity of assets that it uses in patient care, it may be called an investment center.

For each type of responsibility center, the performance measurement criteria are different:

• A profit or revenue center evaluator might be a profit measure, such as a contribution margin
• A cost or expense center evaluator might be an assessment of whether the operating budget of expenses was met
• An investment center evaluator might be a return-on-investment indicator

To evaluate each center's performance, the center's manager should respond fully to the following questions:

• How did the center perform for the period?
• To what degree did the center meet or exceed its profit plan if it is a profit center, or its budgeted expenses if it is an expense center?
• What factors caused the actual results to vary from the plan or budget?
• If there is a prepaid component to the practice, what criteria should be used to assess performance in this component, and if results are not in alignment with these criteria, why not?

For the medical group with a small prepaid component (less than 25 percent of the total practice), it is probably sufficient to treat the prepaid component as a separate responsibility center. Other responsibility centers in the group that treat prepaid patients would then report fee-for-service equivalent amounts as revenue surrogates for providing this care. The effect of this arrangement is twofold. First, responsibility for treating prepaid patients in a cost-effective manner is diffused throughout the group, and no one manager or responsibility center is clearly accountable for the care of these patients. Second, performance is expressed in terms that are meaningful in the fee-for-service environment, and financial results are monitored in these terms. Note that the prepaid environment requires different performance and outcome criteria that may not be consistent with fee-for-service practice, as indicated below.

When prepaid revenues exceed 25 percent of the total revenues of a group, it may be necessary to change both the reporting format and the reward system for physicians. One option is to switch from crediting individual responsibility centers with fee-for-service equivalents to crediting the centers with a pro rata share of the capitation revenue for physician services. The cost of treating prepaid patients internally as well as the cost of outside referrals would be charged to the responsibility center that had been assigned a share of capitation revenue. On the surface, this may not seem to be a significant shift; however, it represents a shift from the fee-for-service orientation of increasing production to the orientation of managing costs within a fixed income amount. This may lead to the individual physician becoming a responsibility center for cost control. The unit of performance measurement would then be the cost per member per month.

Evaluating Performance Against Goals and Budgets

If a medical group sets a profit goal or some other financial target, there should be a periodic assessment (at least annually) to see if the goal has been attained. If nonfinancial goals and objectives have also been established, measures for comparing actual results to planned outcomes must be developed to evaluate these aspects of performance as well.

The operating budget is the primary tool for evaluating financial performance both organizationally and departmentally. Comparison of actual results with budgeted amounts may show departures from plans or objectives, which may occur for any or all of the following reasons:

- Change in the volume of activity from the planned level
- More or less efficiency in the use of practice resources
- Change in the price of resources purchased
- Change in the amounts of charges used in patient billings

Departures from budget usually cannot be attributed to a single cause. These causes of budget variances are often difficult, if not impossible, to determine. A later section covers variances in more detail.

Profit Center Performance

The manager of a profit, or contribution, center is accountable for both revenues and costs, which produce profits. The term *contribution* is sometimes used for this center since costs reflected here may not represent the total costs assigned to it. Financial performance is measured by the achievement of a budgeted profit or contribution toward common costs, and performance reports should include only those costs and revenues over which the profit center manager has control. Keep in mind, however, that for other purposes, such as fee setting, it may be necessary to include a fair share of indirect costs over which the profit center manager has no control when arriving at the full cost of the center's services.

Table 5–1 shows the operating statement for a contribution center, pediatrics, for the first quarter of 19X5. The report includes the actual results for the quarter, results for the same quarter the previous year, the budget for the quarter, and the variance of actual results from the budget. The $722 variance for fee-for-service gross charges, for example, means that actual fee-for-service production was $722 below the planned level. In analyzing this variance, questions such as the following should be addressed: Are the assumptions underlying the budget valid? Were the operating plans on which the budget was based actually followed? Are there any areas that require immediate corrective action, such as increased promotion of the group's services or of the group itself? Similar relevant questions should be raised for other profit centers as well.

The prepaid revenues shown in Table 5–1 were $954 above the planned level. Apparently there were more prepaid visits than expected. These visits may have been due to increased enrollment, or the prepaid patients may have used more services than planned. Because of the increased level of activity, the supplies expense exceeded the budget by $219. The favorable variance in physician benefits ($450) is due to the cancellation of a conference, which may be rescheduled later in the year.

TABLE 5–1 Operating Statement for Pediatrics

	Actual Quarter 1 19X4	*Budget Quarter 1 19X5*	*Actual Quarter 1 19X5*	*Variance (unfavorable)*
Fee-for-service gross charges	$52,011	$57,682	$56,960	$(722)
Adjustments and allowances	(3,120)	(3,461)	(3,418)	43
Fee-for-service net revenues	$48,891	$54,221	$53,542	$(679)
Prepaid revenues (fee-for-service equivalent)	0	663	1,617	954
Total revenues	$48,891	$54,884	$55,159	$ 275
Operating expenses:				
Physician salaries	$34,500	$37,800	$37,800	$ 0
Physician benefits	7,590	9,450	9,000	450
Staff salaries	8,100	9,000	9,000	0
Staff benefits	1,620	1,800	1,850	(50)
Supplies	3,110	3,181	3,400	(219)
Equipment rental	300	300	300	0
Professional liability insurance	1,800	1,800	1,800	0
Total expenses	$57,020	$63,331	$63,150	$ 181
Contribution to common costs and income	$(8,129)	$(8,447)	$(7,991)	$ 456
Patient visits (fee-for-service)	3,110	3,140	3,200	60
Patient visits (prepaid)	0	41	100	59

Total Group Performance

Another important measure of progress is the operating statement for the entire practice. Table 5–2 shows a typical operating statement for a medical group, the Western Clinic. Total operating expenses are shown for each responsibility center because the emphasis here is on control through responsibility centers (Finkler, 1994). As an alternative, expenses could have been presented in natural expense categories, such as salaries and supplies.

Western Clinic's operating statement is a performance budget report. Note that the static budget in the first column of Table 5–2 has been converted to a performance budget in the second column. When performance is evaluated by comparing it with a static budget, changes in activity as well as changes in efficiency or prices may contribute to variances between actual performance and budgeted amounts. However, when performance is compared, as in the table, with a flexible budget in which revenues and costs have been adjusted for activity level, the variances reflect changes only in price and efficiency, not in volume of activity. This makes the performance budget report a more useful performance evaluation tool.

The Western Clinic must also prepare a responsibility center operating statement for the prepaid component of its practice. The statement must relate capitation payments to the fee-for-service equivalent, for both service provided inside the medical group and outside referrals. The prepaid practice operating statement shown in Table 5–3 reveals a loss of $242 overall for the first quarter 19X5.

Cost Center Performance

Cost centers do not generate revenue, although they support the revenue-producing responsibility centers or the group as a whole. Examples of cost centers include

TABLE 5–2 Operating Statement for the Western Clinic: Actual vs. Performance Budget

Quarter 1, 19X5

	Budget	Performance Budget	Actual	Prices and Efficiency Variance (unfavorable)
Fee-for-service gross charges	$663,616	$639,418	$640,000	$ 582
Adjustments and allowances	(39,817)	(38,365)	(39,680)	(1,315)
Fee-for-service net revenues	$623,799	$601,053	$600,320	$ (733)
Capitation (inside services)	7,495	8,896	8,896	0
Capitation (outside referrals)	5,224	6,200	6,200	0
Total revenues	$636,518	$616,149	$615,416	$ (733)
Expenses by responsibility center:				
Family practice	$180,433	$179,833	$180,000	$ (167)
Internal medicine	67,487	67,087	68,000	(913)
Pediatrics	63,331	63,450	63,150	300
Obstetrics/gynecology	84,738	84,390	82,000	2,390
Laboratory	59,426	58,906	60,000	(1,094)
Radiology	42,002	41,552	41,500	52
Prepaid practice (outside referrals)	5,224	6,200	6,500	(300)
Reception and appointments	9,600	9,600	9,650	(50)
Medical records	16,755	16,555	17,000	(345)
Occupancy	66,600	66,600	66,600	0
Administration	60,674	60,175	61,000	(825)
Total expenses	$656,270	$654,448	$655,400	$ (952)
Net income (loss)	$ (19,752)	$ (38,299)	$(39,984)	$(1,685)

TABLE 5–3 Operating Statement for the Western Clinic's Prepaid Practice: Actual vs. Budget

Quarter 1, 19X5

	Budget	Actual	Variance (unfavorable)
Revenues:			
Capitation (inside services)	$ 7,495	$ 8,896	$ 1,401
Capitation (outside referrals)	5,224	6,200	976
Total revenues	$12,719	$15,096	$ 2,377
Expenses:			
Inside services to prepaid patients (fee-for-service equivalent)	$ 6,963	$8,838	$(1,875)
Outside referrals	5,224	6,500	(1,276)
Total expenses	$12,187	$15,338	$(3,151)
Contribution to common costs and income	$ 532	$ (242)	$ (774)

TABLE 5–4   Medical Support Group Operating Statement

	Profit Plan 19X2	Changes in Activity 19X2	Performance Budget 19X2	Actual 19X2	Variances (Other than Activity) 19X2 (unfavorable)
	19X2 ($000 omitted)				
Salaries, RN	$ 11		$ 11	$ 11	
Salaries, other nursing	103	$ (3)	100	100	
Salaries, receptions and appointments	57		57	57	
Salaries, secretarial	40		40	40	
Salaries, medical records	50		50	51	$ 1
Drugs expense	20	(1)	19	21	2
Medical supplies	39	(1)	38	39	1
Linen expense	1		1	1	
Other	13		13	12	(1)
Total	$ 334	$ (5)	$ 329	$ 332	$ 3
Patient visits (excluding ancillary departments)	112,339	(3,139)	109,200	109,200	—

the medical support group, data processing department, occupancy and use center, and administration. Frequently, cost centers are referred to as support centers.

An example of a cost center performance report is presented in Table 5–4 for the medical support group of the Western Clinic. The static budget (labeled "profit plan" in the table) has been adjusted for activity level changes to yield a flexible budget of costs (the performance budget), against which actual expenses are compared. The variances shown are the differences between actual costs and the performance budget. As indicated on the last line of the table, actual patient visits were less than planned patient visits (by approximately three percent). Other expenses, such as nursing salaries, drugs, and medical supplies, are largely variable and have been reduced proportionately. The resulting performance budget indicates that actual expenses of this cost center are almost on target.

In cost centers where the relationship between fixed and variable costs cannot be determined, the budget becomes a maximum authorization to spend. In these cases, performance reports are used to assure that the centers do not go over budget without prior approval. The reports are not designed to assess the efficiency of the centers' operations. When the reports are used to assess efficiency, the staff may be motivated to spend less in order to report favorable variances, potentially leading to budget padding or reductions in the quality of patient care.

Evaluating Performance with External Sources

Another dimension of analyzing operations entails comparing current group data with information about other medical groups. The Medical Group Management Association offers an extensive comparative report, called the *Performance Efficiency Evaluator Report* (PEER), which provides financial, productivity, and efficiency statistical standards. PEER provides trend data, budget comparison, and an external comparison with peer groups on over 160 performance indicators, enabling medical groups to monitor their performance over specified time periods, including historical and concurrent periods; compare their actual performance with budgeted projections; and compare their current performance with that of similar group practices.

The indicators published by PEER are revised and augmented periodically to keep them current. Data are collected from participating medical groups in the following areas:

- Group production and financial performance
- Group staff performance
- Group compensation and fringe benefits
- Group nonphysician expenses
- Prepaid services
- Laboratory and radiology procedures and expenses
- Department production and financial performance
- Department prepaid service costs
- Department staff performance
- Department facilities and ancillary services

KEY OPERATING REPORTS AND INDICATORS

Being successful in the health care environment requires that financial managers are aware of current operating results and trends. Large medical groups may have a sophisticated financial management information system and staff to prepare a variety of operating reports and analyze financial data. Smaller practices may have just one individual—the administrator or business manager—to manage all operations of the practice, both financial and nonfinancial. Regardless of group size, however, familiarity with and the ability to use various operating reports are prime requirements for the financial management role.

Operating Reports

The following list of operating reports is a representative sample of the types of financial and nonfinancial information that may be produced by the financial information system and used in the management of the practice. The reports may be produced by fee-for-service-only groups and groups that have both fee-for-service and prepaid components. Only the re-

ports that fit the specific needs of the group should be produced. Every report on the list may not be necessary for all groups.

- Income statement (actual)
- Operating budget (actual vs. budget)
- Balance sheet
- Cash report
- Cash flow statement
- Accounts receivable analysis (by type)
- Accounts receivable analysis (by age)
- Incurred-but-not-reported claims (IBNR)/lag report
- Utilization: medical report
- Utilization: lab report
- Utilization: X-ray report
- In-house referrals report
- Outside referrals report
- Hospitalization report

Income Statement

This statement, which was introduced in Chapter 3, assists in comparing the current period (month, quarter, year) with the same period a year earlier. If the statement shows the monthly or quarterly results, there should also be additional columns showing the year-to-date totals, both for the current and the prior year.

Large medical groups with several locations may need to prepare a separate income statement for each location and a combined income statement for the entire practice. Small medical practices may need to prepare only simple, one-page financial statements that also contain operating statistics. In the latter case, a formal income statement may not be necessary, with a summary of key elements from the statement, such as net revenues, significant expenses, and net income, satisfying informational needs.

Operating Budget

An operating budget is a quantified financial expression of the practice's operating plan for the next year. It serves as a basis for determining the practice's ability to attain predetermined goals. It also provides a tool for monitoring progress and evaluating operating performance. A comprehensive operating budget consists of a series of informal projections and a number of formal statements. Components may include a profit plan (with detailed breakdowns of revenue and expenses), cash budget, capital expenditures budget, and projected balance sheet.

Once an operating budget has been developed, approved, and disseminated within the medical group, it becomes the blueprint for action, to be followed by group members in planning and carrying out their activities. Periodically (each month or quarter) a report is prepared comparing actual with budgeted amounts to determine whether operations are on target with the plan. Such a comparison enables management to alter the activities of the group or adjust its plans in order to achieve the desired outcomes. Refer back to Chapter 4 for samples of operating budgets.

Balance Sheet

The balance sheet represents the financial condition of the practice at the end of the year. A balance sheet that has columns showing the comparable period for the prior year and the percentage increase (decrease) provides even more information. The simplified balance sheet used by most medical groups, on the other hand, does not contain many individual accounts, so it may not be as important as the income statement.

Cash Flow Statement

This statement provides a picture of cash flows in the medical group for a specific time period (the last month, quarter, or year). On the statement, cash inflows and outflows are classified by operations, investing, and financing, as explained in Chapter 4. Prior-period cash flows can be used as the basis for predicting future cash flows, so cash flow statements are vital tools in cash management.

Cash Report

The cash report is very important to the financial manager. It is usually issued daily, and it serves as a sensitive indicator for monitoring the adequacy of cash

available for forthcoming monetary obligations. The report shows the sources of cash receipts and the types of cash payments that were made for that day. The beginning and ending balance of cash are also shown, together with checking account balance(s). The daily cash report can be compared with the forward-looking cash plan, and deviations from the planned cash flows can be identified. A cash shortage requires action, such as transferring cash from one bank account to another, selling short-term investments, or borrowing short-term debt from a line of credit.

Accounts Receivable Analysis

Two types of reports are very helpful in analyzing and keeping track of accounts receivable balances. One type is a listing of all accounts and their balances, arranged by type of payer (such as patients, insurance companies, Medicaid, and contractors). The second type is the same listing arranged by an aging of each balance (such as 0–30 days, 31–60 days, 61–90 days, and so on). Both types of reports can be prepared at any time as needed by the financial manager. However, the accounts receivable listing of balances by type usually is issued at the end of each month, and the listing of account balances by age usually is issued at the end of each quarter, if not more often.

Incurred-But-Not-Reported (IBNR) Claims/Lag Report

This report lists charges from referred health care providers (nongroup physicians, hospitals, and laboratories) that have not yet been reported by the providers to the referring medical group nor to the prepaying organizations (HMOs) to which the patients belong. The charges are classified by source. Methods for estimating the charges were covered in Chapter 4. The lag report is used to accrue expenses and liabilities by the medical group and HMOs.

Utilization Reports

These reports present a summary of the various services provided by the group to its patients for a given period of time. Three major areas covered by utilization reports are medical services, laboratory testing, and X ray. In the reports, details of the services are shown, such as patient identification information, type of medical procedure or treatment rendered, responsible physician, type of test, and, if appropriate, applicable costs. The report design may reflect summary data only or it may show greater details, depending upon the use of the report. The reports may also present year-to-date cumulative totals for each service area and previous totals for comparative analysis.

Referral Reports

Patients who are referred to other physicians within the group should be listed on an in-house referral report. Patients referred to outside health care providers should be included on an outside referral report. Both of these reports should include patient identification information, name of referring physician, type of treatment or procedure ordered by the group, services received from the referred party, and any applicable charges for the provided services.

Hospitalization Report

This report contains a summary of the hospital services provided to the group's patients for specific periods of time. Information included on this report should include patient identification data, referring physician, surgical services performed, hospitalization duration, and the delineation of all types of charges by source.

Major Indicators of Performance

Beyond the operating reports described above, there are several key indicators that highlight the performance of significant areas or aspects of the practice. Some of these indicators are financial in nature, others are nonfinancial. Their importance rests with the fact that they are single-number measures that can be used in several ways. For example, they can be tracked over time to reveal trends for the practice. The key indicators can also be compared with local, regional, and national statistics, such as those published in the MGMA

Cost Survey or Physician Compensation Survey (Medical Group Management Association, 1996), to ascertain how the practice compares with other medical practices of similar size or make-up.

A Note on FTE

In certain indicators described below, the term *FTE physician* is used. FTE means "full-time equivalent," and it is used to standardize comparisons among medical practices. One full-time equivalent, or 1.0 FTE, is equal to one full-time physician, that is, a physician who works the number of hours that the medical group is normally open each week—usually 35 to 40 hours. A physician cannot be counted as more than 1.0 FTE regardless of the number of hours worked. The FTE of a part-time physician is computed by dividing the time the physician works for the practice by the length of a normal work week for the practice. For example, a part-time physician working 20 hours in a practice for which a normal work week is 40 hours would be classified as 0.5 FTE.

Financial Indicators of Performance

Financial indicators of performance are summarized in Figure 5–1. They are based on financial performance, nonphysician expenses, or accounts receivable. It should be noted that practices using the cash or modified cash basis of accounting will report different values for the financial indicators shown in the figure than practices using the accrual basis. This is because of differences in the timing of revenue and expense recognition. Therefore, when comparing financial indicators among practices, the basis of accounting used by each group must be considered.

Financial indicators of financial performance include total gross charges per FTE physician, total net revenue per FTE physician, and total nonphysician expenses per FTE physician. Each of these indicators is defined in Figure 5–1. Total gross charges per FTE physician identifies the average amount of gross charges generated per group physician, providing an overall

Financial Indicators of Performance

$$\frac{\text{Gross Fee-for-Service Charges} + \text{NonMedicare Patient Prepaid Charges} + \text{Medicare Patient Prepaid Charges}}{\text{Total FTE Physicians}}$$

$$\frac{\text{Total Net Revenue}}{\text{Total FTE Physicians}}$$

$$\frac{\text{Total Nonphysician Expenses}}{\text{Total FTE Physicians}}$$

Nonphysician Expenses

$$\frac{\text{Total Nonphysician Expenses}}{\text{Equivalent Gross Fee-for-Service Charges} + \text{Equivalent NonMedicare Prepaid Patient Charges} + \text{Equivalent Medicare Prepaid Patient Charges}} \times 100$$

$$\frac{\text{Total Nonprovider Salary Expenses}}{\text{Total FTE Physicians}}$$

$$\frac{\text{Total General and Administrative Expenses}}{\text{Total FTE Physicians}}$$

Accounts Receivable

$$\frac{\text{Accounts Receivable}}{\text{Total FTE Physicians}}$$

$$\frac{\text{Adjustments}}{\text{Gross Fee-for-Service Charges}} \times 100$$

$$\frac{\text{Bad Debts Due to Fee-for-Service Activity}}{\text{Gross Fee-for-Service Charges}} \times 100$$

FIGURE 5–1 Financial Indicators of Performance

picture of the financial productivity of the group. Gross charges include fee-for-service charges and fee-for-service equivalent charges for services provided to Medicare and nonMedicare prepaid plan patients.

Total net revenues per FTE physician identifies the average amount of actual revenue per group FTE physician. Total revenue includes revenues from all medical sources. This indicator is an important measure of the financial stability of the group. It also provides a means of comparing relative productivity among practices.

Total nonphysician expenses per FTE physician identifies the average amount of nonphysician expenses incurred to provide patient care, per FTE physician. It

can be used to monitor efficiency and cost effectiveness of operations. When used with other indicators, it can identify the potential financial resources available for physician income and/or group profits.

Nonphysician expense indicators of performance include total nonphysician expenses as a percent of gross charges, total nonprovider salary expenses per FTE physician, and total general and administrative expenses per FTE physician. Formulas for calculating these indicators are also given in Figure 5–1.

Total nonphysician expenses as a percent of gross charges identifies the percentage of gross charges that are being consumed by nonphysician expenses to provide patient services. The indicator allows the group to budget for necessary gross charges to cover nonphysician expenses. It also gives a sense of the efficiency with which nonphysician resources are being deployed.

Total nonprovider salary expenses per FTE physician identifies the average nonprovider salary expense per physician. It indicates how cost efficient the group is in establishing employee salaries. When used with other indicators, the indicator can identify what proportion of nonprovider expense is attributed to nonprovider salaries. It can be used to determine whether salary expenses are being recouped by the group.

Total general and administrative expenses per FTE physician identifies the average general and administrative expenses attributable through cost accounting to each physician. It can be used to assess whether these costs are reasonable. When used with other indicators, it can help identify what proportion of nonphysician expenses is attributable to administrative and general expenses and whether these expenses are being recouped by the group.

Accounts receivable indicators of performance include accounts receivable per FTE physician, adjustments as a percent of gross fee-for-service charges, and bad debts due to fee-for-service activity as a percent of gross fee-for-service charges.

Accounts receivable per FTE physician provides an average measure of the group's billed charges that are outstanding per FTE physician. When used with other financial indicators, this information can assist in determining potential problem areas in the group's billing and collection procedures.

Adjustments as a percent of gross fee-for-service charges identifies the percentage of gross fee-for-service charges that will not be collected for rendered services due to adjustments. This percentage figure is the result of adjustments made by third-party reimbursing agencies, charitable adjustments, or free service. The indicator assists the group in estimating its future collections and in monitoring and controlling the extent of services for which it will not be reimbursed.

Bad debts due to fee-for-service activity as a percent of gross fee-for-service charges provides information identifying the percentage of total gross charges that will not be collected for rendered services due to allowances and bad debts on fee-for-service activity. This indicator

assists the group in monitoring and controlling its ability to collect payment for services already rendered.

Nonfinancial Indicators of Performance

Nonfinancial indicators of performance are summarized in Figure 5–2. They are based on patient data or data on the medical or administrative staff.

Ambulatory patient encounters per FTE physician measures overall group physician productivity by identifying the average number of outpatient encounters by FTE physician.

Hospital admissions per FTE physician identifies the average number of inpatients admitted by each physician. When used in conjunction with another indicator—hospital inpatient professional service gross charges as a percent of total gross charges—it also provides a general indication of the extent that clinical practice occurs in the hospital.

Ambulatory surgery admissions per FTE physician provides the average number of ambulatory surgery admissions per group FTE physician. New patient registrations per FTE physician is an important indicator of survival of a group practice, which usually depends on attracting new patients. This indicator allows a group

Patient Data

$$\frac{\text{Physician Ambulatory Patient Encounters}}{\text{Total FTE Physicians}}$$

$$\frac{\text{Hospital Inpatient Admissions}}{\text{Total FTE Physicians}}$$

$$\frac{\text{Ambulatory Surgery Admissions}}{\text{Total FTE Physicians}}$$

$$\frac{\text{New Patient Registrations}}{\text{Total FTE Physicians}}$$

Medical/Administrative Staff Data

$$\frac{\text{Total FTE Medical Support Staff}}{\text{Total FTE Physicians}}$$

$$\frac{\text{Total FTE Administrative Staff}}{\text{Total FTE Physicians}}$$

FIGURE 5–2 Nonfinancial Indicators of Performance

practice to monitor the amount of services attributable to new patients. It also provides some basis for examining productivity data, because new patients tend to require more provider time than returning patients.

Total FTE medical support staff per FTE physician identifies the utilization of the group's medical support staff. Total FTE administrative staff per FTE physician identifies the utilization of the group's administrative staff to perform administrative, business office, and maintenance activities.

Prepaid Services

Prepaid services include services to both non-Medicare and Medicare contracts. Indicators of prepaid services are based on numbers of, or revenues from, prepaid contracts. They are summarized in Figure 5–3.

Average number of prepaid plan members identifies the average number of prepaid plan members for the reporting period. This information allows a group to monitor the growth or decline of membership in the prepaid plan.

Net prepaid contract revenue as a percent of total net revenue identifies the percentage of total net revenue attributable to prepaid revenue. This information can help the group identify how much of its operational cash flow is dependent upon prepaid revenue for each reporting period. This information can be used for budgeting and planning activities.

$$\frac{\text{Number of Prepaid Plan}}{\text{Members at Beginning of Period}} + \frac{\text{Number of Prepaid Plan}}{\text{Members at End of Period}}$$
$$2$$

$$\frac{\text{Net Prepaid Contract Revenue}}{\text{Total Net Revenue}} \times 100$$

$$\frac{\text{Net Prepaid Contract Revenue}}{\text{Average Number of Prepaid Plan Members}}$$

$$\frac{\text{Prepaid Patient Charges (FFS Equivalent)}}{\text{Average Number of Prepaid Plan Members}}$$

$$\frac{\text{Net Prepaid Contract Revenue}}{\text{Prepaid Patient Charges (FFS Equivalent)}} \times 100$$

FIGURE 5–3 Prepaid Services Indicators of Performance

Net prepaid contract revenue per member per month identifies the average revenue per prepaid member per month. This information can be used to determine whether prepaid subscription (capitation) fees are appropriate. It also can be used for budgeting and planning activities.

Prepaid patient charges (FFS equivalent) per member per month identifies the average monthly gross charges (fee-for-service equivalent) generated per prepaid member. This information, when used with revenue/membership-related indicators, can help determine if capitation fees are appropriate. It also can be used for negotiation of capitation fees between the group and the HMO.

Net prepaid contract revenue as a percent of prepaid patient charges (FFS equivalent) identifies the relationship between prepaid income and the work performed, measured as fee-for-service equivalent gross charges, on behalf of prepaid plan members. If this percentage is greater than 100 percent, there is greater prepaid income than FFS equivalent charges. This indicates that capitation payments, copayments, and risk-sharing revenues exceeded the charges for care provided to prepaid plan members. If this percentage is less than 100 percent, FFS equivalent charges are greater than prepaid income. When used in conjunction with the two preceding indicators, this indicator can help determine if capitation payments, copayments, and risk-sharing contracts are appropriate for the care provided to prepaid plan members.

Case Study 5–1 analyzes operating results for the Western Clinic using some of the indicators described in this section.

RESOURCE-BASED RELATIVE VALUE SCALE

Relative value units (RVUs) and resource-based relative value scales (RBRVS) are useful for evaluating the performance of physicians within a group or of the total group relative to others. RBRVS came into prominence under the Omnibus Budget Reconciliation Act of 1989, which established a Medicare fee schedule (MFS), to be phased in from 1992 through 1996,

---

CASE STUDY 5–1

ANALYZING OPERATION RESULTS

The family practice department of the Western Clinic has experienced substantial growth during the last five years. Dr. Marcia Mistee, department head, wants to determine the factors that brought about this growth. She has contacted Paul Palmer, controller of the clinic, for advice. His department has compiled the following information (dollar amounts in thousands).

Family Practice	19X5	19X0
Total revenue	$ 2,556	$1,454
Discounts and bad debts	245	164
Net revenue	$ 2,311	$1,290
Direct expenses	1,905	1,455
Net earnings before indirect expenses	$ 406	$(165)
Practice-days	635	432
Patient encounters	12,772	9,066
Physician salaries and fringes	$ 1,117	$ 823
Staff salaries and fringes	$ 475	$ 364
Physician-FTE	6.00	5.46
Staff-FTE	14.12	11.36
Occupancy expenses	$ 194	$ 196

Case Discussion Question

1. Using the above information, prepare a report for Dr. Mistee that summarizes the most significant reasons for growth in her department.

---

replacing the current "customary, prevailing, and reasonable" (CPR) payment scheme. The MFS has three components:

1. A relative value component that adjusts relative payments among services, using RBRVS
2. A geographic component that adjusts premiums among areas, using geographic factors that measure area differences in the cost of living and in physician practice costs
3. A conversion factor that transforms relative value units into dollars

Although RBRVS were developed to set fees paid by Medicare to physicians for health care services, they also provide important data about the resources consumed and work expended in delivering specific services. Thus, the RVUs underlying the fee schedule also provide a way to measure financial performance. For example, RVUs can be used to evaluate the relative contributions to profits made by individual physician's activities and by office staff productivity.

Medicare-Based Relative Value Scales

The RBRVS developed for the Medicare system can be used to construct a relative value scale for use in evaluating performance. Medicare's RBRVS divide resources into three parts:

1. Physician work, which involves time, technical skill, physical strength, mental effort, judgment, and stress; and total work
2. Practice expenses (such as rent, support staff, and supplies), which vary by physician gross revenues, mix of services provided, and practice location
3. Malpractice expenses, which vary by specialty

The Medicare RBRVS use relative values for approximately 7,000 current procedural terminology codes (CPT–4). The relative values for procedure codes reflect the relative weights of physician work, expenses, and resource usage for the various procedures. The RBRVS are a master listing of relative values by CPT–4 codes.

One use of the Medicare RBRVS is to determine the total relative value units (RVUs) performed by a medical group for a given time period. First, procedure code data are extracted from the practice's billing system. Then, these data are multiplied by the relative values for each procedure from the Medicare RBRVS, as follows:

$$\begin{array}{c}\text{Total procedures}\\\text{performed, by code,}\\\text{for period}\end{array} \times \begin{array}{c}\text{Relative values}\\\text{for each code}\end{array} = \begin{array}{c}\text{Total relative}\\\text{units}\\\text{for period}\end{array}$$

Table 5–5 illustrates this use of Medicare RBRVS for a sample orthopedic practice. Case Study 5–2 shows how relative values can be used in cost determination.

Once developed, the total relative value units provide a basis for evaluating the performance of physicians and staff as well as for other internal uses. For example, the RVUs can show how changes in physician work and in the efficiency of the office staff directly affect the group's profit. RVUs can also indicate how incentive payment should be distributed to the physicians, based on their contribution to the work of the practice and its profitability. In addition, RVUs can show how bonus payments to office employees should be made, based on employee contributions to efficiency. Finally, RVUs can determine the types of changes that must be made in physicians' activities and

TABLE 5–5   Total Relative Value Service Units for a Sample Orthopedic Practice

		Number Performed					Relative
Code	Procedure	Medicare	Blue Shield	Other	Total Procedures	Relative Values[a]	Value Units[b]
20610	Drain/inject joint	45	22	17	84	1.36	114
20663	Application of thigh brace	66	30	28	124	10.82	1,342
27244	Repair thigh fracture	46	44	17	107	35.17	3,763
27253	Repair hip dislocation	66	25	40	131	28.70	3,760
27310	Exploration of knee joint	83	36	13	132	20.41	2,694
27427	Knee reconstruction	70	45	29	144	26.38	3,799
27440	Revision of knee joint	26	25	36	87	24.69	2,148
27448	Incision of thigh	72	53	34	159	26.56	4,223
27487	Knee joint replacement	86	72	63	221	68.48	15,134
27580	Fusion of knee	23	19	8	50	32.44	1,622
99204	Office visit, new	100	88	60	248	2.59	642
99212	Office visit, established	90	76	50	216	0.72	156
99214	Office visit, established	75	52	22	149	1.52	226
99241	Office consultation	66	63	53	182	1.29	235
99272	Confirmatory consult	22	41	18	81	1.75	142
					Total annual relative value service units		40,000

[a]Obtained from the original Medicare RBRVS listing
[b]Relative value service units = total no. procedures × relative value weight

in office expenditures to achieve specific short-term and long-term profitability goals.

Internally Developed Relative Value Scales

In the costing of medical services, many health care organizations have started to use relative value units based on their own, internally developed relative value scales. These internally developed relative value scales reflect differences among procedures in such factors as:

- Time to complete the procedures
- Difficulty in carrying out the procedures
- Quantity and cost of resources used
- Training and education costs involved
- Malpractice insurance costs incurred

An internally constructed relative value scale requires a special study to determine the relative weights of the factor chosen as the basis of the scale. If the quantity or cost of resources is the basis chosen, for example, then the study determines the resources consumed by each procedure. For example, assume a radiology laboratory conducts three types of tests, W, A, and P, and a special study produces the following results:

Test	Costs	Volume	Average Unit Cost
W	$80	8	$10
A	60	3	20
P	48	4	12

The relative value scale is established by selecting any one of the tests as the standard and assigning it an index value of 1.0. If test W is chosen as the base unit and assigned an RVU of 1.0, for example, then test A, which costs twice as much as test W in the base period, will be assigned an RVU of 2:

$$\frac{\text{Test A base cost}}{\text{Test W base cost}} = \text{Test A RVUs, or } \frac{\$20}{\$10} = 2.0$$

Similarly, test P will be assigned 1.2 RVUs:

$$\frac{\text{Test P base cost}}{\text{Test W base cost}} = \text{Test P RVUs, or } \frac{\$12}{\$10} = 1.2$$

Once an RVU scale has been constructed, it can be used to determine the cost of each test in any subsequent period. For example, assume in a later period that testing costs aggregate $220, with patient testing volume as follows:

> Test W: 2 tests
> Test A: 8 tests
> Test P: 2 tests

Using the RVU scale, one can convert the volume in this subsequent period into total RVUs:

Test	RVUs	×	Volume	=	Total RVUs
W	1.0		2		2.0
A	2.0		8		16.0
P	1.2		2		2.4
					20.4

The cost per RVU can then be determined by dividing the total cost, or $220, by the total RVUs, or 20.4, to yield a cost of $10.78 per RVU. The next step is to calculate the cost for each type of test by completing the following table:

Test	RVUs per Test	Cost per RVU	Cost per Test	Volume	Total Cost
W	1.0	$10.78	$10.78	2	$ 21.54
A	2.0	10.78	21.56	8	172.60
P	1.2	10.78	12.94	2	25.86
					$ 220.00

This application provides a fairer reflection of the relative costs of each test. In the example above, total costs were $220 and total number of tests was 12, an increase in total costs and a decrease in volume from the base period. Although the increase in cost of each type of test was modest (test W went from $10.00 to $10.78, test A from $20.00 to $21.56, and test P from $12.00 to $12.94), there was a substantial shift in volume toward the most expensive type of patient test (test A).

For internally developed RVU scales to be reliable, the original data must be accurate and relative costs must remain stable. In the example, it is assumed that test A remained twice as costly as test W. If there were a change in technology or procedure that affected costs, the relative values would have to be adjusted accordingly.

OTHER TYPES OF PERFORMANCE REPORTING

As medical groups acquire greater sophistication in financial management approaches and enhanced capabilities with information systems, two other types of performance reporting can be used. They involve variance analysis associated with flexible budgets and standards of performance.

Flexible Budget Variances

Flexible budgeting is a valuable tool for reporting on performance. As defined earlier, a flexible budget is one that is adjusted for the actual level of volume achieved in the reporting period. Some costs are fixed, meaning they do not vary with volume. Other costs are variable, meaning they do vary with volume. Thus, a flexible budget must be based on a knowledge of which costs are fixed and which are variable. A flexible budget is developed on the basis of specific actual volume. Variances are then calculated by comparing actual results with flexed budgeted amounts.

Three-Level Variance Analysis

Figure 5–4 shows three variances that can be calculated as an initial evaluation of results. The difference between the total original budget for line items and the flexible budget is called a volume variance, because it is attributable to a change in volume. The flexible budget is compared with the actual costs incurred to determine the extent of the remaining variance. This remaining variance is divided into two parts, the price variance and the quantity variance. Frequently, these two parts are combined and called a flexible budget variance.

The benefit of breaking the total variance down in this way is that it is easier to isolate problem areas. Also, problems can be prioritized based on the magnitude of their variances. For example, the relative magnitude of their variances may indicate that the purchase price of supplies rather than the amount of supplies used is contributing more to an unfavorable supply-cost variance, providing a basis for investigating the causes of budget departures. Clearly, the ability to detect problems and control them is greatly enhanced by this type of analysis, and the costs of calculating and reporting the additional variances are minimal, once a structure of data accumulation has been established.

In addition to volume, price, and quantity variances for direct labor and materials, or supplies, variances for variable and fixed overhead costs can also be calculated. Variable overhead costs are like direct labor and materials in that, with greater volume, variable overhead costs will be larger and thus generate a volume variance. Price and quantity variances for variable overhead costs can also be calculated. These variances are often called spending and efficiency variances, respectively.

By definition, fixed costs do not change with volume changes. Therefore, for any fixed costs, whether they are overhead costs or direct costs, the expected costs for actual volume are identical to the expected costs for budgeted volume, and there are no volume variances. However, it is sometimes possible to determine price and quantity variances for fixed overhead costs. Assume, for example, that the ambulatory surgery department of the MJP Medical Clinic has budgeted nursing costs for a recent month according to the schedule below. The actual cost and hours, also indicated below, go far over budget. Variances can be calculated and compared to determine why.

	Original Budget	Actual Data
Patient hours	650	700
RN hours per patient-day	7	8.5
RN hourly pay rate	$20	$22
Total RN cost	$91,000	$130,900

CASE STUDY 5–2

USING RELATIVE VALUES IN COST DETERMINATION

Dr. Jan Burnside, medical director of the Western Clinic, is negotiating a contract with Coastal HMO in which the clinic and Holy Fathers Hospital will jointly provide medical services for burn patients. Physicians of Western Clinic will provide the medical treatments, and patients will receive nursing care at Holy Fathers Hospital. In reaching a price for the nursing services in the contract, both the clinic and the hospital realize the necessity of accurately estimating the cost of these services. The hospital presents the following information about the cost of burn treatment nursing services, based on a special study conducted last year of past experience with hospital burn treatment care.

Acuity Level	Hours of Care per Patient-Day	No. of Patient-Days Provided During Past Year
1	2.5	160
2	3.8	280
3	5.1	350
4	7.3	190
5	9.4	110

During the next year, the estimated total costs of nursing for the burn unit at Holy Fathers Hospital will be $198,530.

Case Discussion Questions

1. Prepare an analysis to determine the cost of nursing services, using relative value units as the basis of cost.
2. Assume that an average burn patient had a length of stay of nine days, with the following acuity-level classification of care:

Level 1	2 days
2	4 days
3	2 days
4	1 day
5	0 days

What would be the nursing cost for the average patient?

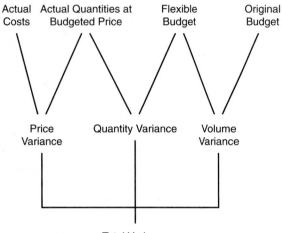

FIGURE 5–4 Price, Quantity, and Volume Variances

The relevant variances can be calculated as follows:

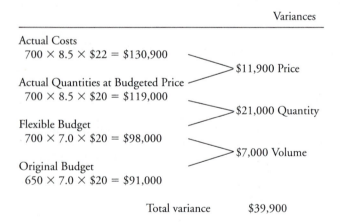

Variances

Actual Costs
700 × 8.5 × $22 = $130,900

$11,900 Price

Actual Quantities at Budgeted Price
700 × 8.5 × $20 = $119,000

$21,000 Quantity

Flexible Budget
700 × 7.0 × $20 = $98,000

$7,000 Volume

Original Budget
650 × 7.0 × $20 = $91,000

Total variance $39,900

The total variance of $39,900 represents the difference between the total original budget ($91,000) and the total actual costs ($130,900). The hourly rate paid nurses averaged $22 per hour, which was $2 per hour greater than the budgeted rate, thus giving rise to the unfavorable price variance of $11,900. The actual nursing hours per patient-day were 8.5 versus the budgeted 7.0, thereby resulting in an unfavorable quantity variance of $21,000. Actual volume of patient hours was 700, which was 50 hours more than the budgeted

hours of 650, thus creating an unfavorable volume variance of $7,000.

It should be noted that a price or quantity variance is considered to be favorable when the actual price or quantity of resource used is less than the budgeted price or quantity. The variance is considered to be unfavorable when the opposite is true. A favorable volume variance denotes an actual volume level greater than the budgeted volume; an unfavorable volume variance denotes an actual volume level less than the budgeted volume.

Four-Level Variance Analysis

A practice may treat exactly the same number of patients or patient-days, but the severity, or acuity, of illness in patients may vary almost continuously on a daily basis. It is useful to isolate the portion of the quantity variance that results from changes in the level of acuity of illness. This requires a patient classification system that can reasonably predict patient-care staffing requirements at different acuity levels.

Suppose, for example, that the MJP clinic determines that the actual incurred acuity level for the indicated month requires the group to pay for 8.0 hours of nursing care per patient-day, rather than the originally budgeted 7.0 hours. Thus, part of the quantity variance is attributable to sicker patients, rather than operational inefficiencies. The question is, how much of the quantity variance is due to this unexpectedly high level of patient acuity?

To answer this question, it is necessary to divide the total quantity variance into two component variances, as follows:

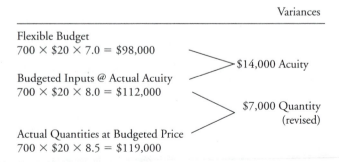

Variances

Flexible Budget
700 × $20 × 7.0 = $98,000

$14,000 Acuity

Budgeted Inputs @ Actual Acuity
700 × $20 × 8.0 = $112,000

$7,000 Quantity (revised)

Actual Quantities at Budgeted Price
700 × $20 × 8.5 = $119,000

The acuity variance ($14,000), which is unfavorable, represents the amount that spending differed from expectations, because patients were sicker than expected. Sicker patients generally require more resources for treatment, as represented by the 8.0 hours per patient-day in the actual acuity budget, versus the 7.0 hours per patient-day in the original budget. The revised quantity variance represents all factors that resulted in consumption of more input per unit of output than budgeted, such as using more hours of nursing care per patient-day than the amount budgeted, irrespective of patient acuity. In sum, a four-level variance analysis yields the following total flexible budget variances for the MJP clinic (all unfavorable):

Price variance	$11,900
Quantity variance	7,000
Acuity variance	14,000
Volume variance	7,000
Total variance	$39,900

Figure 5–5 shows how the acuity variance is related to the other types of variances discussed above.

Use of Standards in Performance Reporting

Group practices are beginning to recognize the value of using standards to measure the quantities and prices of resources needed for patient care. The use of standards requires the establishment of a standard cost system, which delineates how much it should cost to treat certain patients. Setting standards, in turn, involves determining a physical standard of resource usage and a price standard for the cost of each unit of service, such as a procedure or treatment. Usually, the method of developing standards requires the use of technical estimates of labor, supplies, equipment quantity usage, and price of unit cost standards. Once established, standard costs of service units, like procedures, enable comparison of actual costs of services with standard costs. This permits the calculation of variances as departures from desired quantity and price amounts, providing insight into specific activities and applications of patient services, and allowing careful scrutiny of practice techniques and evaluation of changing procedures and protocols to ensure maximum efficiency.

As just described, it is possible to analyze differences between actual and budgeted costs by calculating flexible

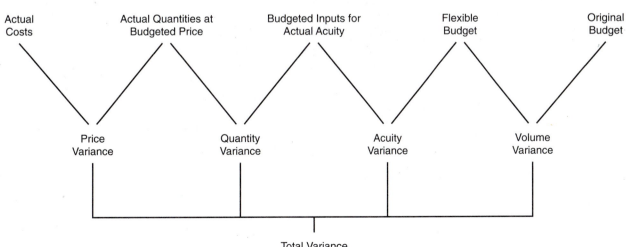

FIGURE 5–5 Price, Quantity, Acuity, and Volume Variances

budget variances. The use of standard costs is yet another approach. Standard costing provides a more definitive and accurate tool than the flexible budget for comparing the efficiency and effectiveness of the application of specific medical procedures and protocol patterns.

Standard costing provides a series of performance reports that show why variances occur and who is accountable. Reports can be prepared in various formats to give management the information needed to evaluate group planning, efficiency, labor rates, and spending. To learn more about these details of standard costing, consult accounting texts or related sources. An example of a summary performance report, in which four types of standard cost variances are displayed, is shown in Table 5–6. Brief comments about each type of variance are presented next.

Volume Planning Variance

This variance shows the difference between the planned number of procedures and the number actu-ally performed. Causes of volume planning variance include changes in physician availability (for example, unanticipated physician absences, additions, or terminations), changes in marketing programs, fluctuations in HMO activity, and the impact of competition

Labor Efficiency Variance

The labor efficiency variance measures labor productivity by assessing the effectiveness of a manager's control over labor resources and their costs. The variance denotes the difference between the quantity of labor hours actually incurred and the quantity that should have been incurred (the standard), given the actual volume of activity. Common causes of labor efficiency variance include managerial ineffectiveness, use of inaccurate standards, and unanticipated changes. The latter might include the adoption of an improved scheduling system that results in fewer delays; cross-training of personnel that reduces idle time; and changes in equipment, technology, or education or skill levels of staff that affect efficiency.

TABLE 5–6   Example of Summary Performance Report

Summary Performance Report for the Period Ending: December 31, 19XX

Responsibility Center	Variance Summary			
	Volume Planning	Labor Efficiency	Labor Rate	Spending
Family practice	$29,390	430 hrs	$ 2,535	$6,926
Internal medicine	2,260	(100)	4,646	440
Pediatrics	(10,564)	846	858	(1,488)
Radiology	(14,525)	530	4,258	(7,920)
Total	$ 6,561	1,706 hrs	$12,297	($2,042)

Responsibility Center	Total Expenses			
	Labor and Spending Variance	Planned Expenses	Actual Expenses	Percent Variance
Family practice	$ 9,462	$217,770	$227,232	4.34%
Internal medicine	5,086	106,000	111,086	4.80%
Pediatrics	(629)	139,650	139,021	(0.45%)
Radiology	(3,662)	147,875	144,213	(2.48%)
Total	$10,257	$611,295	$621,552	1.68%

Labor Rate Variance

The labor rate variance is the difference between expected and actual hourly labor rates. Some causes of this variance are:

- Unforeseen labor market changes forcing the medical group to adjust wages or postpone wage increases
- Turnover of personnel with more or less experience or seniority, resulting in more higher or lower paid personnel
- Personnel working a significant amount of unbudgeted overtime

Spending Variance

The spending variance is the difference between planned and actual nonlabor direct expenses for medical supplies, minor equipment, drugs and medications, and similar purchases. This variance informs management of spending that is inconsistent with strategic or operational plans. Typical causes of spending variance are purchasing and using more medical supplies or drugs than expected, replacing an asset before its anticipated life has ended, adding an asset not included in the budget, spending a different amount than budgeted on equipment or other items, and using an inadequate method to budget capital and other fixed expenditures.

Analytical Software

Developments in computer software are making various analytical tools available to assist financial managers in analyzing financial and clinical data. A useful tool for analyzing physician services and the productivity of medical groups is the Physician Services Practice Analysis (PSPA), personal computer software developed by the Center for Research in Ambulatory Health Care Administration (CRAHCA).

PSPA analyzes physician productivity based on the number and complexity of procedures performed in the practice. Using the medical group's own data as input, PSPA measures physician productivity on a work-performed basis. It weights procedures using a relative value scale so that comparisons of physician productivity can be made (among physicians or groups or over time). Productivity statistics calculated by PSPA include:

- Case intensity (total number of relative values divided by the total number of patients)
- Procedure complexity (total number of relative values divided by total number of procedures)
- Physician productivity (total number of relative values per FTE)

This physician productivity information can be used in negotiating capitation and discounted services, evaluating new reimbursement mechanisms, monitoring utilization, or establishing new methods of compensating physicians based on individual and organizational performance.

ACTIVITY-BASED COSTING

The principles used in costing health care services emanate from the management and cost accounting practices that originated in manufacturing companies. A fairly new development in the manufacturing industry may offer a new approach for costing patient services. It is called *activity-based costing* (ABC), and it is based on the premise that determination of the cost of products (patients) or product lines (groups of similar patients) is improved by more accurately assigning costs on a cause-and-effect basis (Glennie & Terhaar, 1994). In practice, ABC assigns costs first to cost pools of activities, not to departments or cost centers. Then, it assigns the activity costs to outputs using cost drivers, which are activities that cause the costs to be at a certain level for a given amount of activity. The identification of cost drivers requires an analysis of all activities performed throughout the organization, the resources used to perform each activity, and factors that drive costs to be at a certain level.

To illustrate this approach, consider the activities typically performed in purchasing materials (supplies):

- Determining material requirements
- Selecting vendors
- Ordering materials
- Receiving and inspecting incoming materials
- Stocking materials
- Maintaining inventory records
- Accounting for payables
- Issuing materials to operations

The cost of a particular purchasing activity may be driven by the number of units handled, the number of orders, the value of the materials, or other variable(s). The analyst must decide which cost drivers are the best indicators of the cost relationship. These drivers must then be used as the basis for assigning the amounts in each activity cost pool to the output (in health care, the patient). Prior to ABC, the cost of purchasing would be assigned to patient-rendering departments with a single non-activity cost driver, such as number of patients served. Note, however, that under ABC, there may be several activity cost pools within the purchasing department and several activity cost drivers used to assign their costs to patients.

The use of ABC results in more accurate costing, because ABC clearly identifies the costs of different activities performed in the department. ABC also assigns the costs of activities to outputs using measures that represent the types of demands that individual outputs place on these activities. Another advantage of ABC is that it shows more clearly how resources are being consumed throughout the organization. Many costs previously treated as overhead can be treated, with ABC, as direct costs of products or services, and organizations can discover for the first time why overhead has grown.

However, the real benefit of ABC comes from identifying which activities add value to the product produced or service performed. Costs that do not add value are candidates for reduction or minimization in the overhaul of the production or service process. ABC helps discern ways to perform activities more efficiently, such as substituting less expensive activities for more expensive ones, redesigning operating processes to eliminate certain activities entirely, or designing products or processes that make fewer demands on activities.

Activity-Based Costing in Health Care

The ABC approach has the potential to improve substantially the accuracy of costing in health care. Yet, ABC is not an entirely new technique; it still uses the basic cost allocation principle. However, ABC expands this principle by introducing cost drivers and activities as elements of the basic allocation technique. Costing results are more accurate with ABC because the process makes sharper distinctions in assigning indirect costs by activities, rather than by a global single allocation base, usually related to volume. And, ABC enhances accuracy by using a greater number of allocation bases in assigning costs to the end product, the patient. By focusing attention on activity-driven costs rather than on volume-driven costs, the possibility of overallocating overhead to high-volume products and underallocating overhead to low-volume products is avoided.

Readers interested in discovering more about ABC are urged to consult management accounting texts for a fuller treatment of the subject. Consult the health care journals for case studies illustrating its application.

IMPROVING OPERATIONS

Controlling medical practice operations today means finding ways to carry out patient care services more efficiently while maintaining high standards of quality. The movement toward efficiency and equality has been characterized as *total quality improvement* (TQI). It is found in all industries. TQI has been used in various abbreviated forms in health care in three major ways: improving productivity, implementing cost reductions, and increasing income potentials.

Improving Productivity

Productivity relates to the way in which resources are used to produce services or products. It is most often assessed in the context of the relationship between inputs and outputs. Typically, productivity is expressed as a ratio between inputs, or resources used, and outputs, or services or products produced, as shown in Figure 5–6. Examples of productivity ratios include nursing time per clinic visit, therapist time (labor) per physical therapy treatment, and medical supplies per ambulatory surgery procedure. Once information about a group's state of productivity has been compiled, management might review operations to develop standards of productivity and monitor achieving these standards.

To monitor productivity, two types of information are needed:

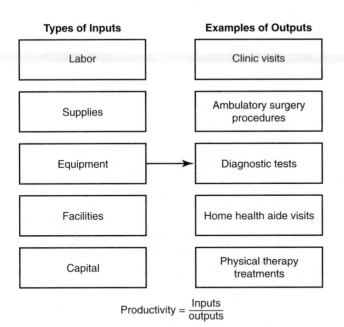

FIGURE 5–6 Inputs, Outputs, and Productivity in Ambulatory Services

1. Trends in the ratio of inputs to outputs
2. Comparisons of actual ratios with expected ratios or standards

Productivity ratios should be calculated and compared with standards on a biweekly or monthly basis.

Operational Reviews

These reviews entail a comprehensive analysis of a specific department, area, or free-standing entity. There are five different types of analysis: organizational, functional, facility, staffing, and material.

Organizational analysis involves an evaluation of the organizational structure of a department or area. This includes evaluation of the responsibilities and roles of all professionals in the area and whether they are appropriate to the area's workload. The purpose of functional analysis is to determine the types of activities being conducted. Each activity is broken down into its various tasks and work steps. A review is made of each of these tasks and steps to determine which ones can be either eliminated or improved in some fashion. The fo-

cus of facility analysis is to assess the appropriateness of size and layout of the physical space in a department or area. Facility analyses should be conducted over a sufficient span of time to ascertain usage during different parts of the week, month, or year. Staffing analysis pertains to estimating the time required to carry out department activities. Past, current, and future staffing levels are reviewed in relation to the workload, and the scheduling of staff is evaluated and compared to the volume of work. Material analysis deals with supplies and equipment. This includes the distribution systems for supplies, the determination of supply inventory levels, and the adequacy and maintenance of equipment.

Areas Where Productivity Gains Can Be Achieved

Productivity improvements involve lowering the ratio of inputs to outputs or raising outputs while keeping inputs constant. Areas where productivity gains can often be attained are:

- Improving scheduling of patients, staffing, and physicians' workloads
- Revising staff support levels to meet expected workloads (rather than past workloads)
- Enhancing the work environment and eliciting ideas from staff for how to increase the efficiency of work flow
- Altering the functional design of facilities to expedite the handling of patient care
- Providing incentives for physicians to be more efficient, through compensation schemes or productivity arrangements
- Installing well-designed systems and procedures to assure that supplies for patient care are available, that billings are made expeditiously and accurately, and that other pertinent work flows can be carried out efficiently

Implementing Cost Reductions

The term *cost management* signifies the continuous process of planning, monitoring, and controlling the cost of operations. Cost management systems use the concepts of responsibility accounting, cost accounting, budgeting, and financial reporting in an integrated fashion to achieve profitable operations, primarily through cost reductions. Cost management can lead to many different changes in the way practice resources are employed and compensated for. Some illustrations are shown in Table 5-7.

Increasing Income Potentials

Increasing income potentials involves the enlargement of revenues to improve operations. Medical groups should view their practices as businesses and adopt broad managerial perspectives in marketing their services. Some medical groups distribute patient brochures advertising the advantages and attractiveness of the medical group's capacities to potential patients and managed-care group audiences. Other medical groups use radio or television advertisements to attract greater patient volume. Market analyses are becoming a necessary tool for assessing the potential patient market to be served in bidding for managed-care contracts.

Other possible directions that marketing strategies might take include:

- Establishing satellite offices or using shared office space
- Creating ambulatory surgical centers
- Increasing production through physician incentives
- Enlarging physician exposure in the local community through public speaking and community work

OUTCOMES MANAGEMENT

Outcomes management is an important component of managed care and competition. It is oriented toward reform and is growing in importance today (Fahey, 1994). Outcomes management addresses the issues of uncontrolled spending and inconsistent quality of care. It does so by redirecting incentives in order to control overuse, underuse, and inappropriate use of medical services. According to Paul M. Ellwood, M.D., one of the principal architects of the managed competition model, outcomes management helps patients, payers, and physicians make rational medical care choices

TABLE 5–7   Examples of Cost Management

Personnel costs:

- Assessing staff levels according to demonstrated need
- Centralizing certain functions, such as appointments, transcription recording, and receptionists
- Matching the duties of various staff members with the skills needed to perform certain functions
- Reviewing the cost of employee benefits and modifying them where appropriate

Clerical and clerical supplies:

- Obtaining discounts by purchasing larger volumes
- Maintaining proper levels of supplies
- Strengthening the accounts payable system by taking available cash discounts
- Keeping supplies locked up during office hours

Facilities and equipment:

- Adapt existing capacity to the current market preference for certain hours to offer services
- Comparison shop for the best maintenance agreements for servicing equipment

Other areas:

- Review telephone costs and compare to other available telephone systems
- Monitor outside laboratory costs and compare to other available sources
- Evaluate the present computer information system and adjust to the needs of the practice

based on better insights into the effects of these choices on patients' lives. Outcomes management analyzes the relationship between medical interventions and health outcomes as well as the relationship between health outcomes and money. It establishes guidelines that physicians can use to select appropriate interventions. In addition, outcomes management routinely and systematically measures the functioning and well-being of patients, along with disease-specific clinical outcomes, at appropriate time intervals. Further, outcomes management pools clinical and outcome data on a national basis, analyzes the results, and disseminates the collected data to health care decision makers throughout the industry.

Several of the predictions from current outcomes management research may be revolutionary in their impact on the mores of health care delivery. Some of these predictions include:

- Patients will be able to select a physician, hospital, or health plan based on a published "batting average," giving patients a more prominent role in health care decisions
- Payers may channel patients to centers of excellence that demonstrate better outcomes
- Employers will be able to use outcomes data to select health plans for their employees
- Physicians will be able to use research-supported data to improve their delivery of services
- Guidelines for effective performance delivery may become standards of medical care in litigation suits
- Physician privileges and credentialing will become largely driven by clinical outcomes, efficiency measures, and patient satisfaction results
- Employer coalitions and managed-care providers will campaign for hospital mortality, length-of-stay, charge, and other outcomes data to rate institutions or physicians on their quality of care

It is clear that outcomes management has great potential for revamping and improving the delivery of quality health care services. Many predict that practices evolving from outcomes management will be the linchpins for establishing accountability standards and upgrading the quality of information about medical services.

EVALUATING PERFORMANCE IN REVIEW

Evaluating the financial performance of medical groups has traditionally centered on the analysis of the activities of responsibility centers and on comparing actual results with the goals of the practice and with the operating budget. A practice can also be evaluated by comparing its performance with that of other groups. Key operating reports include financial statements; departmental financial reports comparing actual results and budgets; and various clinical data relating to utilization, resource consumption, and referrals.

Several significant indicators of performance are another means of evaluation. These indicators assess financial and nonfinancial performance by physician and department and the prepaid component of the practice. Resource-based relative value scales enable managers to develop more refined methods of performance evaluation through consideration of differences in the types of resources expended in various patient encounters. More advanced analyses include the use of flexible-budget and standard-cost variances. A newly emerging cost accounting system, activity-based costing, promises to bring more accuracy to costing patient procedures and treatments. Medical practices should constantly try to improve their operations by increasing productivity, reducing costs, and enlarging the income-raising potential of the group. Outcomes management promises to be an important way to assess the efficiency and effectiveness of operating efforts of health care entities.

REFERENCES

Cost Survey and Membership Compensation Survey (1996). Englewood, CO: Medical Group Management Association.

Faye, P. S. (1994, May/June). Outcomes research—it's not just for academic medicine. *MGM Journal, 41*(3), 16, 18, 62, 64, 66, 68, 70, 72.

Finkler, S. A. (1994). *Cost accounting for health care organizations.* Gaithersburg, MD: Aspen Publishers.

Glennie, S. S. & Terhaar, P. A. (1994, July/August). Activity–based costing. *MGM Journal, 41*(4), 88, 90, 92–94, 96, 98.

Pavlock, E. J. (1994). *Financial management for medical groups.* Englewood, CO: Center for Research in Ambulatory Health Care Administration.

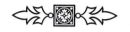

CHAPTER

6

Short-Term and Long-Term Financial Decision Making[1]

Ernest J. Pavlock

CHAPTER TOPICS

Short-Term Investment Decisions
Cost-Volume-Profit Analysis
Long-Term Investment Decisions
Financial Decisions in Review

LEARNING OBJECTIVES

Upon completing this chapter, the reader will be able to:

- Establish an appropriate framework of analysis and select the relevant information for making decisions
- Differentiate between financial data that impact operating costs, volume of activity, and profit levels, and infer meaningful insights from the interplay of these variables in deciding on alternative courses of action
- Calculate the break-even point for a medical practice and for segments of the practice, and evaluate the implications of these results for operating levels
- Apply principles of the time value of money in evaluating long-term investment opportunities
- Identify and assimilate the necessary financial information to assess the desirability of committing funds to various long-term investment options

- Use discounted and nondiscounted cash flow methods of capital budgeting, combined with nonquantitative factors, to arrive at capital investment decisions

Medical practices are faced with many decisions, most of which require a cost-benefit analysis, in which the benefits to be achieved from various alternatives are measured and compared with the costs of pursuing the alternatives. In general, decision making can be envisioned within the investment context of evaluating the possible returns on alternative avenues of investment and selecting the best ones for placing some of the medical group's assets into activities and ventures.

There are two general types of investment alternatives: those involving short-term decisions and those involving long-term decisions. Each type requires considerably different data for analysis. Short-term decisions, that is, those impacting the next few years, involve the use of existing capacity for service delivery. These decisions generally pertain to the volume and mix of services to offer and the fees to charge. Long-term decisions, in contrast, relate to the acquisition or replacement of capacity, and require a long period of time before benefits are fully realized. Long-term decisions generally pertain to the acquisition of buildings, equipment, and, to some extent, key people.

Three major differences characterize short- and long-term investment decisions. First, there is the time frame of analysis, with short-term periods embracing one or a few years and long-term periods embracing longer time spans, such as 5 years, 10 years, or more. The time value of money refers to the fact that a unit of money is worth more today because it is "in hand" than it is worth at some future date because of the interest factor, or a return for use of the money. The time value of money is not an issue in short-term decisions as it is in long-term decisions. Short-term decisions usually entail instead a limited investment and a quick recovery of cash.

[1]Some information in this chapter has been adapted from *Financial Management for Medical Groups* by Ernest J. Pavlock, PhD, CPA with permission of the Center for Research in Ambulatory Health Care Administration, 104 Inverness Terrace East, Englewood, CO, 80112-5306; (303) 799-1111. Copyright 1994.

A second difference between short- and long-term investment decisions is that short-term decisions usually involve repetitive activities whereas long-term decisions may not. Because the immediate future is likely to be similar to the recent past, accounting measurements of revenues and costs are relevant for short-term analysis.

A third distinction between short- and long-term investment decisions pertains to the setting of the decisions. Short-term decisions relate to the types, amounts, and prices of services that will be performed with the existing capacity of the organization. Long-term decisions, in contrast, effect a change in the size of the capacity to provide goods or services.

This chapter covers the approaches used to accumulate and analyze relevant information for both short-term and long-term investment alternatives. Examples are given of typical situations in which these investment evaluations are made. Each example will show the necessity of compiling and using relevant information to reach a decision.

SHORT-TERM INVESTMENT DECISIONS

When making short-term decisions, managers seek the alternative that will most likely accomplish the objectives of the organization.

Framework of Analysis

The thought process in short-term decision making involves the following five steps, which are discussed below:

1. Define the problem
2. Develop possible alternative solutions
3. Measure and evaluate the consequences of each alternative in quantitative terms
4. Identify nonquantitative consequences of each alternative and integrate this information with quantitative elements
5. Reach a decision

Before relevant quantitative data can be compiled, the problem must be clearly defined. This may be the most difficult part of the decision-making process. Even after the problem has been defined, possible alternative solutions may not be obvious. Consider the following example:

A medical group uses an outside laboratory for testing purposes. The group has become dissatisfied with the services provided by the lab. Management sees three alternatives for dealing with the problem of declining outside lab performance: setting up an internal laboratory within the medical group, seeking another outside laboratory and moving the business to this new firm, and meeting with the management of the present laboratory to determine whether any changes can be made to improve services.

In most cases, one alternative is simply to continue what is now being done. This status quo alternative, called the *base case,* is used as the benchmark against which other alternatives are measured. As alternatives are considered, the analysis becomes more complex. Once all possible alternatives have been identified, those that are clearly unattractive should be eliminated to reduce the set to a smaller number.

The financial impacts of each remaining alternative are then expressed in the form of costs and benefits. Stating the effects quantitatively in this way provides a better basis for decision making than if words alone are used in evaluating possible outcomes. For example, assume a financial manager of a medical group states that "If we add another physician, our revenue will increase but so will our costs, and the malpractice insurance premiums will also go up." Such a statement provides no basis for weighing the relative importance of each element of revenue and costs that will change. However, if these elements are quantified (another physician adds $400,000 in revenue, for example, and increases operating costs by $150,000 and insurance premiums by $10,000), this provides a much better basis for arriving at a decision.

Any decision must take into account not only measurable but also unmeasurable differences among alternatives. Even though quantitative data appear definite and precise, nonquantitative elements may have equal importance and must be integrated into the final decision-making process.

After completing the first four steps, the decision maker has two choices: to seek additional information or to make a decision and take action. Many decisions can be improved by gathering more data, if that is possible. But obtaining information always entails effort (which means cost) and time. There comes a point when the manager concludes that it is better to take action than to defer a decision until more data have been collected.

Cost Information Requirements for Different Decisions

Making a decision always involves selecting the proper course of action for the future. Nothing can be done to alter the past. To decide, the decision maker must compare the *relevant* costs and *relevant* benefits of each alternative. The analysis focuses on the difference between relevant costs and relative benefits—a process called differential analysis.

Relevant costs are those expected future costs that differ among alternative courses of action. Relevant benefits are expected future revenues that differ among alternative courses of action. To understand the application of relevant costs and benefits in short-term investment decisions, we need to be able to apply these elements in various situations through the use of three cost concepts: fixed versus variable costs, avoidable versus unavoidable costs, and full costs.

Fixed versus Variable Costs

In many decisions, such as those involving volume and mix of services, some costs are fixed, whereas others change when activity levels change. As stated above, costs that change as activity goes up or down are called variable costs; they include such costs as supply and laboratory costs. Fixed costs are those that do not change as activity levels go up or down. Fixed costs include rent, insurance, and administrative salaries.

Both revenue and variable costs change as activity levels rise or fall. A simple measure of the change in profit as activity levels change is called the *contribution margin,* which is the difference between revenue and variable costs. This measure can be used to evaluate alternatives in reaching a decision. Assuming that fixed costs do not change, management should select the alternative that will maximize the contribution margin.

The types of decisions in which fixed and variable costs play an important role include determining when overall group operations or specific activities reach the break-even point. Another is deciding whether to perform a procedure such as a lab test internally or to purchase it from outside the group. In general, fixed and variable costs are relevant to any decision affected by changes in activity.

Avoidable versus Unavoidable Costs

Another classification of costs relevant to short-term investment decisions is avoidable versus unavoidable costs. An avoidable cost is a cost that can be eliminated as a result of choosing one alternative over another. For example, when an activity such as a laboratory is discontinued, some costs will be eliminated or avoided—those costs that will not be incurred in the future as a result of not operating the laboratory.

Assume a medical practice is considering eliminating its own laboratory and purchasing laboratory services from an outside source. If the equipment for the in-house laboratory is rented on a cancelable lease, the equipment rental expense is eliminated and thus is an avoidable cost in making the decision. However, the rental cost of the space occupied by the laboratory within the office building of the group is not eliminated, because the group will continue renting the facility for its office. This rental cost is an unavoidable cost. In making short-term investment decisions, it is necessary to determine which costs are avoidable under each alternative and which will continue and must be considered as unavoidable costs.

Full Costs

As discussed in a previous chapter, the full cost of a medical procedure or treatment includes both the direct costs traceable to the procedure or treatment and a fair share of all indirect costs that cannot be traced and thus must be allocated to the procedure or treatment. In certain short-term decisions, full costs may not be relevant, but in many other short-term decisions, full costs must be considered when assessing the long-term implications of the short-term decision. Full costs must be considered, for example, when setting fees for services.

Examples of Short-Term Decisions

Examples of short-term decisions that are common to many medical groups include adding a physician, dropping a service, making versus buying a resource, and setting fees for special situations.

Adding a Physician

Many medical practices must decide whether to add a physician to their group in order to avoid outside referrals for services to prepaid patients or to handle increased patient volume. If adding a physician requires additional facilities and equipment, the decision should be evaluated using long-term decision making techniques, which consider the time value of money as well as incremental revenues and costs. If additional facilities and equipment are not required, the analysis can focus on the differential revenues and costs involved in adding the new physician.

For example, assume that the Western Clinic has projected increasing enrollments in its managed-care contracts and is trying to decide whether a general surgeon should be added to the group. Before the financial implications of the alternatives can be considered, there are a number of policy questions that must be answered: Should the group retain its primary care focus? What impact will the addition of a specialist have on the income distribution formula? Will the new physician serve fee-for-service patients as well as prepaid patients? After these basic policy questions are answered, the group must examine the financial implications of the alternatives.

In the financial analysis, the critical data are the incremental revenues and costs due to the expanded capability in providing services. These amounts are derived from membership and utilization projections. The group must determine the point at which capitation revenue for general surgery exceeds the cost of maintaining a general surgeon.

Assume the following incremental cost estimates have been made for the additional physician surgeon:

Salary and benefits . . . . $ 8,333 per month
Support staff and benefits. . . . . $ 2,880 per month
Equipment rental . . . . $ 200 per month
Professional liability insurance . . . . $ 500 per month
Space (1,500 sq. ft. × $1.50 per month) . . . $ 2,250 per month
 Total costs . . . . $14,163 per month
Supplies and other variable expenses. . . . . . $ 5 per patient visit

The flexible budget for the total cost of the general surgeon is $14,163 per month, plus $5 per patient visit. The incremental revenue for the general surgeon is the portion of the monthly capitation payment of the new managed care contract that is for general surgery. Assume that $3.44 of the total monthly capitation payment is for surgery.

Enrollment projections, surgery patient visits (now being referred out), incremental costs, and incremental revenues are presented for the Western Clinic for selected months in Table 6–1. It appears that incremental revenues exceed incremental costs in about the 13th month. This analysis assumes that there is no change in the gatekeeper role of the primary care physician, utilization rates continue as projected, and enrollment projections are reached. This decision emphasizes the importance of accurate planning and projections.

Dropping a Service

Another example of a short-term decision is deciding whether to drop a particular line of service or a certain activity. Assume, for example, that a medical group opened a satellite office in anticipation of contract membership growth in a particular geographic area. The satellite has been experiencing unprofitable operations, and group members now want to know how much will be saved by eliminating this unprofitable location.

The most recent operating statement for the satellite office is presented in Table 6–2. The office has shown

TABLE 6–1 Incremental Costs and Revenues for Adding a Physician to Western Clinic

Month	Surgery Enrolled Members	Patient Visits	Incremental Costs	Incremental Revenues
1	130	1	$14,168	$ 447
3	328	4	14,183	1,128
6	1,875	21	14,268	6,450
9	2,590	30	14,313	8,910
12	3,850	44	14,383	13,244
15	5,330	61	14,468	18,335

TABLE 6–2 Operating Statement for a Satellite Clinic

	Current Month	
Revenues		$12,000
Operating expenses:		
Associate physician's salary	$4,000	
Associate physician's benefits	800	
Staff salaries	2,400	
Staff benefits	280	
Lab and x-ray services	3,000	
Supplies	1,200	
Occupancy	1,400	
Administrative services for main clinic	1,000	$14,080
Net loss		$ (2,080)

an operating loss since it opened because of increased competition from other medical groups, a downturn in the economy in the area, and inability to provide proper supervision of the office. It is doubtful that the satellite office can produce additional revenue without substantial additional resources.

Besides considering variable and fixed costs, the group also must know which costs will be avoided if the satellite office is closed and which costs will continue. Assume that an associate physician's contract is dependent on the continuation of the satellite office and that the staff is working on an hourly basis, only as needed. Space is rented on a five-year noncancelable lease. The best the group can do with the space is to sublease it for

TABLE 6–3   Avoidable and Unavoidable Costs of Closing a Satellite Clinic

Type of Expense	Fixed or Variable	Monthly Costs	Avoidable Costs	Unavoidable Costs
Associate physician's salary	Fixed	$ 4,000	$ 4,000	—
Associate physician's benefits	Fixed	800	800	—
Staff salaries	Variable	2,400	2,400	—
Staff benefits	Variable	280	280	—
Lab and X-ray services	Variable	3,000	3,000	—
Supplies	Variable	1,200	1,200	—
Occupancy	Fixed	1,400	1,000	$ 400
Administrative services	Fixed	1,000	—	1,000
Total		$14,080	$12,680	$1,400

$1,000 per month, thereby losing $400 per month in rent. The administrative services represent allocated costs from the main office, so closing the satellite office will have little, if any, effect on administrative costs. Table 6–3 summarizes the avoidable and unavoidable costs of closing the satellite office. The table shows that $12,680 of the $14,080 total monthly costs are avoidable and $1,400 are unavoidable costs that would still need to be paid out if the satellite office is closed.

Thus, the impact of closing the satellite office is a decrease in revenue of $12,000 per month and a decrease in operating costs of $12,680 per month, yielding a savings in closing the satellite office of $680 per month. In other words, keeping the office open is costing the practice at least $680 per month. The $1,400 of unavoidable costs will continue regardless of what the group decides to do about the satellite office.

In this example, the relevant data are revenues, variable costs, and avoidable fixed costs. Variable costs are always avoidable in decisions of this nature. The occupancy and administrative costs that continue are unavoidable and therefore irrelevant to such decisions.

Other possible alternatives, such as reducing costs or changing staff, might also have been considered. These alternatives might require other cost concepts besides avoidable versus unavoidable costs. However, the analysis would still focus on differential costs, that is, the cost of the satellite operation as it is as compared with the cost of operating the satellite clinic with reduced costs or staff changes.

Making versus Buying a Resource

The most common example of this type is the decision whether to perform all laboratory tests or contract with an outside laboratory for some of the work. Qualitative issues are always a concern in such decisions. For example, will the tests be done properly? Will results be available on a timely basis? Assuming these questions can be answered satisfactorily, quantitative data are used in differential costing to determine which alternative has the lower costs.

Assume, for example, that a medical clinic has its own laboratory, which charges patient treating centers $25 for each test it performs. Monthly fixed costs of the lab are $40,000, and the average variable cost of each test is $15. An outside laboratory offers to perform all the tests for the clinic for a fee of $18 per test. If services are switched to the outside source, the lab will sell its equipment and eliminate $12,000 per month in depreciation expenses and $6,000 per month in other fixed expenses. The remaining fixed costs are unavoidable. The present average volume of tests conducted each month is 8,400.

To determine whether the clinic should continue operating its own laboratory or use the outside service, relevant costs must be compared. The relevant costs are those that differ between the two alternatives. They are summarized in the following table:

	Test Inside	Purchase Outside
Variable costs:		
Inside (8,400 × $15)	$126,000	
Outside (8,400 × $18)		$151,200
Fixed costs:		
Unavoidable	22,000	22,000
Avoidable	18,000	—
Total Cost	$166,000	$173,200

It is clear from these data that it is less costly for the clinic to continue operating its own laboratory. In fact, the monthly costs are $7,200 less. However, this decision assumes that there is no change in the present internal capacity to provide tests. If equipment replacement or expansion becomes necessary, a long-term decision-making process must be followed instead.

Case Study 6–1 provides another example of this type of decision.

Setting Fees for Special Situations

In some medical practices, decisions must be made regarding the appropriate price to charge a third party who controls the utilization of services by a group of patients. For example, suppose that an insurance company requests a medical group to bid on a prepaid basis for its business. The tendency is to base such bids on the average cost for fear that, if customers pay less than the average cost, the business will fail to recover the full costs of operation. However, if new business is attracted by bidding less than the average cost and the capacity already exists to handle the new business, then the group may be better off bidding below the average cost, as long as the bid covers the incremental cost.

A group's profits will increase any time it follows an alternative that generates incremental revenue exceeding the incremental cost of new patients. In the above example, the bid represents the incremental revenue. Typically, extra patients do not generate additional costs at a rate equal to average costs but at a lower rate.

This is because some of the total costs are fixed and do not increase with volume.

These conclusions are valid only in the short term. In the long term, practices cannot afford to replace plant and equipment if all payers pay more than incremental costs but less than average costs. Competition will inevitably lead to some practices being forced out of business. Nonetheless, it is important to recognize that in the short term, a refusal to bid below average cost may cause profits to be lower or losses to be higher. In today's competitive environment, it is likely that another health care organization will cut its price to get the extra business being offered.

There may be other factors, however, that militate against a short-term pricing strategy. For example, bidding low to get a new preferred provider organization (PPO) contract may force the group to lower the price it currently charges other contractors. This reduction of revenues from existing payers may more than offset the incremental profits from the new customer.

COST-VOLUME-PROFIT ANALYSIS

A widely recognized tool of financial analysis involves examining the relationships among cost of resources, volume of operations, and profit levels arising from the interfaces of the first two variables. Known as *cost-volume-profit* (CVP) *analysis,* it is a common method used by management to garner useful information about running a business, such as a medical practice. CVP analysis can be considered both a short- and a long-term way of evaluating the proper scope of operations to generate returns on business investments.

CVP analysis can be used in setting fees, selecting the mix of services to be offered, and choosing among alternative delivery strategies. CVP analysis can also aid in budget development by assessing the impact on costs, volume of service, and profits of changes in any of these three variables. The analysis is complex, however, because the relationships are often affected by forces entirely or partially beyond the control of management. Nevertheless, application of CVP analysis to simple situations can provide insights into possible

CASE STUDY 6-1

PART A: MAKE OR BUY ANCILLARY SERVICES

The Western Clinic has a central laboratory in its facility. The lab charges the patient treating centers in the clinic $20 for each test it performs. The average variable cost of each test is $12, and the monthly fixed costs of the lab are $40,000. The present average volume of tests conducted each month is 7,200.

The Albany Testing Service has approached the clinic and offered to conduct all tests for the clinic for a fee of $14 per test. Dr. Emily Ballet, medical director of the clinic, wonders if she should accept Albany's offer and eliminate the clinic's own lab. If she switches to an outside source, she estimates that she could sell the lab equipment and eliminate $12,000 in monthly depreciation expenses and $6,000 per month in other fixed expenses. The remaining fixed costs would be unavoidable.

Case Discussion Question

1. Should Dr. Ballet continue testing internally or purchase lab services outside the clinic?

PART B: EXPANDING THE PRACTICE WITH PREPAID SERVICES

The urology department of the Western Clinic anticipates that it will treat 6,000 patients next year. The department currently has the capacity to treat 8,000 patients per year. The average variable cost of patient treatment per day is $350. The department's fixed costs are $690,000 per year. Thus, the department is incurring an average cost per patient visit of $465 (6,000 × $350 = $2,100,000 + $690,000 = $2,790,000 / 6,000 = $465). An HMO has approached the clinic and offered a two-year contract to treat 1,000 patient visits per year. It is willing to pay a flat amount of $375 per patient visit. The case mix for the HMO patients would be similar to the current 6,000 patient visits. Dr. Vivian Renner, department head, is not sure whether to enter into this contract.

Case Discussion Questions

1. Would you advise Dr. Renner to accept the HMO business? Why or why not?
2. What assumptions are necessary to support your decision?

results of changes in the cost structure, fee arrangements, and/or volume load of the practice.

Contribution Margin Concept

One relationship between cost, volume, and profit that is very useful in business planning is the contribution margin concept, which provides insight into the profit potential. The contribution margin is defined as the excess of revenue over variable costs and expenses. Operating income or loss is calculated by deducting fixed costs and expenses from the contribution margin. An income statement presented in a contribution margin format is given below.

The Three Sisters Medical Group
Contribution Margin Income Statement

Gross charges	$1,000,000
Variable expenses	600,000
Contribution margin	$ 400,000
Fixed expenses	300,000
Operating income	$ 100,000

The $400,000 contribution margin is available to cover the fixed costs of $300,000. Any remaining amount can contribute directly to the operating income of the group.

Unit Contribution Margin

The unit contribution margin is the amount of money available from each unit of revenue to cover fixed costs and provide operating profits. For example, if the Three Sisters Medical Group's average fee per patient is $40 and the average variable cost per unit is $15, then the unit contribution margin is $25 ($40–$15). The unit contribution margin can provide a useful measure for analyzing the profit potential of proposed new lines of service.

Unit Contribution Margin Ratio

Sometimes called the *profit-volume ratio,* the unit contribution margin ratio is the percentage of each reve-nue dollar available to cover fixed costs and contribute to operating income. For the Three Sisters Medical Group, the contribution margin ratio is 40 percent, as calculated below.

$$\text{Contribution margin ratio} = \frac{\text{Revenue} - \text{Variable costs}}{\text{Revenue}}$$

$$40\% = \frac{\$1,000,000 - \$600,000}{\$1,000,000}$$

To illustrate how this ratio can be used, assume the group's management is evaluating the effect of adding $200,000 in revenue volume. If the ratio of variable cost to revenue and the amount of fixed costs remain the same, multiplying the contribution margin ratio (40 percent) by the change in revenue volume ($200,000) indicates an increase in operating income of $80,000 if this volume is attained.

Break-Even Analysis

Both the unit contribution margin and the contribution margin ratio can be used in analyzing a critical level of operations—the break-even point.

For any business, the break-even point represents that level of operations at which revenues and costs are exactly equal. At this level, a business neither realizes an operating profit nor incurs an operating loss. Break-even analysis can be applied to past periods, but it is most useful when applied to future periods as an aid in business planning, especially when an expansion or curtailment of operations is being contemplated. Because the future is involved in this analysis, estimates of future prospects and financial results are required. The reliability of the analysis is greatly influenced by the accuracy of these estimates.

Two popular methods are used to compute break-even points. One relies on mathematical equations that represent the relationships between revenue, costs, and volume. The other shows these relationships graphically. Although graphs show the effects of changes in the variables more clearly, the use of equations to calculate break-even points adds precision and the capability of dealing with several changes simultaneously. An example of break-even analysis is given in Case Study 6–2.

CASE STUDY 6–2

ANALYZING BREAK-EVEN POINTS AND DEALING WITH PRACTICE CONSTRAINTS

The Saratoga Grove satellite office of the Western Clinic specializes in the treatment of three types of patients, DRG M, DRG J, and DRG P. The operating statistics for patient care of these three DRGs for last year are shown below. They include patient volume proportions, average charges, average variable costs, and the amount of specific fixed costs assignable to each DRG. In addition, the satellite had joint fixed costs last year of $240,000.

DRG	Proportion	Charge	Variable Cost	Fixed Cost
M	50%	$1,700	$1,000	$ 500,000
J	30%	2,600	1,200	280,000
P	20%	900	600	110,000
			Joint Fixed Costs	830,000
	100%			$1,720,000

Dr. Kate Purcell, newly appointed director of the satellite office, wants to know what the break-even points are for each DRG. Dr. Purcell also wants to know which DRG would be the most profitable to promote in expanding the practice of the office. A recent time study she conducted showed that procedures involved in each DRG took the following time: DRG M, two hours; DRG J, five hours; and DRG P, one hour.

Case Discussion Questions

1. Calculate the break-even points, in numbers of treatments, for each type of DRG, using the weighted average contribution margin approach.
2. a. Which DRG should be promoted in an advertising program if the office has excess capacity? Why?
   b. Which DRG should be promoted if the office is almost at maximum capacity in terms of available hours? Why?

Mathematical Break-Even Analysis

The equation for calculating the break-even point, expressed in the volume of units, is fixed costs divided by the unit contribution margin. For example, assume a clinic operates an ambulatory immunization and test center. The center charges $6.00 per test and incurs an average variable cost per test of $2.74. Also assume that the center's fixed costs per month total $9,040. Using the break-even equation yields a break-even point of almost 2,800 tests per month:

$$\text{Break-even point (in number of tests)} = \frac{\text{Fixed costs}}{\text{Contribution margin per test}}$$

$$2{,}773 \text{ tests} = \frac{\$9{,}040}{\$6.00 - \$2.74}$$

Now assume that clinic management wants the ambulatory immunization and test center to contribute $1,000 a month toward the coverage of administrative costs of the clinic, in addition to covering all costs of the center. How many tests would be required to break even under this assumption? The answer can be found as follows:

$$\begin{array}{c}\text{Required number of tests} \\ \text{to generate required} \\ \text{contribution}\end{array} = \frac{\text{Fixed costs} + \text{Allocated costs}}{\text{Contribution margin per test}}$$

$$3{,}080 \text{ tests} = \frac{\$9{,}040 + \$1{,}000}{\$3.26}$$

Graphical Break-Even Analysis

Some people find it is easier to visualize and understand cost-volume-profit analysis graphically. A break-even graph shows much more than just the point at which the practice will break even. It also shows a picture of profit or loss at all levels of activity within the relevant range of activity.

Data for the same ambulatory center as above are shown graphically in Figure 6–1. In the top graph, the break-even point is the point at which the revenue line crosses the total cost line. The vertical dashed lines on the graph represent the relevant range, that is, the range over which the cost-volume-profit relationships are known to be valid. Any projection above or below the relevant range may not be reliable, because there is no experience upon which to base the projections. By reading the graph, it is possible to determine the profit or loss at 4,000 tests (a profit of $4,000), 2,000 tests (a loss of $2,520), or any other level of activity within the relevant range.

Another form of break-even graph is the profit-volume graph shown at the bottom of Figure 6–1. By plotting only the contribution margin, the profit or loss is easy to determine at any level of activity with a single line. At zero activity, the loss is equal to fixed costs. The break-even point, the profit at 4,000 tests, and the loss at 2,000 tests are the same as those shown on the break-even graph.

The benefit of using graphical break-even analysis is apparent from the following example. Assume that the same group described above is dissatisfied with the predicted results of its ambulatory center. There are at least three possible courses of action: increase the fee per test,

increase the volume of tests, or decrease the costs of tests. Figure 6–2 shows the impact of cost and fee changes. In the top graph, the dashed line shows the impact of decreasing fixed costs by $2,000. The break-even point falls to about 2,160 tests. In the bottom graph, the dashed line shows the impact of increasing fees by $0.50 per test (or, alternatively, of decreasing the variable cost per test by $0.50). This increases the contribution margin by $0.50 per test. The slope of the line is steeper, dropping the break-even point to about 2,400 tests.

Cost-Volume-Profit Analysis for a Prepaid Practice

In most prepaid health care plans, patients enrolled in the plan pay a monthly premium to an HMO, which in turn makes a monthly capitation payment to a medical practice. In exchange for the capitation payment, the practice agrees to provide all or certain health care services for the prepaid patients, including medical services originating within the practice, referrals to outside specialists, and hospitalization.

If the measure of activity is the number of prepaid patients, the break-even graph for the prepaid practice will look much like the break-even graph shown above in Figure 6–1. It will show the number of patients at which the plan will break even. It will also show the profit or loss at any level of activity. However, mature prepaid plans tend toward constant enrollment levels. This is shown in the profit-volume graph in Figure 6–3 as a fixed level of revenue, regardless of the number of patients (measured as activity on the horizontal axis). The total cost line includes the fixed costs of the practice, the variable cost per patient visit, and the variable costs of referrals and hospitalization. Because revenue is fixed and cost is increasing as the prepaid patients make more visits, the practice shows a profit below the break-even point and a loss above the break-even point. To change this outcome, either capitation payments must be increased or operating costs must be reduced.

As Figure 6–3 shows, the prepaid practice is rewarded for efficient use of resources. Any effort that minimizes the use of practice resources (while providing quality

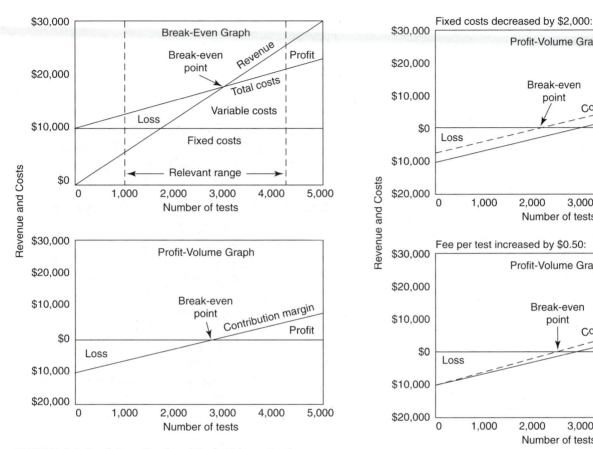

FIGURE 6–1 Break-Even Graph and Profit-Volume Graph

FIGURE 6–2 Impact of Cost and Fee Changes

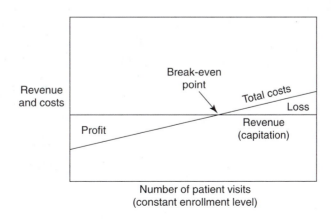

FIGURE 6–3 Break-Even Chart for a Prepaid Practice

care) will increase practice income. In contrast, the fee-for-service practice is rewarded for increased patient visits and, therefore, revenue.

Cost-volume-profit analysis for a combined fee-for-service/prepaid group is complicated by the fact that revenue and cost data are expressed in different terms for the two components of the practice. Capitation payments are on a per-member per-month basis; fee-for-service revenue and cost data are on a per-procedure, per-treatment, or per-visit basis. The following example shows how to deal with this discrepancy when calculating the break-even point.

Assume the Dennell Clinic had a satellite office that contracted with an HMO to provide services to its members. Data pertaining to the contract include the following:

Capitation payment for
  services to be performed
  at the satellite office. . . . . $14.50 per member per month
Cost of operating satellite office:
  Direct costs:
    Fixed costs per month. $40,000.00
    Variable cost per visit . . . . $ 12.00
  Allocated costs from clinic for
    administrationand support
    (15 percent of capitation) . . . . $ 2.18
Expected utilization . . . . 3 visits per member
                                             per month

If variable costs are expressed per member per month, the cost-volume-profit analysis may use the number of enrolled members as the measure of activity. Using the above data, the variable cost per visit of $12.00 translates into $3.00 per member per month (three visits $\times$ $12.00 = $36.00 divided by 12 months). The contribution margin per member per month is then calculated as $9.32 ($14.50 − $3.00 − $2.18). The break-even point becomes 4,292 members as calculated by:

$$\text{Break-even point} = \frac{\text{Fixed costs per month}}{\text{Contribution margin per member per month}}$$

$$4{,}292 \text{ members} = \frac{\$40{,}000}{\$9.32}$$

LONG-TERM INVESTMENT DECISIONS

Long-term investments involve the commitment of funds to the acquisition of assets that provide benefits over a long period of time. Typical long-term investments for medical practices include the acquisition or leasing of buildings or equipment. These investments entail an addition to, or a replacement of, the capacity of a medical practice to render services.

Characteristics of Long-Term Investments

When an organization acquires a long-lived asset, the investment is similar to that made by a bank when it lends money. In both transactions, cash is committed today in expectation of a return of that cash, plus an additional amount, in the future. The additional amount is called the *return on investment*.

For a bank loan, the return on investment is the receipt of interest payments over the life of the loan. For a long-lived asset, both the return of investment and the return on investment are cash earnings generated by use of the asset. If, over the life of the investment, the inflows of cash earnings exceed the initial cost, then the original investment is recovered (return of investment) and some profit is earned (positive return on investment). In other words, an investment may be considered as the purchase of an expected future stream of cash inflows.

Before an organization decides to invest in a new long-lived asset, it must determine whether future cash inflows are likely to be large enough to justify making the investment. Generally, proposals for such expenditures are supported by detailed analyses that contain projections of expected cash inflows and an evaluation as to whether these inflows warrant the initial cash expenditure.

Typical situations in which long-term investments are considered are illustrated by the following examples:

• Should the organization replace existing equipment with more efficient equipment? (Future expected cash inflows in this case are the cost savings resulting from lower operating costs or the profits resulting from the additional volume produced by the new equipment or both)

Year	Investment at beginning of year	Interest earned	Investment at end of year
Year 1	$1,000.00	$80.00	$1,080.00
Year 2	$1,080.00	$86.40	$1,166.40
Year 3	$1,166.40	$93.31	$1,259.79

- Should a new facility be acquired or built? (Future expected cash inflows in this case are the cash profits from the goods and services produced in the new facility)
- Which of several proposed items of equipment should be purchased for a given purpose? (The choice is usually based on which alternative is likely to produce the largest return on the investment; see Case Study 6–3 for an example)
- Should an asset be purchased to perform an operation or activity that is now done manually? (Future expected cash inflows in this case are the savings resulting from lower operating costs)
- Should a new product or new service be added to the existing line? (The choice in this case depends upon whether the future expected cash inflows from the sale of the product or service are larger than the cost of the investment plus the costs required to make or develop and introduce the new product or service)

Traditionally, long-term decisions for medical practices have been made on the basis of medical need. If economic considerations were taken into account at all, simple techniques usually were used. These techniques do not embrace expected future cash flows nor the return on giving up cash today for a larger amount in the future. Because long-term decisions involve investments in assets that yield returns over extended periods, it is important to consider the time value of money in long-term investment decisions.

Time Value of Money

As stated above, the time value of money rests on the concept that cash in hand today is worth more than the same amount of cash in the future. The difference is called the *time value of money*. This concept can be explained by comparing it with the principle of compound interest. Assume we invest $1,000 in a savings account that pays interest at a rate of eight percent compounded annually. "Compounded annually" means that interest earned in the first year is retained in the account and, along with the $1,000 of original principal, earns interest in the second year, and so on for future years. If there are no withdrawals from this account, over time the account balance will grow as shown below:

Future Value and Present Value

There are two concepts that are important in further explaining the time value of money, future value and present value. Future value is illustrated by the example above, which shows that the future value of $1,000, compounded annually at eight percent, is $1,080 at the end of year 1, about $1,166 at the end of year 2, and about $1,260 at the end of year 3.

Present value applies to money that is expected to be received at a specified time in the future. It is the amount that, if invested today at a designated rate of return, would accumulate to the expected future amount. Referring back to the previous example, it can be seen that the present value of $1,080 to be received at the end of one year, compounded at eight percent, is $1,000; the present value of $1,166 to be received at the end of two years, compounded at eight percent, is $1,000; and the present value of $1,259 to be received at the end of three years, compounded at eight percent, is also $1,000. The interest rate (eight percent in this example) in present value problems is commonly referred to as the discount rate, or the rate of return.

The use of future and present values allows comparisons of any two or more dollar amounts that are paid or received at different points in time. The amounts can be measured either in future values (what they will be worth at some future time) or in present values (what they are worth today). Both approaches provide similar results. However, because investments are made in the present, it may be easier to understand and work with present than with future values.

Present Value Tables

Mathematical formulas can be used to calculate present values, but these are complex and cumbersome to use. It is easier to use present value tables, which show the present value of $1 at different rates of interest and at different points in time. Multiplying a given amount of money by the appropriate value in the table yields the present value of the given amount at a particular rate of interest and given point in time.

Present value tables for selected rates of interest are shown in Table 6–4.

Using Present Values in Long-Term Decision Making

Assume a practice wishes to invest in a long-lived asset at an eight percent rate of return. It has the following three investment options:

1. Invest $1,000 now and receive $1,200 at the end of three years
2. Invest $1,000 now and receive $800 at the end of one year, $300 at the end of two years, and $100 at the end of three years
3. Invest $1,000 now and receive $100 at the end of one year, $300 at the end of two years, and $800 at the end of three years

All three investment options involve an initial cash outlay of $1,000 and a total cash inflow of $1,200. However, the timing of the receipt of cash differs among the options. The present value of cash outflows in each case is $1,000 because the cash is paid now. The present value of the cash inflows, however, varies by alternative. It is calculated by multiplying each cash inflow amount by the appropriate value from the present value table as shown below:

Investment 1	Present Value
Year 3: $1,200 × 0.794.	$ 953

Investment 2	Present Value
Year 1: $800 × 0.926 = $741	
Year 2: $300 × 0.857 = $257	
Year 3: $100 × 0.794 = $ 79	$1,077

Investment 3	Present Value
Year 1: $100 × 0.926 = $ 93	
Year 2: $300 × 0.857 = $257	
Year 3: $800 × 0.794 = $635	$ 985

It is clear that only the second investment option is acceptable in having a present value for future cash inflows that is greater than the present value for the present cash outflow, at the desired eight percent rate of

return. This process, in which amounts to be received in the future are discounted to their present values, is called *discounted cash flow analysis.*

Long-Term Decision Rule

The preceding example leads to the formulation of a rule to be used in making long-term investment decisions: A long-term investment option is favorable if the incremental discounted cash inflows attributable to it are equal to or greater than the incremental discounted cash outflows attributable to it.

Present Value of an Annuity

In the preceding examples, future cash inflows were not equal, and the present values of the yearly amounts were computed individually and then summed to arrive at the total present value of cash inflows. When cash inflows are equal, as in annuity, calculation of the total present value of cash inflows is simpler.

For example, assume that an annuity (Investment 4) requires an investment of $1,000 and provides cash inflows of $500 per year for three years. The present value of the annuity can be calculated by multiplying the annual cash inflow of $500 by the appropriate value from Table 6–5. With three years of payments at an eight percent rate of return, the value is 2.577. This yields a total present value for the annuity of $1,289 ($500 × 2.577). Note that the values in Table 6–5 are determined by cumulating the relevant values in Table 6–4.

Information Relevant to Long-Term Decisions

To carry out investment analysis, we need to know when cash is invested (and not available for other purposes) and when cash is recovered and (thus available for other uses). In addition, one needs to know both the amount and the timing of cash flows, which must be estimated as accurately as possible.

For long-term investment decisions, projections of cash flows are the relevant data. To carry out investment analysis, the following important variables are needed:

TABLE 6–4 Present Value of $1 $\left[PV = (1 + r) - 0 = \dfrac{1}{(1 + r)^0} \right]$

Period	2%	4%	6%	8%	10%	12%	14%	16%	18%	20%	22%	24%	26%	28%	30%	35%	40%	45%	50%
1	.980	.962	.943	.926	.909	.893	.877	.862	.847	.833	.820	.806	.794	.781	.769	.741	.714	.690	.667
2	.961	.925	.890	.857	.826	.797	.769	.743	.718	.694	.672	.650	.630	.610	.592	.549	.510	.476	.444
3	.942	.889	.840	.794	.751	.712	.675	.641	.609	.579	.551	.524	.500	.477	.455	.406	.364	.328	.296
4	.924	.855	.792	.735	.683	.636	.592	.552	.516	.482	.451	.423	.397	.373	.350	.301	.260	.226	.198
5	.906	.822	.747	.681	.621	.567	.519	.476	.437	.402	.370	.341	.315	.291	.269	.223	.186	.156	.132
6	.888	.790	.705	.630	.564	.507	.456	.410	.370	.335	.303	.275	.250	.227	.207	.165	.133	.108	.088
7	.871	.760	.665	.583	.513	.452	.400	.354	.314	.279	.249	.222	.198	.178	.159	.122	.095	.074	.059
8	.853	.731	.627	.540	.467	.404	.351	.305	.266	.233	.204	.179	.157	.139	.123	.091	.068	.051	.039
9	.837	.703	.592	.500	.424	.361	.308	.263	.225	.194	.167	.144	.125	.108	.094	.067	.048	.035	.026
10	.820	.676	.558	.463	.386	.322	.270	.227	.191	.162	.137	.116	.099	.085	.073	.050	.035	.024	.017
11	.804	.650	.527	.429	.350	.287	.237	.195	.162	.135	.112	.094	.079	.066	.056	.037	.025	.017	.012
12	.788	.625	.497	.397	.319	.257	.208	.168	.137	.112	.092	.076	.062	.052	.043	.027	.018	.012	.008
13	.773	.601	.469	.368	.290	.229	.182	.145	.116	.093	.075	.061	.050	.040	.033	.020	.013	.008	.005
14	.758	.577	.442	.340	.263	.205	.160	.125	.099	.078	.062	.049	.039	.032	.025	.015	.009	.006	.003
15	.743	.555	.417	.315	.239	.183	.140	.108	.084	.065	.051	.040	.031	.025	.020	.011	.006	.004	.002
16	.728	.534	.394	.292	.218	.163	.123	.093	.071	.054	.042	.032	.025	.019	.015	.008	.005	.003	.002
17	.714	.513	.371	.270	.198	.146	.108	.080	.060	.045	.034	.026	.020	.015	.012	.006	.003	.002	.001
18	.700	.494	.350	.250	.180	.130	.095	.069	.051	.038	.028	.021	.016	.012	.009	.005	.002	.001	.001
19	.686	.475	.331	.232	.164	.116	.083	.060	.043	.031	.023	.017	.012	.009	.007	.003	.002	.001	
20	.673	.456	.312	.215	.149	.104	.073	.051	.037	.026	.019	.014	.010	.007	.005	.002	.001	.001	
21	.660	.439	.294	.199	.135	.093	.064	.044	.031	.022	.015	.011	.008	.006	.004	.002	.001		
22	.647	.422	.278	.184	.123	.083	.056	.038	.026	.018	.013	.009	.006	.004	.003	.001	.001		
23	.634	.406	.262	.170	.112	.074	.049	.033	.022	.015	.010	.007	.005	.003	.002	.001			
24	.622	.390	.247	.158	.102	.066	.043	.028	.019	.013	.008	.006	.004	.003	.002	.001			
25	.610	.375	.233	.146	.092	.059	.038	.024	.016	.010	.007	.005	.003	.002	.001	.001			
30	.552	.308	.174	.099	.057	.033	.020	.012	.007	.004	.003	.002	.001	.001					
35	.500	.253	.130	.068	.036	.019	.010	.006	.003	.002	.001	.001							
40	.453	.208	.097	.046	.022	.011	.005	.003	.002	.001	.001								
45	.410	.171	.073	.031	.014	.006	.003	.001	.001										
50	.372	.141	.054	.021	.009	.003	.001	.001											

Period refers to the interest period and denotes the time span between interest compoundings. *r* refers to to the rate of interest

- Amount and timing of cash outflows
- Amount and timing of cash inflows
- Economic life, or the number of years for which cash inflows are anticipated
- Required rate of return, or the discount rate, used to measure the time value of money

Amount and Timing of Cash Outflows

The relevant cash outflows are the incremental cash outflows directly involved in making the investment. Generally, there will be a large initial cash outlay for acquiring or constructing the asset, such as the purchase cost and shipping, installation, and training costs for a piece of equipment. All additional resources that are related to the investment item and needed to support the higher level of activity must be included in the cash outflows. When these additional resources are recovered (usually at the end of the economic life), they are treated as cash inflows. They may include money invested in working capital (increased accounts receivable and supplies inventory),

TABLE 6–5 Present Value of an Annuity of \$1 $\left\{ PV = \dfrac{[1 - (1 + r)^{-n}]}{r} \right\}$

Period	2%	4%	6%	8%	10%	12%	14%	16%	18%	20%	22%	24%	26%	28%	30%	35%	40%	45%	50%
1	0.980	0.962	0.943	0.926	0.909	0.893	0.877	0.862	0.847	0.833	0.820	0.806	0.794	0.781	0.769	0.741	0.714	0.690	0.667
2	1.942	1.886	1.833	1.783	1.736	1.690	1.647	1.605	1.566	1.528	1.492	1.457	1.424	1.392	1.361	1.289	1.224	1.165	1.111
3	2.884	2.775	2.673	2.577	2.486	2.402	2.322	2.246	2.174	2.106	2.042	1.981	1.923	1.868	1.816	1.696	1.589	1.493	1.407
4	3.808	3.630	3.465	3.312	3.170	3.037	2.914	2.798	2.690	2.589	2.494	2.404	2.320	2.241	2.166	1.997	1.849	1.720	1.605
5	4.713	4.452	4.212	3.992	3.791	3.605	3.433	3.274	3.127	2.991	2.864	2.745	2.635	2.532	2.436	2.220	2.035	1.876	1.737
6	5.601	5.242	4.917	4.623	4.355	4.111	3.889	3.685	3.498	3.326	3.167	3.020	2.885	2.759	2.643	2.385	2.168	1.983	1.824
7	6.472	6.002	5.582	5.206	4.868	4.564	4.288	4.039	3.812	3.605	3.416	3.242	3.083	2.937	2.802	2.508	2.263	2.057	1.883
8	7.325	6.733	6.210	5.747	5.335	4.968	4.639	4.344	4.078	3.837	3.619	3.421	3.241	3.076	2.925	2.598	2.331	2.109	1.922
9	8.162	7.435	6.802	6.247	5.759	5.328	4.946	4.607	4.303	4.031	3.786	3.566	3.366	3.184	3.019	2.665	2.379	2.114	1.948
10	8.983	8.111	7.360	6.710	6.145	5.650	5.216	4.833	4.494	4.192	3.923	3.682	3.465	3.289	3.092	2.715	2.414	2.168	1.965
11	9.787	8.760	7.887	7.139	6.495	5.938	5.453	5.029	4.656	4.327	4.035	3.776	3.543	3.335	3.147	2.752	2.438	2.185	1.977
12	10.575	9.385	8.384	7.536	6.814	6.194	5.660	5.197	4.793	4.439	4.127	3.851	3.606	3.387	3.190	2.779	2.456	2.196	1.985
13	11.348	9.986	8.853	7.904	7.103	6.424	5.842	5.342	4.910	4.533	4.203	3.912	3.656	3.427	3.223	2.799	2.469	2.204	1.990
14	12.106	10.563	9.295	8.244	7.367	6.628	6.002	5.468	5.008	4.611	4.265	3.962	3.695	3.459	3.249	2.814	2.478	2.210	1.993
15	12.849	11.118	9.712	8.559	7.606	6.811	6.142	5.575	5.092	4.675	4.315	4.001	3.726	3.483	3.268	2.825	2.484	2.214	1.995
16	13.578	11.652	10.106	8.851	7.824	6.974	6.265	5.668	5.162	4.730	4.357	4.033	3.751	3.503	3.283	2.834	2.489	2.216	1.997
17	14.292	12.166	10.477	9.122	8.022	7.120	6.373	5.749	5.222	4.775	4.391	4.059	3.771	3.518	3.295	2.840	2.492	2.218	1.998
18	14.992	12.659	10.828	9.372	8.201	7.250	6.467	5.818	5.273	4.812	4.419	4.080	3.786	3.529	3.304	2.844	2.494	2.219	1.999
19	15.678	13.134	11.158	9.604	8.365	7.366	6.550	5.877	5.316	4.843	4.442	4.097	3.799	3.539	3.311	2.848	2.496	2.220	1.999
20	16.351	13.590	11.470	9.818	8.514	7.469	6.623	5.929	5.353	4.870	4.460	4.110	3.808	3.546	3.316	2.850	2.497	2.221	1.999
21	17.011	14.029	11.764	10.017	8.649	7.562	6.687	5.973	5.384	4.891	4.476	4.121	3.816	3.551	3.320	2.852	2.498	2.221	2.000
22	17.658	14.451	12.042	10.201	8.772	7.645	6.743	6.011	5.410	4.909	4.488	4.130	3.822	3.556	3.323	2.853	2.498	2.222	2.000
23	18.292	14.857	12.303	10.371	8.883	7.718	6.792	6.044	5.432	4.925	4.499	4.137	3.827	3.559	3.325	2.854	2.499	2.222	2.000
24	18.914	15.247	12.550	10.529	8.985	7.784	6.835	6.073	5.451	4.937	4.507	4.143	3.831	3.562	3.327	2.855	2.499	2.222	2.000
25	19.523	15.622	12.783	10.675	9.077	7.843	6.873	6.097	5.467	4.948	4.514	4.147	3.834	3.564	3.329	2.856	2.499	2.222	2.000
30	22.396	17.292	13.765	11.258	9.427	8.055	7.003	6.177	5.517	4.979	4.534	4.160	3.842	3.569	3.332	2.857	2.500	2.222	2.000
35	24.999	18.665	14.498	11.655	9.644	8.176	7.070	6.215	5.539	4.992	4.541	4.164	3.845	3.571	3.333	2.857	2.500	2.222	2.000
40	27.355	19.793	15.046	11.925	9.779	8.244	7.105	6.233	5.548	4.997	4.544	4.166	3.846	3.571	3.333	2.857	2.500	2.222	2.000
45	29.490	20.720	15.456	12.108	9.863	8.283	7.123	6.242	5.552	4.999	4.545	4.166	3.846	3.571	3.333	2.857	2.500	2.222	2.000
50	31.424	21.482	15.762	12.233	9.915	8.304	7.133	6.246	5.554	4.999	4.545	4.167	3.846	3.571	3.333	2.857	2.500	2.222	2.000

Period refers to the interest period and denotes the time span between interest compunding. *r* refers to the rate of interest.

in equipment, or in training personnel to operate the equipment.

Amount and Timing of Cash Inflows

The relevant cash inflows are the incremental cash receipts to be received in the future that are directly related to the investment decision. Most cash inflows arise from earnings from the investment or from cost savings that result from putting the new investment into use. If the purchase of a new asset results in the sale of an existing asset, the net proceeds from the sale are also treated as cash inflow. The net proceeds are the asset's selling price less any costs incurred in selling, dismantling, and removing it.

Economic Life

The economic life of an investment is the number of years over which cash inflows are expected from the investment. For an investment in equipment or a facility, the economic life corresponds to the estimated service life of the asset. The estimated service life includes physical life as well as technological considerations that may shorten the physical life estimate.

The end of the period selected for the economic life of an asset is called the *investment horizon,* suggesting that cash inflows cease at this point. Economic life cannot be estimated exactly, but it is important that the best possible estimate be made because of the significant effect the estimate has on calculations. Because of the uncertainties in estimating the economic life of most assets, managers are often conservative in projecting the time period of investment inflows.

Required Rate of Return

The required rate of return, or discount rate, is the desired rate that a particular medical practice expects to achieve from any investment it makes. A rate of return is comprised of three elements: a risk-free, or real, rate of return; a recovery of any inflationary loss; and a portion to cover the risk of losing the principal amount. If inflation is deemed to be a serious factor, future cash flows must be adjusted accordingly. The possibility of losing the principal amount is gauged by evaluating the business risk surrounding the investment, and risks may vary among investments.

There are two ways of determining the appropriate rate of return for measuring the present value of future cash flows. The first uses the cost of capital, the second the opportunity cost of funds to be invested.

The cost of capital indicates the minimum rate of return on a particular investment that an organization needs to obtain in order to cover the cost of acquiring and maintaining the entity's capital resources. It is calculated with the formula:

$$\text{Cost of capital} = \frac{\text{Annual payment to investor}}{\text{Market value of investment}}$$

The *annual payment to investor* might be, for example, the amount of interest paid from a debt instrument. The *market value of investment* represents the current market price of the debt security.

Each source of capital has a different cost arising from the risk associated with the borrower and the return expectation of the provider of funds. The commercial banker, the mortgage banker, and the physician all have different expectations of how much they should earn on the investment in the medical group, and each has a different assessment of the risk involved. The cost-of-capital approach would probably set a lower desired rate of return if the group were able to borrow all or a majority of the money for an investment in facilities and equipment than if the physicians provided the funds. Owners of any business seek a higher rate of return than creditors.

The above formula for computing cost of capital applies to profit-making corporations. The cost of each source of capital is calculated, and a weighted average cost of capital is computed. The following example illustrates this approach.

Assume a company has a cost of debt capital (for example, bonds) of 7 percent and a cost of equity capital (for example, common stocks) of 18 percent. Its capital structure is 40 percent debt capital and 60 percent equity capital. The cost of capital for this company is calculated as follows:

Capital		Weighted	
Type	Cost	Weight	Cost
Debt(bonds)	7%	0.4	2.8%
Equity (stock)	18%	0.6	10.8%
Total		1.0	13.6%

Thus, the total cost of capital for the company is about 14 percent.

The cost-of-capital approach to estimating the rate of return is difficult to apply in practice. It requires careful reflection and estimates of future market conditions and it may involve personal preferences. For instance, the group may decide to seek to earn a reasonable rate of return on all assets employed rather than a higher rate. It may also decide to seek to recover just the cost of its investments in facilities and equipment and to compensate the physicians out of charges for professional services.

The second way to estimate the rate of return is the opportunity-cost approach. This entails members of a group, individually and collectively, determining the next best opportunity for obtaining a return on the funds invested. Generally, the comparison is made between retaining cash in the practice versus what return physicians may obtain from investments outside the practice. This decision will differ for each group and will change over time.

In the final analysis, management must decide on the rate of return it deems desirable. Generally, the return demanded varies with the investment's risk. An investment with greater-than-average risk generally requires a higher rate of return than an average-risk investment. Conversely, an investment with below-average risk requires a lower rate of return.

Many organizations must make another type of investment, called *nondiscretionary,* about which decisions are made based on the necessity, rather than the profitability, of the investment. Examples include the purchase of pollution-control equipment and the installation of devices to protect employees from injury. These nondiscretionary investments use capital but provide no demonstrable cash inflows. As a result, discretionary investments must not only provide a satisfactory return on their own capital, but they also must carry the capital-cost burden of these nondiscretionary investments. To compensate, many companies use a required rate of return that is higher than the cost of capital.

Impact of Taxes on Cash Flows

Most medical groups are taxable entities, and any amounts paid out for income taxes must be considered as cash outflows in the investment analysis process. The amount of income taxes owed by a medical group is dependent on the tax code, which is very complex. The impact of income taxes on cash flows in the discounted cash flow framework may be demonstrated without detailed coverage of the tax code.

One of the major areas in which income taxes affect cash flows is through the deduction of depreciation expense to arrive at taxable income. Current tax regulations specify precise methods of depreciation and list the economic life for individual classes of depreciable assets, in a system called *The Modified Accelerated Cost Recovery System* (MACRS).

Table 6–6 shows the tax impact of the acquisition of a piece of equipment, which costs $25,000. Although the equipment has a five-year life for tax purposes, the group expects to replace it at the end of three years. The equipment will reduce annual operating costs by $8,000 per year, over the three years. Any salvage or residual value is expected to be equal to removal costs, and all undepreciated cost at the end of year three will be expensed in that year. Assuming a 34 percent income tax rate for a professional service corporation, Table 6–6 presents both before-tax and after-tax cash flows.

The before-tax cash flows include the investment of $25,000 now and cash inflows of $12,000 in each of the next three years. The after-tax cash flows change by the refund (cash inflow) in year one of $1,105 and by tax payments of $2,754 in year two and $2,091 in year three. Different depreciation strategies would result in different cash flows.

Table 6–7 applies the long-term decision rule to the before-tax cash flows from Table 6–6. Because

TABLE 6–6 Impact of Income Taxes on Cash Flows

	Now	*Years* 1	2	3
Before-tax cash flows				
Cash outflows:				
1. Payment of $25,000 for equipment	$(25,000)			
Cash inflows:				
2. Annual cost savings		$ 4,000	$ 4,000	$ 4,000
3. Additional patient billings		8,000	8,000	8,000
Total cash flow by year	$(25,000)	$12,000	$12,000	$12,000
After-tax cash flows				
Cash outflows:				
1. Payment of $25,000 for equipment	$(25,000)			
2. (Payment) refund of income taxes*		$ 1,105	$ (2,574)	$(2,091)
Cash inflows:				
3. Annual cost savings		4,000	4,000	4,000
4. Additional patient billings		8,000	8,000	8,000
Total cash flows by year	$(25,000)	$13,105	$ 9,246	$ 9,909
*Computation of income taxes:				
Additional patient billings	$8,000	$ 8,000	$ 8,000	
Annual cost savings	4,000	4,000	4,000	
Total	$ 12,000	$12,000	$12,000	
Depreciation				
First-year expensing	(10,000)			
Year 1: $15,000 × 35%	(5,250)			
Year 2: $15,000 × 26%		(3,900)		
Year 3: $15,000 − ($5,250 + $3,900)			(5,850)	
Taxable income (loss)	$ (3,250)	$ 8,100	$ 6,150	
Income tax payment (refund) (34%)	$ (1,105)	$ 2,754	$ 2,091	

Table is taken from Ross, A., William, S.J. & Schafer, E.L. (1991). *Ambulatory Care Management* (2nd ed). Albany, NY: Delmar Publishers.

discounted cash inflows exceed discounted cash outflows, the project is favorable and should be accepted. The long-term decision rule is applied to the after-tax cash flows in Figure 6–8. Although it is smaller now than before taxes were considered, there is an excess of discounted cash inflows over discounted cash outflows, indicating a favorable investment. Expensing $10,000 of the equipment in the first year and using the declining balance depreciation method in MACRS instead of straight-line depreciation results in a postponement of taxes. Any postponement of cash outflows (or advancements of cash inflows) increases the present value of the investment and makes it more favorable.

Clearly, determining the effect of taxes on an investment project is a very complex process. The important point to remember is that taxes affect cash flows and therefore must be considered in the analysis of investments. However, a fuller discussion of the impact of

TABLE 6–7 Computation of Present Values of Before-Tax Cash Flows for Investment

Present value of cash outflows: . . . . ($25,000)
Present value of cash inflows:

End of Year	Cash Inflows ×	Present Value Factor =	Present Value
1	$12,000	0.893	$10,716
2	$12,000	0.797	9,564
3	$12,000	0.712	8,544
			28,824

Excess of present value of cash inflows over present value of cash outflows . . . . $3,284 ($28,824 − $25,000)

Table is taken from Ross, A., Williams S.J. & Schafer, E.L. (1991). *Ambulatory Care Management* (2nd ed). Albany, NY: Delmar Publishers.

TABLE 6-8 Computation of Present Values of After-Tax Cash Flows for Investment

Present value of cash outflows:...................... ($25,000)
Present value of cash inflows:

End of Year	Cash Inflows ×	Present Value Factor =	Present Value
1	$13,105	0.893	$11,703
2	$ 9,246	0.797	7,369
3	$ 9,909	0.712	7,055
			26,127

Excess of present value of cash inflows over present value of cash outflows...................... $1,127 ($26,127 − $25,000)

Table is taken from Ross, A., Williams S.J. & Schafer, E.L. (1991). *Ambulatory Care Management* (2nd ed). Albany, NY: Delmar Publishers.

taxes on long-term investment decisions is beyond the scope of this book.

Capital Budgeting Techniques

To assure that long-term investment decisions affect operations favorably for many years, a system for planning, evaluating, and controlling these investments must be developed and implemented. Most businesses adopt a (formal or informal) capital budgeting process. A written proposal may be required for each potential long-term investment project, setting forth the expected benefits and costs involved in the project. There may also be a designated flow of proposal preparation and documentation, a review procedure for each proposal, and a final approval process by the governing body.

Two types of techniques are widely used in business to evaluate investment prospects: techniques that satisfy the long-term decision rule and techniques that do not satisfy this rule. The basic difference between the two types of techniques is the use of the concept of time value of money. As mentioned above, the long-term decision rule is based on this concept.

Techniques that satisfy the long-term decision rule include the net-present-value method and the internal-rate-of-return method (sometimes called the adjusted-rate-of-return method). Two techniques that do not satisfy the long-term decision rule are the payback-period method and the average-rate-of-return method (sometimes called the unadjusted-rate-of-return or the accounting-rate-of-return method).

Each method has both advantages and limitations, and some of the computations can become rather complex. In some firms, including some medical groups, management uses a combination of methods in evaluating various aspects of long-term investment proposals.

Net-Present-Value Method

As stated above, an investment in equipment or a facility may be viewed as the acquisition of a series of future net cash inflows that are composed of two elements: recovery of the initial investment and income from the investment. The value of the investment is determined by the period of time over which the net cash inflows will be received and the rate of return used to discount these inflows.

The net-present-value method uses present-value concepts to compute the present value of the cash flows expected from a proposed investment. To be acceptable, the investment's discounted cash inflows must equal its discounted cash outflows. Discounted cash

TABLE 6–9 Recovery of an Investment

Year	Investment at Beginning of Year	10% Return on Beginning Balance	Balance of $1,000 Annual Cash Inflow	Investment at End of Year
1	$3,170	$317	$683	$2,487
2	2,487	249	751	1,736
3	1,736	174	826	910
4	910	91	909	1*

*Nonzero balance due to rounding error

outflows are deducted from discounted cash inflows to measure the net present value. If the net present value is zero, this indicates that exactly the desired rate of return will be earned from the cash flows. If the net present value is positive (that is, discounted cash inflows exceed discounted cash outflows), more than the desired rate of return will be earned. Conversely, if the net present value is negative (that is, discounted cash outflows exceed discounted cash inflows), less than the desired rate of return will be earned.

For example, assume a piece of equipment may be purchased for $3,170, and it will generate cost savings of $1,000 each year for four years. If taxes are ignored and a desired rate of return of 10 percent is assumed, is this a good investment? To answer this question, the net present value of the investment is calculated as follows:

Present value of cash outflows...	$(3,170)
Present value of cash inflows ($1,000 × 3.170).............	3,170
Net present value..	$ 0

The zero net present value indicates that the investment will produce exactly a 10 percent return. To verify this, examine the investment return and the recovery of the initial investment amount over a four-year period, as shown in Table 6–9. Observe that a portion of each $1,000 cash inflow represents a recovery of the investment and a return of 10 percent (based on the amount of investment at the beginning of each year).

As another example, recall the four investments discussed on page 136. Each investment involved a cash outflow of $1,000 and a total cash inflow of $1,200. The only difference among the investments was the timing of the cash inflows, as summarized below:

Investment	Initial Investment Amount	Cash Inflows by Year		
		1	2	3
1	$1,000	–	$1,200	–
2	1,000	$600	400	$200
3	1,000	200	400	600
4	1,000	400	400	400

The net present value of each investment, assuming a desired rate of return of 10 percent, is shown in the following table:

Investment	Present Value of Cash Outflows	Present Value of Cash Inflows	Net Present Value
1	$(1,000)	$ 991	$(9)
2	(1,000)	1,025	25
3	(1,000)	963	(37)
4	(1,000)	994	(6)

In no case is the net present value exactly zero; thus, none of the investments would earn exactly 10 percent. If 10 percent is the cutoff rate for investing or not investing, only the second investment should be accepted, because this is the only investment with a positive net present-value at that rate of return.

The net-present-value method has distinct advantages over other methods. It is simple and does not involve repeated calculations, which may be necessary in the internal-, or adjusted-, rate-of-return method. The net-present-value method can be used in any situation, regardless of whether cash inflows are equal or unequal or whether competing projects have equal or unequal economic lives. In summary, using the net-present-value approach involves the following seven steps:

1. Selecting a required rate of return for all investment proposals (this rate will apply to proposals deemed to be of average risk and may be adjusted for proposals deemed to be well above or below average risk)
2. Estimating the economic life of the proposed project
3. Estimating the net cash inflows for each year during the project's life
4. Finding the net investment or net cash inflows pertaining to the project
5. Finding the present value of all cash inflows identified in step three by discounting them at the required rate of return (using Table 6–4 for single amounts and Table 6–5 for a series of equal annual amounts)
6. Finding the net present value by subtracting the present value of the net cash outflows from the present value of the net cash inflows (if the net present value is zero or positive, the proposal is acceptable in monetary terms)
7. Considering nonmonetary factors related to the proposal and reaching a final decision that is based on both monetary and nonmonetary factors (more will be said about nonmonetary factors in a later section)

Internal-Rate-of-Return, or Adjusted-Rate-of-Return, Method

This method also uses present values but takes a different approach than the net-present-value method. The rate of return is computed by equating the present value of cash inflows with the amount of net investment or the present value of cash outflows. In other words, the internal or adjusted rate of return is the rate that makes the net present value equal to zero.

To make the investment decision, the internal rate of return is compared to the required rate of return, which is sometimes called the *cutoff rate.* Any investment project earning less than the cutoff rate should be rejected, and any investment project earning at or above the cutoff rate should be accepted. The cutoff rate may be in-creased or decreased to reflect the availability of funds and other factors such as risk.

The internal rate of return may be computed in two different ways. The way that is used depends upon the timing of the cash inflows. If the cash inflows are in a stream of equal receipts (that is, an annuity), the internal rate of return may be determined by use of present value tables. If, on the other hand, the cash inflows are unequal, a trial-and-error method must be used.

Consider this example. The initial cost of an investment is $32,740, and the cash inflows are $10,000 per year for five years. The first approach to calculating the internal rate of return for this investment involves two steps: determining the present value factor (PVF) that equates the initial cash outflow with the cash inflows and finding the computed PVF in Table 6–5. In this example, the PVF that equates the cash inflows and cash outflows is 3.274, determined as follows:

$$\$32,740 = \$10,000 \times \text{PVF}$$

$$\text{PVF} = \frac{\$32,740}{\$10,000}$$

$$\text{PVF} = 3.274$$

In Table 6–5, the PVF in the five-year row (because the project has a five-year life) that is nearest 3.274 is the PVF in the 16 percent column. Thus, the internal rate of return is 16 percent. (If the computed PVF falls in between two values in the table, it is necessary to estimate the internal rate of return by interpolating between the two columns in the table.)

Next consider the four investments described above that varied in the timing of their cash inflows. The internal rates of return for investments one and four may be determined from present value tables. Investment one involved a single receipt of $1,200. The PVF that equates the two cash flows for this investment is 0.833, determined as follows:

$$\$1,000 = \$1,200 \times \text{PVF}$$

$$\text{PVF} = \frac{\$1,000}{\$1,200} = 0.833$$

In Table 6–4, 0.833 falls between the 8 percent and 10 percent columns. By interpolation, the internal rate of return is found to be 9.54 percent:

Internal rate of return = 8% + 2% [(0.857 − 0.833)/(0.857 − 0.826)]
= 8% + 2% (0.77)
= 9.54%

Investment four involved cash inflows of $400 per year for three years. The PVF that equates the cash flows for this investment is 2.500, determined as follows:

$$\$1,000 = \$400 \times \text{PVF}$$

$$\text{PVF} = \frac{\$1,000}{\$400} = 2.500$$

In the three-year row of Table 6–5, the PVF of 2.500 falls between the 8 percent and 10 percent columns. The internal rate of return is therefore found by interpolation as follows:

Internal rate of return = 8% + 2% [(2.577 − 2.500)/(2.577 − 2.486)]
= 8% + 2% (0.85)
= 9.70%

If the cash inflows over the lifetime of an investment are not equal and a trial-and-error method must be used, net present values of the cash flows at different rates are computed until a zero net present value is achieved. Consider investment two from above. In earlier calculations, this investment was found to have a rate of return above 10 percent. If 12 percent is used, then the net present value can be computed as follows:

Present value of cash outflows. . . . . . . $(1,000)
Present value of cash inflows:
Year 1 $600 × 0.893 = $536
Year 2 $400 × 0.797 =   319
Year 3 $200 × 0.712 =   412
                                 997
Net present value $(3) ($997−$1,000)

Because the net present value is very close to zero, the practice may accept 12 percent as the adjusted rate of return for this investment.

Considering investment three from above, the internal rate of return may be determined by computing the net present value at 8 percent:

Present value of cash outflows. . . . . $(1,000)
Present value of cash inflows:
Year 1 $200 × 0.926 = $185
Year 2 $400 × 0.857 = 343
Year 3 $600 × 0.794 = 476
                                1,004
Net Present Value . . . .$ 4 ($1,004−$1,000)

The net present value for this investment is very close to zero, so an internal rate of return of 8 percent may be accepted.

In summary, the internal rates of return for the four investments are:

Investment	Internal (or Adjusted) Rate of Return
1	9.54%
2	12.00%
3	8.00%
4	9.70%

If the cutoff rate is 10 percent, only the second investment is acceptable. This is the same decision as the one reached under the net-present-value method.

Payback-Period Method

The payback-period method is the simplest method and the one that is used most widely by businesses, including medical groups. As the name implies, the payback-period method is based on the payback period, or the number of years over which the investment outlay will be recovered, or paid back, from the cash inflows (assuming that the correct estimates have been made). If the payback period is more than, equal to, or slightly less than the economic life of the investment project, then the proposal is unacceptable. If, on the other hand, the payback period is considerably less than the economic life, then the project may be acceptable.

Payback periods for the four investment projects cited earlier show a range of from 1.8 to 2.7 years, as shown in the following table:

Investment	Investment Amount	Period 1	Period 2	Period 3	Payback Period
1	$1,000	$ 0	$1,200	$ 0	1.8 years
2	1,000	600	400	200	2.0 years
3	1,000	200	400	600	2.7 years
4	1,000	400	400	400	2.5 years

If the payback period for the return of the initial investment is less than two years, only the first investment would be accepted. Note that investment two, which was evaluated as the most profitable when using the net-present-value or internal-rate-of-return methods, is rejected when the payback-period method is used and a payback period of less than two years is the decision criterion. Similarly, the first investment, which was found unacceptable by the net-present-value method, is evaluated as the best investment under the payback-period method.

The major drawback in using the payback-period method is that neither the profitability nor the life of the investment beyond the payback period is considered. For example, consider the following two investments. Both have the same payback period, but they have substantially different rates of return.

	Investment X	Investment Y
Initial investment	$10,000	$5,000
Annual cash inflow	$ 5,000	$2,500
Estimated useful life	2 years	5 years
Payback period	2 years	2 years

The payback-period method provides an excellent supplement to the net-present-value or internal-rate-of-return method. This is especially true when there is a high degree of risk associated with the investment or when the rate of obsolescence is high. In these cases, the best investment is the one that is paid back first.

Average-, or Unadjusted-, Rate-of-Return Method

This method, sometimes called the accounting-rate-of-return method, does not use cash flows in computing the rate of return on an investment. Rather, accounting income, or the income amount derived by the application of generally accepted accounting principles, is used in the calculation. This rate of return is calculated as follows:

$$\text{Accounting, or unadjusted, rate of return} = \frac{\text{Average annual accounting income}}{\text{Initial investment}}$$

Because the average accounting income is used, all investments with equal lives, equal total income, and equal initial investments are evaluated the same, regardless of their cash inflows.

Consider the following example:

Investment	Average Inflows	Straight-line Depreciation	Annual Income	Initial Investment	Unadjusted Rate of Return
1	$600*	$500	$100	$1,000	10.0%
2	400	333	67	1,000	6.7%
3	400	333	67	1,000	6.7%
4	400	333	67	1,000	6.7%

*$1,200 / 2 years = $600

Like the payback-period method, the unadjusted-rate-of-return method evaluates investment one highest because of its shorter life. Note that the remaining investments have identical unadjusted rates of return because their total cash revenues and total costs for the three-year period are the same.

Because the accounting, or unadjusted, rate of return uses accounting measurements, it is consistent with the accounting records. Practices that use this method

---

CASE STUDY 6–3

DECIDING ON AN ALTERNATIVE INVESTMENT

Dr. David Dunn, head of the radiology department of Western Clinic, is adding a new piece of diagnostic equipment to the departent. Two similar models are offered by two different vendors, and both models would serve the needs of the clinic. Both also have an estimated useful life of five years, with no salvage value at the end of five years. The only difference between the two models is in the cost and estimated annual labor savings, as shown below:

	Model A	Model B
Cost, including installation	$120,000	$110,000
Estimated annual labor savings	$ 40,000	$ 32,000

The straight-line method of depreciation is used on the books. Senior management of the clinic has established a target rate of return of 15 percent for all equipment with a useful life of over two years and a desired payback period of three years.

Case Discussion Questions

1. Which model should Dr. Dunn purchase? Make your decision based on an evaluation of the alternatives using the following techniques (and ignoring income taxes):
    (a) Payback method
    (b) Net present value
    (c) Internal rate of return
2. Assume that an income tax rate of 40 percent applies to Western Clinic. Using the net present value method and incorporating the effects of income taxes, prepare an evaluation showing what your decision would be in this case.

---

typically do so because it is easily understood and uses available accounting information. Conceptually, however, this method does not provide the best way to evaluate new investment proposals.

Nonmonetary Considerations

Before making the final decision on a long-term investment prospect, nonmonetary factors should be evaluated. For example, assume that monetary data indicate that the acquisition of a new scanner is likely to be profitable. Also assume that a new governmental regulation may set limits on the number of scanners that

are permitted in the practice's geographical region. This regulation may become an overriding factor, leading to a negative decision regarding acquisition of the scanner. In other instances, nonmonetary factors may involve environmental regulations that negate an otherwise profitable investment prospect, as indicated by the quantitative analysis of monetary factors.

In conclusion, the decision rules and techniques presented here should be used to determine the economic feasibility of proposals for acquiring assets to increase the capacity to serve. However, the rules and techniques should not replace the judgment of the financial manager and the governing body of the practice. Nonmonetary factors often outweigh economic ones, and noneconomic criteria must also be considered in making long-term investment decisions.

FINANCIAL DECISIONS IN REVIEW

Most decisions facing a medical practice, whether short- or long-term, can be addressed through the use of a cost-benefit analysis framework and the application of a traditional problem-solving model. For short-term decisions, it is necessary to sort out relevant variable and fixed costs and to determine which costs are avoidable and which are unavoidable. The application of differential cost and revenue analysis can be useful in deciding upon adding another physician to the group, adding or dropping a service, making or buying a resource, and setting fees for special situations. The concept of contribution margin can be helpful in analyzing cost-volume-profit relationships and determining the break-even point and its implications for a practice and components of a practice.

Because long-term investments require a commitment of funds for a long period of time, these decisions require a different set of considerations. The time value of money is important, as well as estimations of amounts of expected cash flows, duration of flows, and expected rates of return, when evaluating various opportunities for long-term investments. Medical practices use several different methods of capital budgeting, including approaches that discount cash flows (net-present value and internal-rate-of-return methods) and a nondiscounting approach (payback-period approach). After quantitative methods are used to estimate the likely profitability of investment possibilities, nonmonetary factors should be considered before a final decision is made.

REFERENCES

Pavlock, E.J. (1994). *Financial management for medical groups.* Englewood, CO: Center for Research in Ambulatory Health Care Administration.

Ross, A., Williams, S.J. & Schafer, E.L. (1991). *Ambulatory care management.* (2nd ed.). Albany, NY: Delmar Publishers.

CHAPTER

7

Physician Compensation Systems

Vinod K. Sahney and Thomas C. Royer

CHAPTER TOPICS

LEARNING OBJECTIVES

Upon completing this chapter, the reader should be able to:

- Explain the necessity for exploring new group practice physician compensation plans
- Identify the characteristics and operational implications of various compensation models
- Compare the various models using major criteria for acceptance

Nothing has more potential to polarize a group of physicians than a new compensation plan. Indeed, compensation plans are a source of dissatisfaction in most organizations, and physician group practices are no exception. In fact, in medical groups, physician compensation distribution plays an especially important role because the revenue is generated by the physician members of the group, and compensation differences are a major reason that many medical groups break up. Because each physician has a different potential to generate revenue and the marketplace sets different hourly reimbursement rates for different specialists, division of the net earnings of a group is a complex undertaking. Large groups, such as the Mayo Clinic, Henry Ford Medical Group, and Kaiser Permanente, traditionally have compensated their physician members with a base salary, which is established by taking into account differences in specialty as well as marketplace factors. It is this salary process, with its inherent fiscal security, which has attracted many physicians to large group practices.

The compensation process has been complicated by the advent of managed care. Groups accepting capitation must develop very different methods of compensating physicians. Under a fee-for-service model, most small groups, especially those groups not involved in teaching and research, compensate members of the group based on the percentage of net revenues they generate. Under a managed-care model, in contrast, a group is paid on the basis of capitation, and distribution is production-based, creating a care-inhibiting system of incentives. In order to reach the productivity standards required in managed care in an efficient and effective way, groups are moving to bonus and risk/reward compensation plans, which attempt to align incentives with work plan strategies, for example, by using approaches that reward productivity or cost control oriented decision making. Although changing the compensation plan is one of the most difficult and, often, most risky undertakings of a group's leadership, most physician leaders agree that the way in which physicians behave is related, at least in part, to how they are paid (Enthoven, 1978).

Over the last decade, demand shifted from specialist to primary care, and starting pay for primary care doctors increased. Physician pay is now leveling off, however, and with managed care and government restructuring of reimbursement, boom times may be over. The ability to maintain a guaranteed straight salary with annual increments is decreasing, replaced by the growth of variable compensation models.

To facilitate the process of restructuring compensation plans, physicians must be given a clear understanding of the negative consequences of maintaining the status quo (Advisory Board Company, 1966). While doing this, leadership must also focus on the value of patient care (providing the highest quality of care at the lowest cost), as well as on any other goals inherent in the group's mission statement, such as academic medicine and research. In addition, leadership must be aware of the profile of the majority of younger physicians, because recruiting and retaining young physicians is necessary for the group's future success. Younger physicians appear to be less entrepreneurial and more security-minded and to place more emphasis on family and lifestyle than physicians before them. These are also the attributes of group practice that may be jeopardized by an incentive salary plan, unless it is developed and implemented correctly.

COMPONENTS OF A COMPENSATION PLAN

Before specific compensation models are discussed, the general goals and components of all plans should be understood. The compensation plan should ultimately align physicians and provider teams with group objectives. The plan should foster desirable physician behavior, including (Sahney, 1995) cost-effective care, high-quality care, external customer focus (i.e., insurers, employers), internal customer focus (i.e., practice employees), teaching/research participation (if this is part of the group's mission), and contribution to organizational improvements. Clearly, to be successful today, a physician often must see more patients; be comfortable with more nonphysician providers; reduce unnecessary utilization of hospitals, laboratories, and radiology resources; and utilize the most cost-effective pharmaceuticals. These tasks must be accomplished while maintaining a level of quality of care and services that will assure that patients and their families maintain their confidence in the health care system.

In order to foster these positive physician behaviors, a compensation model must have certain characteristics. These include (Sahney, 1995):

- Ease of communication
- Fair and equitable perception
- Low-cost implementation
- Sensitivity to improvements in performance
- Capability of physician productivity
- Reward system for achievement of organizational goals
- Ability to enhance physician recruitment and retention
- Capability of improving job satisfaction

Once the general characteristics and goals of a compensation plan are understood, specific models can be proposed for the group. Tools must be developed to implement the plan, such as physician profiling of the agreed-upon parameters of performance. It is important to note that compensation plans and tools should not be used for discipline. Rather, it is meant to assist physicians and management in working together to build and maintain an organization that will survive the fiscal challenges of the changing market. The transition process in compensation is challenging, because most large group practices have a mixture of fee-for-service and managed-care patients. The confusion of this mixed system can be managed by the development of group goals, aligned with the compensation plan, which foster the concept that managed care is a style of practice and not a payment mechanism. Thus, managed care will be seen as a total practical and philosophical approach.

WHY USE INCENTIVE PLANS?

Increasingly, group practices that traditionally used a straight salary model are switching to new compensation plans that use incentives. The reason for this switch is the belief that incentives create a more rapid alignment of goals by motivating people to reach performance standards. They "pull" rather than "push" people to change, and they change attitudes from "reluctant compliance" to "commitment." The product is care and although the group's cohesiveness and collegiality must be maintained, the core event in health care has been and always will be the physician–patient encounter. Thus, it is reasonable that the physician is the

focus of reward. Also, group changes occur one physician at a time, and incentives help facilitate this process.

WHAT CAN YOU EXPECT FROM INCENTIVE PLANS?

Like all compensation plans, incentive plan salary models have pros and cons. On the positive side, incentives foster self-motivation of the individual physician. Physicians become more attentive to key performance goals as well as to group goals when they are rewarded with incentives, and they more rapidly develop an aggressive, winning attitude. On the negative side, incentives may lead to neglect of nonreward areas, such as development of clinical protocols, and they may dampen efforts to reach group goals if the focus on the individual becomes too intense and overrewarded. Also, total quality improvement efforts depend on a cohesive team, and they are easily jeopardized by incentives unless the incentives are appropriately structured. Balance—between process and outcomes, and between listening and acting—is essential in medical leadership today. In compensation planning, there must be a balance between the individual and group performance, and this is a major challenge.

WHY DO INCENTIVE PLANS FAIL?

Some form of incentives seems to be a requirement of successful physician compensation models in today's health care environment. Nonetheless, incentive plans sometimes fail. The reasons for failure include lack of goal setting, lack of top management participation and review in goal setting, and failure to set challenging goals. Incentive plans also may fail because the incentives are unrelated to key organizational goals, the incentive formula is too complicated to understand, the incentive amounts are too small, there is poor communication about the incentive plan, or incentives are paid without objectives being achieved.

Clear action plans must be delineated by medical leaders to avoid each of these potential causes of failure of their incentive plans. This is true whether the group's compensation plan follows a pure incentive or a risk/reward model.

ALTERNATIVE COMPENSATION MODELS

Four basic compensation models are used in the majority of medical groups in mixed fee-for-service and managed-care markets: straight salary, production-based payments, capitation and subcapitation, and base salary plus incentives.

Straight Salary

In the straight salary model, one of the more traditional models, compensation is based on established ranges for each specialty, where ranges are determined by market surveys. Annual merit raises are based on performance evaluations and annual raises on the budget process.

Practices following a straight salary model tend to have lower physician productivity and higher overhead cost of physician management. Patient access problems are also often encountered. There tends to be higher participation by physicians on organizational teams and increased participation in teaching, research, and other nonrevenue-generating activities. Under a straight salary model, merit raise implementation is not handled effectively in a uniform and equitable manner. There is often constant medical group discussion on patient contact hours, production, and access, with difficulty reaching consensus. With this model, there may also be difficulty maintaining uniform compliance with service standards and the required high level of maintenance.

Production-Based Payments

Another traditional model, production-based payments are a fee-for-service model, in which compensation is based on the fees generated by each member of the group. For example, members may receive 50 percent of their billings. Practices following a production-based payments model tend to have high physician productivity and fewer problems of patient access. Physicians in these practices typically have low participation in teaching and research and on organizational teams. The model is also associated with low medical group overhead costs. With production-based payments, however, intergroup conflicts are likely, especially between primary care physicians and specialists. There also is likely to be continuous medical group discussion regarding the appropriate overhead and compensation ratio.

Capitation and Subcapitation

In capitation and subcapitation models, physicians are compensated by professional capitation fees ranging from $30 to $60 per member per month (PMPM) (Goldfarb, 1992; Advisory Board Company, 1996; Sahney, 1995). There are five capitation submodels, differing in their method of distributing the capitation to primary care physicians and specialists. These differences are summarized in Table 7–1.

Base Salary Plus Incentives

In a base salary plus incentives model, each physician is responsible for the total health care management of a portion of the group's patients. Physicians are compensated with base pay plus a percentage of salary at risk, which is based on performance (Sahney, 1995; Griffith et al., 1995). To act as an incentive, the risk amount must be meaningful. Usually 25 to 30 percent of compensation is recommended. Incentives should be based on one of the following variables:

TABLE 7–1   Five Capitation Submodels

Submodel	Primary Care Physicians	Specialists
Submodel A	Discounted fee-for-service utilization managed by plan	Discounted fee-for-service utilization managed by plan
Submodel B	Capitation for primary care services, but sharing in specialty pool savings	Discounted fee-for-service
Submodel C	Capitation for all professional services but management of specialty referral	Discounted fee-for service
Submodel D	Fee-for-service	Capitated
Submodel E	Capitation for all professional services	Capitated

- Utilization/cost criteria, such as in-patient days/ 1000, PMPM cost (professional), ancillary costs, or specific utilization management initiatives
- Panel performance, which is based on quality of care indicators such as mammography and immunization rates
- Patient satisfaction, which is measured by market surveys, voluntary panel turnover, and number of patient complaints and compliments
- Panel size, which should be weighed according to patient disease, using severity criteria appropriate for ambulatory patients

COMPARISON OF COMPENSATION MODELS

The four compensation models reviewed above, including submodels B and E of the capitation model, are compared in Table 7–2. In the figure, each model is graded from A (excellent) to D (minimally effective) on eight criteria, which are considered most important for compensation models to be successful (Sahney, 1995). The eight criteria were listed above on page 151, and they appear in the first column of Table 7–2. Note that the comparison in the table is based upon a market with

TABLE 7–2   Comparison of the Compensation Models against Eight Criteria*

Eight Criteria for Success of Model	*Straight Salary*	*Production-Based Payments*	*Capitation and Subcapitation, Submodel B*	*Capitation and Subcapitation, Submodel E*	*Salary and Incentives*
Ease of communication	A	A	B	B	B
Fair and equitable perception	C	A	B	A	A
Low-cost implementation	A	B	B	B	B
Sensitivity to improvements in performance	D	C	B	A	B
Capability of improving physician productivity	D	A	B	A	A
Reward system for achievement of organizational goals	C	D	B	A	A
Ability to enhance physician recruitment and retention	B	B	B	A	A
Capability of improving job satisfaction	B	B	A	A	A
Overall relative grade under managed care	C	D	B	A	A

*This evaluation assumes a market with at least 30 percent of the patients covered by an HMO.

at least 30 percent HMO patients. The models would be rated differently in a pure fee-for-service market or in a market with a low rate of managed care.

COMPENSATION SYSTEMS IN REVIEW

As payment mechanisms in the managed health care environment move to an increase in capitation payments and a decline in fee-for-service revenues, a change in physician compensation plans is inevitable. Four compensation models, including the two more traditional ones, have been reviewed and compared. It is clear from the comparison that there is no perfect compensation system. Each system has negative aspects.

The most important objective of any compensation system is to maximize alignment with group goals while minimizing the negative aspects of compensation. To be successful with physicians, a compensation plan must be simple and easy to understand. Constantly changing plans or adding complexity to existing plans may cause uncertainty and mistrust. Initially, group practices should use the salary as the basic platform for compensation on which to build a few specific organizational and individual goals in an incentive process. Two commonly used areas for goal setting are utilization (days/1000 members) and customer satisfaction.

Compensation plans are never a panacea for a practice's problems, and they do not replace management.

Incentive pay plans do not relieve medical group leaders of dealing with unacceptable practice issues. Perhaps the most important aspects of any plan are the dialogue, education, involvement, and implementation processes, not money.

REFERENCES

Advisory Board Company. (1996). *Reworking cost effective Medicare: Aligning physician incentives under managed care.* Washington, DC.

Dreams and Nightmares: Designed for Integrated Health Care System. Joseph T. Ichter and John J. Byrnes, MD Chair.

Enthoven, A.C. (1978). Shattuck lecture: Cutting cost without cutting the quality of care. *New England Journal of Medicine, 298,* 1229.

Goldfarb, N.I., (1992). Method of compensating physicians contracting with managed care organizations. *Journal of Ambulatory Care, 15*(4), 81–92.

Griffith, J.R., Sahney, V.K. & Mohr, R.A. (1995). *Reengineering health care: Building on CQI.* Ann Arbor, MI: Health Administration Press.

Sahney, V.K. (1995, July). *Contracting and physician compensation strategies.* Paper presented at *Dreams and nightmares: Design for integrated health care system.* Santa Fe, NM.

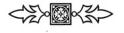

PART THREE

OPERATIONS MANAGEMENT

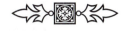

CHAPTER

Facilities Design and Operations

Phillip A. Kieburtz

LEARNING OBJECTIVES

Upon completing this chapter, the student should be able to:

- Explain how to initiate, conduct, and evaluate a facilities construction project
- Assess project performance and documentation, and evaluate alternatives for project financing
- Assess alternatives for the selection of key players, such as architects and contractors
- Understand how to operate, open, and maintain a facility

From the moment an organization decides to construct a facility to the point when the project is completed and occupied, there are multiple opportunities for conflicts and problems. As long as there is uncertainty about the economics and future form of health care, many groups will find facility questions to be some of the most divisive issues they face. They must answer such questions as: How can we afford a new facility? Why do we need it? Where should it be? Should we develop a satellite? How will a new facility affect my income? Do I have to personally guarantee payments?

The stress and strain associated with project construction or extensive renovation may be a leading factor contributing to administrative turnover or fragmentation of the group. The intent of this chapter is to identify the key issues and sequence the decisions required to complete a project successfully with the fewest possible conflicts and problems. The chapter identifies ways to eliminate or reduce the risks inherent in any facility-development project. The more predictable the process and outcome, the less administrative stress and conflict there should be. The chapter is not intended as a detailed guide to facilities design and operation. Rather, it stresses the importance of retaining competent assistance to guide a project through to a successful conclusion.

INITIATING A PROJECT

Initiating the facility-development process is like the building itself. A well-conceived, stable, and level foundation eliminates future problems. Anything else invites disaster. Considerable background preparation is especially important in developing new facilities. Important factors that the administrator must be aware of in initiating a project are discussed in this and the following sections.

Before initiating any project, every group needs a written plan, whether it is called a game plan, a business plan, or a strategic plan. The plan should state the principles of the group, the goals and objectives it wishes to achieve, and a strategy for achieving the goals and objectives. The plan may require four typewritten sheets, two three-ring binders, or just be on the back of a restaurant place mat. Once the plan is written, the

more widely it is dispersed and agreed upon the better. Parts of the plan may be confidential, but the more clinical physicians and employees that buy into the plan the better.

In developing a new facility, someone is needed (either in-house or in a consulting capacity) who has the experience and expertise to determine the size and scope of the project. This could be an architect, consultant, or space planner. It also could be an individual in a large firm or sole proprietorship. The important thing is that the individual has a track record of assisting on similar projects. Then a preliminary program and budget must be developed that accurately reflect a realistic, affordable solution. Information, depicting the scope and nature of the project, should be approved by the management team before the design and construction firms that actually produce the facility are hired.

SELECTING A DESIGN AND CONSTRUCTION APPROACH

Several different approaches can be used for the design and construction of a facility. Some of these are presented next.

Traditional Design/Bid/Build Approach

As the name suggests, this is the traditional approach to designing and constructing a facility, in which an architect is retained, who completes working drawings; contractors are asked to submit bids; and the lowest bidder is awarded the contract to build the project. The main advantage of this approach is that it assures competition among general contractors and the lowest price for the architect's design. In this approach, the architect is the key player. This person serves as the owner's agent, developing detailed specifications and drawings, and theoretically, serving as a monitor to assure that the contractor is meeting those specifications.

The design/bid/build approach has tremendous pitfalls for the unwary administrator. As the name implies, the design/bid/build process is sequential. As a result, it not only takes more time to complete the process, but it also results in the client receiving information in a

CASE STUDY 8–1

GETTING STARTED

The Elwood Clinic is a 25-person internal medicine and primary care group in a rural midwestern community. There are two hospitals in town, St. Swithen's and Memorial Medical Center. Historically, most of the doctors in town have worked at both hospitals. However, Memorial's new administrator, Wayne Smiley, is far more aggressive than his predecessor. He convinces Dr. Elwood, Elwood Clinic's medical director, that both Memorial and the clinic would be stronger with a closer working relationship. Dr. Elwood has long felt a new location might help keep his group together once he retires. The group's location is old, parking is inadequate, the doctors are crowded without enough examining rooms, and the building has been remodeled several times, which has only added to its inefficiency.

The hospital administrator has offered Dr. Elwood a site for the clinic on his 52-acre campus. From the administrator's standpoint, this is a no-lose opportunity. Not only will Memorial get 100 percent of the business of the largest internal medicine and primary care group in town, it also will get lease income from previously unused ground. From Dr. Elwood's standpoint, the project will not only keep the group together but also allow it to grow. They tentatively agree on the plan, and both go back to inform their management teams.

Dr. Elwood reports to his people that the hospital is so eager to get the clinic on campus that Memorial will virtually guarantee their future viability by building them a new building.

Fred Bright, Elwood Clinic's administrator, and other members of the management team at the clinic see a lot of merit in the plan but also some potential pitfalls. Team members realize they have not updated their business plan since a third partner came on board 17 years ago. They have several unanswered questions, such as: How big do they want to be? At how many hospitals do they intend to practice? Do they want to remain independent? And what would happen to the present building, which the clinic owns but has not yet paid for? They realize that they cannot possibly decide on Mr. Smiley's proposal until they answer such questions.

The group uses two consultants and spends six months and thousands of dollars to address the questions. As a result, one doctor quits, although two smaller groups in town approach Fred about becoming part of the Elwood medical group. Most importantly, however, when Fred meets with Mr. Smiley, he will be ready to ask relevant questions.

At the same time the new plan was developed, Fred set up a new facility committee, established a new column in the in-house monthly newsletter, wrote an open letter to the local newspaper discussing the planning process they went through and why they felt a new facility would help them better serve the community. The intent of the letter was to minimize alienating colleagues, the other hospital, and patients, and also to create a positive atmosphere before rumors and assumptions fueled skeptics in the community.

Case Discussion Question

1. What are some questions the new facility committee at Elwood Clinic should address before reaching a final decision?

sequential manner. For example, using this approach, the client does not know how much the project will actually cost until it is bid, which is some time after working drawings are completed. Nothing could be worse than finding that a project is 30 percent over budget after spending a year or two designing it, arranging the financing, and finally being ready to break ground.

The design/bid/build approach was once the overwhelming favorite of the architectural community. However, more and more architects now prefer other approaches that retain the role of the architect as a design and engineering professional but provide both the architect and the client with better and more timely cost and construction information with which to make decisions.

Fast-Track Approach

An alternative approach is to overlap the separate steps of the design/bid/build process. This is often referred to as the fast-track approach. With this approach, major decisions have been made concerning the footprint (area covered) of the building; they are not usually changed during the later design development phase. This means that contractors can be selected to start foundation work and major construction while detailed planning of the interior design continues.

This approach should be used with great caution. Although it has the potential to reduce the overall time necessary for design and construction, and thereby minimize the effect of inflation, it is likely to result in an excessive number of change orders. It often requires the over-design of such elements as footings and foundations, structural systems, mechanical systems, and plumbing systems in order to accommodate design decisions that have not yet been made.

In practice, the only time most design or construction professionals advise an aggressive, fast-track approach is when the cost is insignificant compared to the completion or move-in date. This is not to say that some overlapping of design and construction tasks cannot be used effectively in other types of projects. In fact, in some jurisdictions the permit process is so cumbersome that it requires a modified fast-track approach.

Nonetheless, it should be used only with experienced professionals who are accustomed to working together.

Design/Build Approach

The design/build approach was created as a direct response to the perceived inadequacies of the traditional design/bid/build approach. Whereas the traditional approach is sequential and requires a great deal of time, the design/build approach emphasizes a coordinated team effort during both design and construction, with maximum overlapping and minimal sequencing of activities. The design/build approach also has another advantage. The fact that standard, or stock, details are more commonly used and working drawings do not have to be prepared for an open competitive-bid market with the design/build approach means that drawings, specifications, and other documents require less preparation time and cost. Finally, whereas the traditional approach keeps project cost a mystery until the end of the bid period, the design/build approach emphasizes keeping to a budget established during the conceptual planning of the project. The involvement of the contractor or estimating division of the design/build firm from the first phase of design to completion, with authority to maintain the budget, is the absolute strength of the design/build approach.

The integration of discipline and authority that is the strength of the design/build approach is also its greatest potential weakness. The architect, traditionally the owner's agent, is now the employee of the contractor. Under a design/build approach, it may not be clear to the administrator who represents the group's interests.

The design/build process has proven to be very satisfactory in instances where the design/build firm developed a specialized project that had been used successfully elsewhere. Significant cost savings associated with this approach are realized only if each new use of a design minimizes customizing. For example, assume that a large multispecialty group practice in an urban setting wishes to establish a satellite clinic but realizes that a family-practice primary care setting has different needs than its present specialty–tertiary care urban setting. It may turn to a design/build firm to produce a building to fulfill the new function. In doing so, the practice parent organization may recognize that it does not have the expertise to contribute to the final custom details and may be willing to accept a model that has been developed and used successfully elsewhere. Thus, although the design/build process is highly integrated and faster than the traditional approach, it does not allow as much customizing or as much control by the owner.

Another potential problem with the design/build approach is the way its costs and fees are usually quoted to a client. Most design/build firms prefer to quote one figure, which includes the actual cost of construction plus design engineering services and the company's overhead and profit. This means the client never knows whether the building costs $80-per-square foot, with an additional $10 per square foot for professional services and $10 per square foot for the firm's overhead and profit; or the building costs $70 per square foot, with $8 per square foot for professional services and $22 per square foot for overhead and profit. In each case, the total cost is $100 per square foot, but in the first example the overhead and profit are 13 percent and in the second they are 31 percent.

Turn-Key Approach

Like the design/build approach, the turn-key approach emphasizes the integration of services as its strong suit. Design/build firms that use the turn-key approach advertise that all the owner has to do is "turn the key, open the door, and go to work". In addition to design and construction services, these firms include an array of other development and financing services in their packages.

The greatest weakness of the turn-key approach is the lack of diverse opinions and recommendations that are normally expressed by independent contractors, architects, engineers, and consultants. Under the turn-key approach, all these normally independent agents are agents of the contractor. There are other weaknesses as well. Some turn-key firms have been criticized for sharing cost savings on the project with the project manager rather than with the owner. This type of arrangement, which enhances the project manager's compensation, can lead to cost savings that are not in the owner's best interest. Also in attempts to convince prospective clients that they are truly competitive and knowledgeable, many turn-key (and design/build) firms stress that their prices are "guaranteed." Too often, however, close inspection or thorough review of the footnotes or fine print reveals that many of the guaranteed costs are actually allowances. Therefore, the guarantees are meaningless.

Construction Management Approach

Construction management, as an approach, refers to instances in which the owner employs an individual or firm experienced in the construction process to represent the owner's interests in working out specification details and arrangements with both the contractor and the architect. The construction manager in this approach truly represents the owner. For example, if the architect designing the facility does not have the owner's best interests at heart when it comes to economizing or designing cost-effective structures, the construction manager employed by the owner can serve as an auditor to raise questions concerning specifications. The manager communicates directly with the contractor to negotiate changes in design that will work to the owner's benefit without compromising the design.

A major drawback of the construction management approach is that it adds an extra layer of administrative cost that is unnecessary unless the project is extremely complicated and requires a multitude of specialized contractors and subcontractors, such as would be needed to build a new manufacturing facility or airport. A modification of the construction management approach that eliminates this drawback is to have the general contractor also act as the construction manager. Under this modified approach, the contractor not only bids portions of the work to subcontractors but also has his own firm bid on portions of the work that he wants it to perform. The construction manager/general contractor often works for a stipulated fee in what is referred to as "open book" accounting, which entitles the owner to review construction costs at any time.

Professional Team Approach

The final approach is an attempt to take the best from all of the above methods while minimizing their weaknesses. It is often referred to as the professional team approach, or the project management approach. Like the construction management approach, the professional team approach assumes that the owner employs an experienced representative to protect the owner's interests. In this approach, however, the representative's title and duties are expanded from construction manager to project manager. Rather than just focusing on the design and construction process, the project manager, or project management firm, focuses on the total project, from inception to completion.

Ideally, the project manager assists the owner in conceiving the proposed project so that the initial program, budget, and schedule are realistic in view of the group's mission and strategic plan. The project manager can also help the client with site analysis and acquisition, selection of other team members, (including architects, contractors, and engineers), analysis of funding sources, negotiation of loan terms, and oversight and coordination of the design and construction process. Rather than restrict the owner's options, the project management professional team approach allows maximum flexibility regarding the selection of design and construction professionals and the choice of approach to delivering services.

As the project manager is totally independent of the architect and contractor, so are his or her fees, which are typically quoted on an hourly or lump-sum basis rather than as part of the actual cost of construction.

MANAGING THE PROJECT

The steps necessary to complete a project successfully include the following:

1. Determination of needs
2. Preparation of a program description (program document)
3. Preparation of preliminary budget and proformas to determine the feasibility of the project
4. Approval of the project concept and proposed financing by the governing board
5. Final selection of the architect and consultants
6. Development of schematic drawings
7. Estimate of construction costs by a professional source other than the architect
8. Submittal of the schematic drawings to the governing board for approval
9. Authorization by the governing board of the working drawings and budget
10. Submission of the working drawings and specifications to the contractor for final prices
11. Completion of contract negotiations
12. Final approval by the board and initiation of construction
13. Staging, supervision, and completion of the project
14. Final evaluation report to the board on the performance of the parties involved (consultants, architects, and contractors)

Many of these steps are elaborated upon in the sections that follow.

Project Responsibility and Documentation

Before selecting the architect, contractor, and other consultants, careful consideration should be given to appointing an internal building committee whose members are charged with adequately describing the functions to take place within the new facility. The composition of the building committee should include, ideally, a mixture of disciplines. In addition to appropriate administrative involvement, it is important to involve physicians or other practitioners who have an interest in following the project through to its completion. However, care should be taken to avoid loading the committee with individuals with too many vested personal interests. For example, if there is competition for space, thought should be given in advance to how issues of space or resource allocation will be resolved.

Building committees always should function in an advisory capacity to an executive committee or board of directors. There should be a clear line of administrative responsibility concerning the project, and a single individual, the project administrator, should be charged with project implementation. It is the administrator's responsibility to steer the course from beginning to end, while assuring that appropriate individuals are involved.

CASE STUDY 8-2

DEVELOPING A PROJECT

Ray Bullet is the assistant administrator in charge of developing a 40-doctor full-service satellite for the East Coast Medical Group. The group's strategic plan coupled with recent demographic data indicate that the area around St. John's Hospital, just south of town, is ideal for the group's expansion plans. In addition, a number of doctors with practices in that area have joined the group over the last few years and were told that a new, consolidated facility was in the planning stage.

Ray leases a site from St. John's and then plans to hire an architect. Although the clinic has a firm they have used several times before, this is Ray's project and his brother-in-law works for a firm with tremendous health care experience. The firm's brochure says they have designed two major VA hospitals and several other major hospitals and government projects around the country. The firm's representatives are interviewed and hired. After three and one-half months of programming, the firm is ready to discuss the project with Ray and his management team. Using computer-generated graphics, they display the results of their work—a 120,000 square-foot facility costing over $23 million. Ray's CFO anticipated a project cost somewhere in the neighborhood of $5 million, and that is what he had used for the proformas and projections he sent to the main office downtown.

How could the project be so far off budget? Ray was correct in assuming he needed information with which to make decisions. What he didn't need was an architect whose expertise was in the design of VA hospitals.

In his haste, Ray had hired a firm with "health care experience" that had never designed a medical office building, much less a group practice facility. Their program consisted of interviewing doctors, department supervisors, and administrators and then turning that "wish list" into conceptual drawing using statistical information from their hospital data base. They had then given the schematic drawings to their in-house estimator, who used the same pricing approach used on VA hospitals. To compound the problem Ray's CFO's estimate, based on contractor's opinions, was equally erroneous.

Ray has decided he can afford no more mistakes. So far, his mistakes have wasted only a few months and a few thousand dollars. The CEO of the main clinic now suggests that Ray use one of the experienced firms they have worked with before, but that still leaves Ray with several options.

Case Discussion Question

1. What approach should Ray use for the design and construction of the facility?

The members of the building committee should be identified early, and, once involved, they should serve as advisors in the selection of the architect and other consultants. This committee, in concert with financial advisors, should review preliminary budgets and proformas so that the group is assured that the project is economically viable before large sums are committed.

Financing

Prior to proceeding with any significant project, the economics and financing of the project must be understood fully by the group. This means that a complete project budget must be developed and the implications, risks, and requirements of financing accepted.

In the past, financing a group practice facility was relatively easy. Most lenders, whether small savings and loan associations in rural committees or major insurance companies or pension funds in urban areas, considered doctors, or their employing group practices as extremely good risks. Even though the financing was usually for single-purpose real estate in locations that otherwise might not be commercially viable, doctors were considered to be almost recession proof and therefore desirable borrowers. This often resulted in loans greater than the cost of the project. Coupled with tax laws that were favorable toward real estate owners, it was the rare exception when a doctor or group of doctors did not own the facility in which they worked.

The economics of real estate ownership have changed dramatically, and the economic realities of health care have made lenders wary. Conventional loans in excess of 80 percent of value or cost (whichever is less) are now virtually nonexistent. Personal recourse (i.e., loan guarantees) is often required, and highly favorable tax treatment no longer exists. With many groups already strapped for capital, the idea of coming up with equity equaling 20 or 25 percent of the project cost, from either the group or the individual doctors, usually is not an acceptable alternative.

The result is that many groups are using new and innovative approaches for funding projects. Terms such as *securitization, beneficial occupancy agreements,* and *synthetic leases* are used to describe approaches to capital acquisition that have been used in other industries for years but not in health care until now. Some of these approaches involve a soft guarantee with a hospital or health care system which helps the group negotiate favorable rates and terms with the lender but does not affect the hospital's balance sheet. Another approach for groups trying to generate or preserve capital is long-term leasing. This is used for both proposed and existing buildings.

In many cases, the objective is to change the loan from a real estate loan to a credit loan. The advantages to the borrower of a credit loan are twofold. First, the group can borrow a higher percentage of the project cost (often in excess of 95 percent), which means the group needs less equity and perhaps no longer needs to seek an equity investor. Second, the funds are borrowed at a substantially lower rate, often 200 basis points under a conventional real estate loan.

The disadvantages of a credit loan are also twofold. First, for all but the largest and strongest groups, a credit loan is available only with some sort of support or assistance from a major hospital or health care system. Whether this support or assistance is acceptable to the institution should be investigated at the inception of the project. Second, fees for a credit loan typically are slightly higher than for conventional real estate financing. However, considering the potential results, the advantages of a credit loan usually outweigh the disadvantages.

Programming

In addition to determining needs, it is very useful for the institution's representatives to design a program document. A program document includes descriptive material on the functions that will be based in the new building or addition. The program document should furnish the architect with preliminary estimates on the number of physicians (or other practitioners), practice patterns (such as number and types of examination and consultation rooms required per physician), type of practice (for example, specialty/tertiary or primary care), ancillary support services (such as laboratory,

X-ray, electrocardiograph, physical medicine, or other special requirements), and administrative and service-area needs (for example, business office, record storage, and switchboard areas). It is not necessary to design a program document in an architectural layout or design sense but simply to describe what will take place in the new structure. Developing a program document also serves as an integrative force for the building committee, medical staff, and others involved, because it clarifies participants' understanding of the scope of the project.

There is a tendency to develop floor plans reflecting particular styles of practice. A difficult task for the building committee is to determine where standard layouts for exam rooms, consultation rooms, and lobbies should be used and where specially designed treatment facilities should be used instead. Special requirements might include, for example, the design of an otolaryngology unit with acoustical sound rooms or an ophthalmology section with eye lanes for examination.

As a general rule, care should be taken to make the best prediction regarding potential future section expansion, so that special facilities can be expanded later if necessary without having to redo the total section or floor area. Conforming to standard plans has the advantage of flexibility in future growth of sections; as practitioners are added, additional rooms can be reassigned from one section to another without moving the entire section to a different floor.

At some point during this design process, the building committee should listen carefully to the architect as the design begins to unfold. Keeping in mind that it is the owner's option to establish the final design, the committee should question the architect regarding floor plan relationships, mechanical support systems, and other building features with which the architect has demonstrated success elsewhere. A facility that operates well when completed is one that has been designed by a team effort, with owner representatives who are generally interested and involved in the details as well as in the overall scheme.

One approach that is highly recommended relates to the design of standard rooms, such as exam rooms and offices. It is the mock-up approach, in which a room is built to the exact dimensions of the proposed room but with plywood walls and doors. Furniture is then placed in the mock-up room to see whether the design actually works. It may cost several thousand dollars to design and built the mock-up room, but being able to actually see a room as important as an exam room may well be worth the time and effort, particularly because it allows everyone to see the relationship of the exam table, sink, cabinets, and other equipment.

When the plan calls for designing special features (for example, automatic front doors in a lobby), representatives of the organization, in consultation with architects, should, whenever possible, visit sites with similiar features and ask about maintenance or other problems. Although the number of elevator manufacturers is limited, vertical transportation—whether it be elevators, pneumatic tube systems, vertical lifts, or other systems—is so critical in the day-to-day operation of health care facilities that it must be evaluated carefully well in advance of commitment.

Supervision

In larger projects it may be highly desirable to consider employing a "clerk of the works," who is retained by the owners to represent their interests in monitoring development of plan specifications during the design stage. This individual may also make continual on-site visits during construction to assure that the quality of the construction meets the specifications. (This is a modification of the professional team approach reviewed earlier). Although the architect still shares responsibility for supervision, it is important to have an owners' representative available to serve as an intermediary in contract negotiations and related matters.

The owner's representative (perhaps the administrator) already carries a heavy burden of day-to-day operations and seldom has sufficient time to oversee the total project in great detail. The clerk of the works can serve a vital function by assisting the administrator and overseeing the total project. This person is in a position to raise

---

CASE STUDY 8-3

DECIDING WHETHER TO CENTRALIZE OR DECENTRALIZE

The new Graystone Memorial Clinic facility houses 50 specialists. The old clinic building was located in a gradually decaying portion of the city, and the group decided to build a new facility to allow for expansion of the staff and to better serve the population, which has shifted away from the original location.

During the course of planning for the project, a number of decisions regarding functions were made. One important decision was to centralize the nursing station on each floor, with approximately twelve physicians housed in each unit and three to four in each subspecialty section. This was done in order to increase efficiency. Although the physicians' offices and the exam rooms all had telephones, telephone calls to the floor were to be handled centrally within the nursing section. Other duties of the nursing and office staff were also to be shared. As a patient was brought back from the central reception area with the chart, the chart was to be placed in a pocket outside the patient's exam-room door, and the flag indicator moved to alert the physician that this was his or her next patient.

The move was completed over a weekend, and the doors of the new facility opened to patients for the first time on the following Monday. Within an hour, utter chaos reigned. The chief of medicine became so upset that he threatened to resign. The problem was that the physicians did not accept the centralization of the nursing staff because they felt they could not operate without having their own personal assistant.

Somehow the clinic floundered through the first week, with growing tension among employees, professional staff, and administrators. The following Monday, a special meeting of the partnership was called to consider the design problems of the new building.

Case Discussion Question

1. Assume that you are the administrator of the Graystone Memorial Clinic. What went wrong, and how would you correct the problem?

---

appropriate questions of a design, specifications, and construction with both the architect and the contractor.

Such a person should not be selected with the intent of placing him or her in an adversarial relationship, and appointing a person for this capacity should be done with the full knowledge of the architect and the contractor, both of whom should normally welcome this addition to the team. If either the architect or the contractor discourages the owners' employment of such a person, the matter should be followed up. This is because, whenever a clerk of the works is involved in a project, the person should have total access to all building committee meetings and other internal and external activities of the project.

Project Insurance

Building insurance brokers should be informed of potential projects. It is important to establish clearly insurance responsibilities of the existing insurer and the contractor's insurance company, both for purposes of fire protection on the project and for hazard liability protection.

Questions occasionally arise concerning the bonding ability of the contractors. Generally, it is wise to insist that the contractor has a bond on the project to assure performance. In some cases, for example, with a very prominent and well-established contractor, bonding may be avoided, but generally the cost of bonding is not large enough to offset the value of the protection it provides.

SELECTING TEAM PLAYERS

Obviously, selection of the architect, contractor, and consultants is a key factor in facility planning. Historically, one of the first tasks, if not the first, in initiating a project was to select the architect. However, with the present array of approaches to design and construction that were reviewed above, many groups facing the challenge of developing a new facility first select an approach before interviewing specific firms to be part of the team. For example, if the group adopts the design/bid/build approach, it might interview architects A, B, C, and D. If, however, it adopts the design/build approach, it might interview firms D, F, G, and H. Only firm D would be appropriate under either approach.

Another option appropriate with either the traditional design/bid/build approach or the design/build approach is to select the contractor first and the architect second. How and why this is done will be clear later in this section.

Selecting the Architect

The process of selecting the architect begins early in the project. The architect can be useful in advising the owners on site selection and the many design options that face the builder. In most cases, the architect's work (including both the design and the permitting process) is the basis for the critical path taken prior to construction; therefore, this team member is most often the initial one to be selected.

The architect selection process is of prime importance. Although the group initially may review the credentials of ten or twelve firms, a final group of no more than three of four firms should be considered for interviews, or "short-listed". If the group has decided to use the professional team approach, the firm or individual who acts as project manager should be helpful in soliciting proposals from appropriate architectural firms and assessing their merits.

It is often necessary to visit projects the architect has already completed and to discuss with the architect's prior clients their evaluation of the architectural services. Particular emphasis should be placed on the architect's previous projects that are similar in size and type to the project that is being considered. A group interested in a facility for a four-person, orthopedic practice, for example, probably would short-list an entirely different group of architects than those who would be short-listed for a 70-person, multispecialty, group-practice facility. Architects or firms that are not specific about their relevant experience and only claim to have "extensive health care experience" should be considered with caution. Their experience may be with hospitals, nursing homes, or any other type of health care facility, and it may have no bearing on the project under consideration. In addition, it should be determined whether the specific people in the architectural firm who have experience with projects similar to the one under consideration are still with the firm and would be assigned to the proposed project.

Two common methods of selecting the architect are through competition and by interview. Interviews are used by most group practices. The competition method is normally reserved for government work or larger, more complicated projects, such as hospitals.

In the interview part of the selection process, the architectural firm is invited to meet with the building committee to discuss the firm's experiences and qualifications. This allows the building committee an opportunity to ask many specific questions. Questions might relate to the architect's selection and use of consultants, experience with similar projects, and history of performance with regard to square-foot costs and completion dates. Other questions might relate to the date the architect could actually begin the project, the role the group's professional and ancillary staff would play in assessing equipment and other needs, the level of the architect's professional liability insurance, the architect's professional compensation schedule, and even an early discussion of the architect's design philosophy.

If the group has adopted the design/build approach, it should pay particular attention to the architect's experience with builders and developers. Architects who are unfamiliar or uncomfortable with the design/build approach may make poor team members and add unnecessary difficulty to the design and construction process. On the other hand, architects who prefer the design/build or professional team approach not only understand what is expected of them, but often have lower fees, particularly if they have previous experience working with the other team members.

The project is usually divided into phases (design, working drawings, and project supervision), and it should be clear who on the architect's staff will be involved in each phase of the project. Failure to ask questions about these matters can lead to problems later on in the process. For example, it is not uncommon for the sales presentation to be made by a senior architect, whose performance leads to the selection of the firm, and then for junior representatives of the organization to be the ones actually assigned to one or more phases of the project. If there is a discrepancy in performance between the senior architect and the junior architects actually assigned to the project, disappointment and problems may result.

Clarification of the role of consultants is necessary in order to determine whether the cost of the consultants is included in the basic architectural service fee. In a complex medical project, there may be several consultants involved, including communication experts, technical medical equipment consultants, traffic consultants, and a variety of others who specialize in heating, plumbing, structural concerns, elevators, electrical components, and landscape design, among other areas. It is important to determine well ahead of time who these consultants will be and also what their degree of involvement will be.

In some cases, an administrator may select an architect who has virtually no experience with the type of project being considered. Instead, his or her experience in a particular locality or with a particular contractor or developer may outweigh the lack of experience with the particular type of project. There may be other political or nonarchitectural reasons for such a selection. In these cases, it may be necessary to combine a firm or individual experienced in medical space planning with the less experienced but otherwise preferable architectural firm. This can be done with very acceptable results.

In the case of a hospital developing an ambulatory unit, where the architectural firm has been employed for previous hospital construction, the process of selecting the architect may be simplified. Nonetheless, care must be taken to assure that the hospital architect fully appreciates the differences between ambulatory and hospital care and group practice care.

The worst situation is when neither the client nor the architect realizes the level of expertise that is required for the project. Some architects (even large firms with extensive health care experience) do not realize the level of sophistication involved in a good group practice design. If the client is equally unaware of what to expect from an experienced group practice designer, the client may settle for a second-rate result and never even know the difference. For example, the design might use more space than is actually required, leading to higher occupancy costs, higher personnel costs, and an overall lack of efficiency. On the other hand, a design that uses less space than is actually required can limit even more the number of patients a doctor can see in a day or the efficiency of ancillary or support personnel.

The architect should be asked not only about square-foot costs and completion dates of recent projects, but also about the level of change orders and costs added to the basic bid figures. However, a competing architect is unlikely to report that he or she seldom hits the budget or has projects that are usually behind schedule, so these are questions that are better asked of references and other professionals in the construction industry.

The question about change orders is especially important because the answer can reveal whether or not the architect has been operating conservatively in estimating costs. The number of change orders can reflect a lack of foresight by the architect. Alternatively, it could reflect a lack of decision making by the physician-owners or management. Nonetheless, the question still should be posed.

Yet another question relates to the priority of the project in the architect's schedule. The firm should state not only when it would actually be able to begin the project, but it should also provide an estimated progress schedule. This establishes the priority the architect will attach to the project.

Although architects often quote compensation schedules that are based on a percentage cost, these fees are often negotiable. They are based on the complexity of the building, the confidence the architect has in the type of information that will be received from owners and managers concerning design requirements, and the backlog of work the firm has on its books.

Another question that is very important to administrators and professional staff relates to the architect's attitude toward involving the organization's professional and ancillary personnel. If the architect does not want a direct interface and promotes instead a package program, this could lead to additional work on the part of the organization to adapt to the configuration of the building. Close communication is essential, because the latest information on new equipment to be housed and used in the new facility usually will come from the professionals who will use the equipment rather than from the architect.

Although the architect's willingness to listen to owners and owners' consultants in designing detailed areas is important, the owners or owners' representatives should be careful on their part not to reinvent the wheel. This means that communication should flow in both directions. The experienced architect will not just listen; he or she will have state-of-the-art information and be able to make a positive contribution.

Another issue relating to the selection of an architect is whether the architect carries adequate professional liability insurance. These days, not only physicians tend to be sued for malpractice, but also attorneys and architects.

A final question concerning the selection of an architect relates to the architect's design philosophy. The best way to determine the architect's design philosophy is to examine carefully the end result of the architect's work. This requires visits to project sites, with thoughtful and thorough reviews of the buildings, their layout, and their functional success. The architect's willingness to conform to the owners' interests is worth investigating, because an architect with a predisposition to create unique architectural structures may not relate to the needs of the owners. The architect's willingness and ability to pick up on the sensitivities of the owners can be determined only through careful interview and examination of the relationship between the architect and previous clients.

Selecting the Contractor

Traditionally, contractors have been selected by the bid process. In an open bid, all interested contractors receive bid documents (including working drawings and specifications) and are asked to submit their bids on a given date. Although this process may assure the client of the lowest price for the project, in reality it often means that the contractor with the lowest bid has made an error in the estimate, was not sufficiently knowledgeable or experienced to submit a proper bid, or is likely to lose money on the project when it is completed. In some instances, an open bid actually reduces the number of qualified contractors who respond. This is because it is likely that an inexperienced or unqualified contractor will submit a low bid that does not represent the true cost of the work to be performed.

Although the idea of getting the lowest possible price may seem desirable, if that price does not include a fair margin or profit for the contractor, then the contractor may become the owner's adversary for the duration of the project and possibly even for the duration of the guarantee period following project completion. The ultimate disaster is when a low bid results in the contractor going bankrupt trying to complete the project.

A partial solution to this problem is the select, or closed-bid, list, which limits the number of firms submitting bids to those who have been prequalified. Bonds may also be required of bidders, and this may help limit the number of respondents. However, even a closed-bid approach does not preclude the development of an owner-contractor adversarial relationship, because this is inherent in the bid process. In essence, the owner says to the contractor: "You were hired because you promised to deliver the same work product as the other contractors submitting bids but at a lower cost." In return, the contractor says: "That is true, but I am going to look for every opportunity to save every dollar I can and still fulfill the requirements of the contract, because I get to keep the dollars I save, and they will increase my profit." Although this situation does not necessarily mean there will be problems with the contractor, it should be assumed that the contractor's motives and the owner's objectives do not necessarily coincide.

Another problem with the bid process is that it does not take advantage of the contractor's experience and expertise during the preconstruction phase. The building industry generally acknowledges that more money can be saved during the first half of the design period than during the second half of the design period. Clearly, a competent experienced contractor should know more about construction costs, cost-effective systems, and alternate approaches to solving construction problems than anyone else involved. However, the bid approach does not include the contractor as part of the team until the design is complete and ready for construction.

Selecting a contractor on the basis of negotiations and interviews is intended to solve some of the problems created by the traditional bid process. Although there is no set method for selecting a contractor using this approach, the following describes in general how the process works.

First, based on a predetermined project scope, the contractor to be considered is asked to submit a fixed fee to be paid over and above the actual cost of the work to be performed. The contractor is also asked to submit a fixed amount for "general conditions," based on a stipulated time period. Interviews are then conducted and the contractor selected coincidentally with the selection of the architect, so the contractor becomes a team member at the very inception of the design process.

Because 80 percent of the total cost of most projects is supplied by subcontractors who are selected on the basis of bids, the general contractor is also required to bid any portion of the work to be supplied with the contractor's own crew. This results in competitive pricing on virtually all aspects of the project, except for miscellaneous labor, general conditions, the contractor's fee, and miscellaneous permits and taxes.

Although there are many variations, the most basic contract form is cost plus fixed fee, possibly with stipulated contingencies for unexpected events. Some contractors or construction managers may request a separate payment for preconstruction services. Others may request payment only if the project is canceled. Still others may provide the service at no cost or risk to the client prior to signing the final construction contract.

Whereas almost any selection method can be used successfully, optimum results can be achieved only if all parties have a clear understanding of objectives and priorities relating to such factors as total cost, timing, and risk.

FACILITIES OPERATIONS

Many of the issues in this section are of special concern in the development of new facilities. However, they also are relevant to the renovation of existing facilities and to changes in the way existing facilities are used.

Facility Ambience

The ambience of a facility should be considered carefully when the facility is being designed. A lobby and office area that meet the needs and desires of the owners or board of directors may not promote patient access. Patients tend to judge services based on the physical surroundings. For example, a richly furnished entrance area may suggest to patients that the services rendered are expensive. A crowded, congested lobby may suggest a lengthy wait to see the doctor.

All seats for waiting patients should be within sight of receptionists. On occasion, waiting patients may require special attention or be unable to tolerate the wait until their scheduled appoint time. A feeling of caring can be communicated by receptionists who are sensitive to patient needs.

Patients also draw conclusions about the caring attitude of the staff based on the dress and grooming of receptionists, the willingness of receptionists to maintain eye contact as opposed to paper contact alone, the age and condition of the magazines, the availability of coffee service or cafeteria access, the ease with which cars can be parked, and a great number of other factors, all of which contribute to the ambience of the facility and the patient's perception of it. Larger practices, for example, should seriously consider having attendants at the door to assist patients who are being dropped off and need wheelchair assistance or help with belongings. Clinics with remote parking structures should consider adopting valet parking.

The appropriate ambience in the group's main facility may differ from that in a satellite clinic serving a different population. Some patients, for example, may consider visiting the physician to be a social activity and find waiting rooms that are conducive to easy interpersonal communications most attractive. Other patients may feel uncomfortable with close physical proximity and desire more isolation and separateness in waiting rooms.

Decorating Issues

Like the frosting on a cake, the interior decor of a facility is very important, and it contributes a great deal to the ambience. Interior design consultants, in coordination with architects and owners, should work to establish the appropriate interior setting for the organization. There are a number of issues to consider in interior design. One is the choice of furniture. Owners may feel they can overlook patient comfort when selecting furniture and concentrate instead on the appearance of the furniture and how it fits into a lobby or exam room. However, owners should keep in mind that some patients (for example, those with bad backs) may have difficulty getting in and out of overstuffed couches or soft chairs that do not provide firm support or sufficient height.

The choice of colors can do much to soothe or agitate patients. Artwork also should be chosen with care. Physicians may select art work that appeals to them but not to patients. Generally, patients seem to prefer artwork that can be recognized as such.

The number of clinics built prior to the Americans with Disabilities Act that do not have accommodation for wheelchairs in restroom facilities is astounding. Adequate lighting levels for patients waiting in lobbies is still often overlooked. Drinking fountains, paper cup dispensers, restroom facilities, and other items need to be convenient for patients. They should also be addressed early so they are not add-ons and therefore aesthetically unappealing.

Equipping the Facility

Equipping the facility involves taking a careful inventory of existing equipment that might be moved into the new or remodeled facility and determining what to keep and what to discard. Careful attention to the budget is important at this point, because there is a tendency to overspend. Sometimes completely adequate items of equipment are discarded in the rush to start anew. The budgeting of the project includes not only construction of the facility but also appropriately equipping it, and the executive committee or board must always be aware of the total budget and not focus too much attention on just the building construction budget.

Equipment lists should be prepared very carefully on a room-by-room basis and checked against the blueprints. Equipment should be categorized as to whether it is fixed or movable. Fixed equipment consists of items that are permanently attached to the walls and structure. Movable equipment are desks, chairs, exam tables, and countless other such items.

Equipment lists should be developed early in the project because of the time required for delivery and so that special power requirements, grounding, waste disposal, and protective shielding can be incorporated into the design. Lead time is also needed in order to categorize the equipment into types for purposes of bidding. Administrators should maximize the use of shared purchasing arrangements and other practices that can achieve substantial savings.

Regulatory Issues

Added costs and time delays of weeks, months, or even years can result from the actions of city, county, or state regulatory agencies. In some areas, in addition to the traditional plan check or building permit fee, mitigation fees and other charges can add substantially to the project costs. The administrator should have early conversations with consultants and representatives of all regulatory agencies that oversee the project in an effort to ascertain how these charges will affect the project's total cost.

Added time may be even more troublesome than added cost. The cause of delays in the regulatory review and approval process varies from community to community. In some instances, delay is due to concern on the part of neighborhood and citizen groups. In other instances, the regulatory agency has inadequate staff to handle the volume of applications. In yet other instances, jurisdictions use an application/hearing/permit process, which slows the approval process and limits new development. For example, one county may hold only two meetings a year during which applications for changing land use can be heard. It is likely that the agenda of the first meeting will be filled six months before the meeting is held, which means that a proposed project could be delayed for a year before approval to use the site—much less approval to build—is granted. As with added costs, the best an administrator in charge of a project can hope for is early detection of problems that may cause delays so their impact can be minimized and planned for.

OPENING A FACILITY

As the time to open a new facility approaches, a different sort of management process must be put in motion. First, the timing of the move should be set well ahead of time, and professional staff and employees should be organized into groups to manage the many details that are necessary for a smooth transition into the new building with its new systems. Different teams may be used: one for constructing and completing the facility, another for planning the move. Overlapping membership on these teams is essential.

As the project nears completion, careful attention must be given to the details associated with finishing the project. All systems need to be checked, detailed sign-offs on the quality of the finished work must be received from the architect, and a multitude of other assignments must be listed and checked off from the master completion schedule.

Decisions must be made concerning advance publicity, such as whether to use brochures or other public relations pieces to announce the opening; and whether and when to hold an open house and how to communicate an open house to the public. Lead time is required if a new location is involved in order to notify patients of the change in location. New telephone numbers or new listings in telephone directories must be provided months ahead of the time when the new numbers are to be activated.

The purpose of this recitation is not to provide a list of all the events that must take place when opening a new facility, but to convey to the reader how complex the process is. Physicians or administrators involved in the process of opening a new facility might benefit greatly from the lessons learned by other administrators who have already gone through this process. It may be very helpful to spend time interviewing such individuals.

Final Preparations

The date of occupying a new facility should be established conservatively in anticipation of delays. Final building inspections must be undertaken before the facility can be occupied, and the architect must finish the final checklist to assure that all construction details have been completed satisfactorily. Window treatments and other furnishings must also be installed before the facility is ready to open for business.

When moving day arrives, furniture in an existing plant should already have been marked for its new location. Older furniture that needs refinishing before being moved into the new facility should be ready. Even if all the items are not ready, the basic equipment required for the physicians and other professionals to function must be operable before the facility opens.

Moving day should be scheduled to produce the least possible interruption of patient flow, because the continuation of patient activity is particularly important when a new facility is opening up and there are higher cash demands. As many of the furnishings as possible should be moved before the main move is undertaken to minimize the interruption of services. Well in advance of the move, lead staff personnel should become very familiar with the actual operation of the new building, including its electrical, communication, and transportation systems. Personnel and staff also must be alerted well in advance of the need for their involvement in the move. Administrators and managers in particular should be prepared to spend extra hours assuring that the move is accomplished with as little disruption as possible.

FACILITIES MAINTENANCE

Careful attention must be paid to the design of the building to assure that floors, bathrooms, and service facilities can be maintained easily. Colors for carpeting, walls, and upholstery should be carefully selected with ease of maintenance in mind. Very light or very dark colors and solid colors tend to require more maintenance to remain attractive than do intermediate colors and earth tones. It should be noted that graphics and special symbols painted on walls are costly to repaint.

Only limited variation in color and design should be used so that offices and exam rooms are easier to repaint or refurnish. Rooms should be color-coded and maintenance records should be kept, starting with the opening of a new facility.

Wooden parquet floors in elevators are easier to maintain than carpeting. Vinyl and other synthetic materials require less maintenance than cloth upholstery on furniture. These and dozens of other factors must be considered during the specification and construction phase. Although maintenance is not always a primary consideration, it is a factor that should be considered when making decisions. Carpeting in lobbies has an acoustic effect and creates a different ambience than hard finishes.

New facilities always should be designed with energy conservation in mind. Fluorescent lighting, carefully designed, can often produce as comfortable a feeling as incandescent lighting, which creates heat and is less efficient. The lighting over work areas needs to be bright, but not too bright. The location of lighting relative to work surfaces is important so that employees are not constantly working in their own shadows. Architects have been known to over-design lighting in reception

---

CASE STUDY 8–4

THE CASE OF THE BURNED-OUT LIGHT BULBS

Elizabeth S. McQueen, the clinic administrator of a 20-physician group practice located in upstate New York likes to get to work early. Each morning she visits the employee lounge for a cup of coffee and passes through a second-floor lobby area. Because early morning procedures are done on this floor, the first receptionist is already at work. Ms. McQueen notices on a number of occasions that, although the reception desk lights are always on at this time, there are only one or two fixtures lighted in the waiting area, so the patients are sitting in semidarkness.

She approaches the receptionist and asks whether the lights should not be turned on. The receptionist says that the bulbs in two of four lamps have been burned out for about 10 days, even though she has reported it to the maintenance head at least twice.

Case Discussion Question

1. Whose responsibility is it to ensure that the ambience of a reception room is maintained? How would you suggest that Elizabeth McQueen go about correcting the problem described above?

areas, which tends to overemphasize the difference between the patient's seating area and the receptionist's.

The smooth functioning of a practice depends on the accessibility of medical records, so the vertical or horizontal transportation system must be chosen very carefully. Administrators and practitioners who are part of the building committee should visit other installations personally to check on the degree of maintenance required with different systems, the effectiveness of the systems as perceived by current users, and other relevant factors. It is usually unwise to skimp on funds used for elevators or vertical and horizontal lift systems, because these are such critical support systems in a busy ambulatory setting.

Security

All facilities should operate with employee and patient security in mind. Fire alarm systems, smoke detectors, and other security equipment should be installed and maintained. Power outages can adversely affect laboratory specimens, cause substantial damage to linear accelerators, and create computer crashes that result in the loss of stored financial and clinical data. Thus, backup power generators may be essential.

Employees who work second or third shifts in ambulatory settings when very few people are around should be in a protected environment. Switchboard operators, for example, should be in an enclosed area where doors can be locked. External and internal night lighting should be considered with the safety of employees and patients in mind.

Fire and disaster plans should be prepared in writing, and fire drills should be conducted periodically. Top management must demonstrate visible support of these drills for them to be effective. Clinics that are attached to hospitals need to pay particular attention to fire protection systems. Although ambulatory patients can be removed easily from a hazardous area, hospital patients cannot. It is also the responsibility of the administrators to assure that fire doors are not locked or propped open, exit lights are replaced when burned out, and employees understand the need for security and safety. Internal security involves taking measures to protect employees' and patients' belongings from pilferage and theft.

Of growing concern in many urban settings is the security of parking areas. There are a variety of solutions depending upon the nature and extent of the problem. The most obvious is lighting. Some areas may need to be fenced or walled off from public access. The ultimate in secured parking is usually considered to be an enclosed, well-lit parking structure that is gated and guarded. An alternative is valet parking, which is often an economical solution where other security options are not practical.

Facility Touring

The management challenge is to assure an overall high level of maintenance of the structure. Many employees are job-focused and specialized. As such, many maintenance problems fall between the cracks because employees fail to observe and report burned-out light bulbs or other conditions that detract from the overall safety or appearance of the building. Administrators tend to become office bound, especially as day-to-day pressures grow. That is why regular facility touring is so important.

Touring the facility by administration involves viewing the whole environment and not concentrating on single aspects of it. As the administrator moves through the building, he or she should note its level of cleanliness, the adequacy of lighting, the condition of paint and fabrics, the overall impression made by employees' dress and grooming, and, most importantly, the nature of interrelationships among employees, patients, and professional staff.

It is important for the administrator to tour not just the building's public areas but also its service areas, including exam rooms and offices. Employee lounges especially should be monitored, because it is here that poor maintenance patterns are likely to occur first. If the employees' lounge is well maintained and employees cooperate in helping to assure that the setting is clean, their pride in their surroundings will carry over into their work environment. If, on the other hand, management ignores these areas, it is difficult to expect employees to care much about their working environment.

Much can be learned by simply observing the interactions between the various parties occupying an area. It is not the responsibility of the administrator to intervene personally in any problems. However, the administrator can demonstrate leadership by being on the look out for problems and bringing them to the atten-tion of supervisors, who may be too specialized or busy to view the whole picture.

More experienced administrators should demon-strate to less experienced administrators the building-touring process. They are designed to remind employees and supervisors of problem areas and to serve as a con-tinuing maintenance audits. Administrators should also set examples in building maintenance.

CHAPTER

Communication Systems within a Medical Practice

Deborah Duncan and Jeffrey B. Milburn

LEARNING OBJECTIVES

Upon completing this chapter, the reader should be able to:

- Describe different types of telephone systems and their features
- Identify personnel needs and explain the necessity of physician-approved protocols
- Describe the scheduling needs of a practice
- Distinguish between manual and automated scheduling systems
- Explain the importance of scheduling policies and procedures

Good communication is critical to quality patient care. An effective communication system complements and supports all aspects of a successful practice operation. A practice must have the ability to exchange information effectively, and this requires appropriate staffing, training, equipment, and procedures. Because verbal communication generally is the fastest and the most cost-effective type of communication, this chapter addresses the systems, equipment, and procedures that support verbal communication in a medical practice.

The telephone system is the cornerstone of a practice's communication channels, and the analysis and choice of a telephone system and its features are extremely important. A major objective of this chapter is to give the reader an overview of the components of an effective telephone system. The balance of the chapter addresses verbal communications that are supported by the phone system but that are also dependent upon adequate staffing, training, and procedures. These communication systems include patient scheduling, phone-answering procedures, nurse triaging, and delivery of medical information.

Medical practitioners should be familiar with the various communication systems used in practices and understand the need for adequate equipment, trained staff, and comprehensive procedures that support patient care delivery functions. The case studies in this chapter give the reader an opportunity to use this information to solve typical problems in practice management.

TELEPHONE COMMUNICATION SYSTEMS

The telephone communication, or telecommunication, system is a primary component of any successful medical practice. It supports the communication needs of the practice in the same way that the computer system supports the information needs of management. An effective telephone system facilitates communication for physicians, patients, and staff, and supports a well-functioning working environment in which quality medical care and service can be provided. The well-planned system improves employee efficiency and provides better patient service. A poorly functioning telephone system, in contrast, cannot support quality care. It also creates frustration for everyone using the system, projects a poor image, wastes time, and is a source of endless complaints. Excessive hold times, busy signals, and call-routing problems are frustrating to patients, physicians, staff, and outside referring physicians and are barriers to effective, quality medical care. Especially in today's environment of cost effectiveness and provider efficiency, it is imperative that the telephone communication system functions effectively.

Physicians have the responsibility to be accessible to their patients. Ultimately, it is the responsibility of the physician to assure that the telephone system is functioning properly. Physicians have been subject to disciplinary action because of inaccessibility and failure to respond to the needs of patients. This liability creates another imperative for operating an effective telephone communication system.

A telephone system is a combination of people and equipment that is adequate to serve the communication needs of the organization, as illustrated in Figure 9–1. For a telephone system to function at the optimal level, necessary equipment and adequate staffing must be provided to process the volume of calls needed to serve the patients of the practice. Appropriate selection of the telephone system, as well as appropriate design of the operational system (staffing and protocols), are necessary to assure successful practice communications. The remainder of this part of the chapter is meant to help guide the health care administrator in the selection and

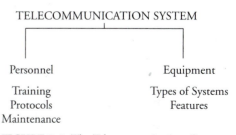

FIGURE 9–1 The Telecommunications System

implementation of an effective telephone communication system.

Staffing

Staffing is key to the development and implementation of a successful telephone system. Staff members should be thoroughly familiar with system features as well as with the telephone image the practice wishes to convey. The first contact a patient has with a practice should convey an image of a competent, caring staff. Patient satisfaction is the primary responsibility of each and every staff member in the practice. The expectation for performance in a staff member is courteous and friendly behavior while performing job duties effectively and efficiently. The practice exists to serve patients, and they must always be treated with courtesy and respect. Emphasis on both system features and communication styles allows the equipment and staff to complement each other toward this end.

Communication styles are an important factor in an office staff training program. Often training time is allotted to explain the mechanical features of a telephone system but not the verbal communication styles the staff should use. The ability to communicate effectively helps provide patient satisfaction (Jones, 1990). Ineffective communication leaves patients feeling angry and frustrated, and they carry away a perception of lack of service and support. The office staff should understand that the success of the practice depends on quality customer service. A professional image from the office staff gives the patient confidence in the ability of the staff to provide adequate access to the necessary medical care. For example, patients appreciate the efforts of staff to accommodate scheduling and information needs that are presented in the telephone encounter.

The volume of calls coming into a practice is a critical determinant of the design of the telecommunication system. Adequate staff as well as equipment are necessary to process the volume of calls in a timely and efficient manner. Both the number of physicians and the volume of patient calls should be reviewed in the analysis of appropriate staffing needs. Survey data from the Medical Group Management Association

(MGMA) can be utilized to analyze practice staffing and compare it to staffing in similar practices. MGMA produces annual statistics of participating medical practices concerning practice procedures and costs, including physician compensation and production and management compensation, for both private and academic practices.

Appropriate additional staffing may consist of part-time employees or employees cross-trained to cover telephone lines during peak times for incoming calls. Often, peak calling times are low-volume periods for other departments. For example, medical assistants may be able to help cover telephone lines during an early morning peak calling time while waiting for the physician to arrive. Part-time employees may provide flexible coverage for peak calling times as well as coverage for sick time and vacation time of regular staff. The most expensive equipment will not be cost effective if it is not supported by the appropriate number of adequately trained staff.

Protocols

In addition to adequate staffing, protocols for answering telephone calls are important to the flow of information. Every practice needs written policies and protocols for routing callers and messages. Items that should be addressed in such a protocol are listed in Table 9–1 and

TABLE 9–1 Items To Be Addressed in a Protocol for Answering Telephone Calls

1. ALL Telephone Calls
   a) Answered with desired greeting
   b) Initial request of caller noted
2. Emergency Calls
   a) Transferred directly to nursing personnel/physician
   b) Never placed on hold or told to call back
3. Calls from hospitals
4. Calls from other physicians
5. Calls to schedule appointments
6. Calls from patients requesting medical information
7. Business office/billing inquiry calls
8. Personal calls

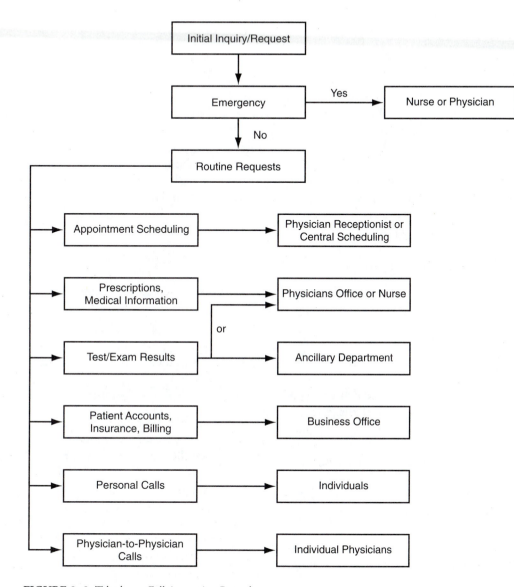

FIGURE 9–2 Telephone Call Answering Procedures

shown schematically in Figure 9–2. A written protocol also supports training for new employees. The plan should address who is to answer medical and nonmedical questions, how patients are to be scheduled, how messages for physicians and staff are to be handled, when physicians should be interrupted, what constitutes an emergency, and how personal calls are to be handled. A

telephone triage system, addressed later in this chapter, should also be part of the plan for routing callers.

Telephone Triage and Medical Advice

Because communication with the patient is critical, telephone nurse triage/medical advice systems to support

---

CASE STUDY 9-1

TELEPHONE STAFF ATTITUDES

Suzanne Jones has been a valuable and loyal employee of a growing medical practice for the past ten years. She is responsible for scheduling patients and has always had a warm, friendly manner with them. Patients have come to have confidence in her abilities. Due to increasing patient volume, however, Suzanne has become more irritable at work. She has been interacting with patients in an abrupt manner, and patients have been complaining about the lack of service in the practice. Suzanne is aware of patient complaints but seems to be unable to adapt her work practices to the increasing patient volume. With the growing number of complaints, the stress for Suzanne continues to grow. The physicians are complaining that something must be done about Suzanne's attitude and the way she treats patients.

Case Discussion Question

1. How would you analyze this situation? What solution would you recommend?

---

patient communications are becoming more common in medical practices. Almost every nurse practices telephone nursing by answering questions and delivering information from the physician. Successful triage/advice systems include written protocols, thorough training, careful documentation, and quality assurance. Specifically, a nurse triage/advice system should include the following:[1]

- Physician-approved guidelines (protocols) for assessing, triaging, and referring patients
- Training and education for communication skills, ethical and legal issues, and distinguishing among emergent, urgent, and nonurgent problems
- Organizational support for clinical consults, policies, and procedures
- Procedures and forms for documentation of calls (see Figure 9–3)

- Quality assurance monitors to assure proper standards of care
- Adequate telephone equipment and work space

A structured system with policies and protocols for nurses provides better telephone care to patients and helps reduce the risk of physician malpractice suits by providing quick identification of problems or education to patients about their condition and care. Telephone nursing systems can deliver high-quality, cost-effective care by decreasing the use of emergency rooms for nonemergent care, increasing accessibility to the practice, matching patients with appropriate physician/provider services, and increasing patient satisfaction through quicker response times (Conklin, 1994). The telephone triage system also greatly enhances physician efficiency by eliminating unnecessary telephone calls and allowing time to be spent more productively.

A telephone triage/advice system must operate with policies and protocols to assure the consistency of information provided. Using established protocols, the triage nurse can answer and resolve the majority of medical telephone calls coming into the practice. A sample protocol for assessing patients is shown in Figure 9–4.

[1]Reprinted with permission from Matherly, Sandra and Shannon Hodges, *Telephone Nursing: The Process.* The Center for Research in Ambulatory Health Care Administration, 104 Inverness Terrace East, Englewood, CO, 80112-5306; (303) 799-1111. Copyright 1992.

DATE _____   HOW HEARD: ☐ RADIO   ☐ PRINT AD

TIME _____   ☐ MD OFFICE   ☐ YELLOW PAGES

TIME RETURNED _____   ☐ BROCHURE   ☐ _____

PATIENT INFORMATION

PATIENT NAME_____ AGE_____ SEX: ☐ M ☐ F

PHONE: _____ (home) _____ (work)

ADDRESS _____ CITY _____ STATE_____ ZIP_____

CALLER NAME (if different) _____

RELATIONSHIP _____ REASON FOR CALL _____

PATIENT HISTORY

ALLERGIES _____

CHRONIC DISEASE _____

☐ PREGNANT? ☐ MEDICATIONS? _____

CURRENT PHYSICIAN _____ MD#_____

CHIEF COMPLAINT/REASON FOR CALL
(SOAP notes)

_____
_____
_____
_____
_____
_____
_____
_____
_____
_____
_____
_____

RECOMMENDATIONS

SIGNS/SYMPTOMS TO OBSERVE _____

HOME TREATMENT/TEACHING (diet, activity, etc.)_____

CALLER'S RESPONSE _____

FOLLOW-UP
(Note time and/or date after each item checked)

☐ ER REFERRAL _____   CONTACT PERSON _____

☐ HOME HEALTH REFERRAL _____   CONTACT PERSON _____

☐ ER PHYSICIAN NOTIFIED _____   ☐ CLIENT CALL BACK _____

☐ CLIENT TO CALL MD _____   ☐ NOC TO CALL MD _____

☐ NOC TO CALL _____   ☐ OTHER DATE_____

☐ PLACE IN MEDICAL RECORDS   ☐ HOLD IN OFFICE (release date _____)

FIGURE 9–3 Sample Form for Documentation of Telephone Calls

Specific Questions	*Disposition/Advice*

Emergent/Urgent Symptoms

Third Degree
- Absence of pain, loss of skin?
- Third degree in excess of 10% body surface?
- Third degree in excess of 3% body surface (child)?
- Third degree of face, hands, feet, or groin?
- Second degree in excess of 20% (child), 30% (adult)?
- White, dark, charred appearances?
- Degree, Percentage, Location, Complications, Age?

ED/MD in 0–2 Hours

- Immed. apply cool (not ice) water × 10 min
- Wrap in clean wet sheet or plastic wrap
- Transport to ED

Semi-Urgent Symptoms

Second Degree
- Red, mottled color, blisters, extreme pain?
- Facial, neck, genitals, hands, feet?
- Deep sunburn?
- Uncomplicated second degree of 10–20% (child)?
- "Moderate Burn" + High Risk Factor (Saved)?
- Age: 0–5 years, 60+ years = Thin skin, low immunity?

First Degree (Poss. fatal if 2/3 surface involved)?
- Degree, Percentage, Location, Complications, Age?
- Infectious process requiring antibiotics?
- Painful conditions requiring prescription drugs?
- Failure to improve after 48 hours on Antibiotic?

MD/Appt in 2–24 Hours

- Immed. apply cool (not ice) water × 10 min
- Wrap in clean wet sheet or plastic wrap

Routine Symptoms

First Degree
- Red, mild swelling, moderate pain, no blisters?
- Sunburn?

MD/Appt in 24 Hours to 2 Week

- Immed. apply cool (not ice) water × 10 min
- Remain at home and begin treatment
- Call back if symptoms become markedly worse or fail to improve with treatment within 48 hours

FIGURE 9–4 Sample Protocol for Assessing Burn Patients

Protocols must be well designed and comprehensive so that appropriate information can be delivered to the patient and necessary referrals made. The telephone nurse's roles and responsibilities are subject to various rules and regulations, but may include gathering information, assessing severity and urgency of the problem, developing a plan of action, identifying appropriate resources, giving the patient criteria to evaluate the outcomes of his or her actions, and documenting the call (Matherly & Hodges, 1990).

Telephone Systems Equipment

Functional equipment is a critical component of a successful telecommunication system. The equipment must support the needs of the practice, so its selection demands an adequate investment of time and money to assure that the right choice is made. A survey of the staff prior to reviewing the system can identify the needs of the personnel who work with the existing system. A sample survey questionnaire is shown in Figure 9–5. Time, energy, and money can be saved through the selection of a system that adequately meets the demands of the practice not only for today but also for the foreseeable future.

When choosing a telephone vendor, installation, training, and maintenance are critical issues. The ongoing service the vendor provides can make the difference between a successful or failed system. It may be beneficial to employ a telephone system consultant as an independent party to provide support in the

Questionnaire for Staff
Assessment of Telephone Needs

	Don't Know	Never	Seldom	Sometimes	Usually	Always
1. Do people ever mention that they get a busy signal when they try to call the practice?	_____	_____	_____	_____	_____	_____
2. Do callers ever mention that they had to wait too long on "hold"?	_____	_____	_____	_____	_____	_____
3. Should your department be able to receive outside calls directly, without going through the switchboard?	_____	_____	_____	_____	_____	_____
4. If adequate staffing is available, would it ever help if there were more lines in your area?	_____	_____	_____	_____	_____	_____
5. How often does it happen that calls you receive have already been transferred once or more than once?	_____	_____	_____	_____	_____	_____
6. How often do urgent calls to or from a hospital *not* get through quickly enough?	_____	_____	_____	_____	_____	_____
7. Are there times when you could make good use of an intercom line to some person or office not now connected to your phone?	_____	_____	_____	_____	_____	_____
8. If you now have an intercom line, how often do you use it?	_____	_____	_____	_____	_____	_____
9. Do you ever have need for a hands-free phone?	_____	_____	_____	_____	_____	_____
10. How often do you need a speakerphone?	_____	_____	_____	_____	_____	_____

Other Comments: _____

FIGURE 9–5 Telephone Assessment Instrument

selection process. The telephone consultant not only can provide initial advice but also can assist with ongoing system operation issues. The expertise of the consultant helps the practice utilize current technology in the most cost-effective and efficient way.

The true cost of a system includes the cost of equipment, service and maintenance, and staff training, plus any savings realized from implementing additional features. A system with advanced features often can expand employee productivity and help control overhead costs by increasing efficiency. However, the cost of a sys-

tem also increases with its complexity and the number of advanced features. The appropriate cost is determined through a cost-benefit analysis of the system's ability to meet the needs of the practice. Caution should be utilized not to overbuy or underbuy a system. With the speed of changes in technology, however, a system must be reviewed for its ability to be expanded and upgraded as necessary. For example, any system should have the ability to expand with additional equipment, lines, and features. Sometimes it may be necessary to overbuy to anticipate growth.

Types of Systems

The following, in order of complexity, are the basic types of telephone systems: two-line systems, key service unit systems, key systems, private branch exchange systems, hybrid systems, and computer-telephone integrated systems.

Two-line systems use a standard telephone with two phone lines. Pressing a key allows the selection of a line. Calls can be placed on hold and picked up at another extension. This system usually is used in small offices.

In key service unit (KSU) systems, all features are operated within each individual telephone set, and the telephones are wired together. An attendant is not required with this system, and it does not require a central processing unit. It accommodates two to three incoming lines with up to six extensions, but it has limited capabilities for expansion.

Key systems are used in small-to-medium offices with five to fifty users, and they may have the capability to expand to up to a hundred users. Key systems require a central processing unit with extensions for each user. Calls on hold can be picked up by any extension. Each user must have a feature telephone set that displays all extensions. A feature telephone has special keys for each line and feature.

Private branch exchange (PBX) systems require an attendant to answer all incoming calls and to transfer each call to the appropriate extension. To obtain an outgoing line, the caller must press nine. PBX systems are used in large offices.

Hybrid systems have features of both key systems and PBX systems, but they are usually based on key systems. As noted above, key systems require feature telephones that display all extensions, whereas PBX systems can use single-line telephones at extensions. The hybrid system can save money by not requiring each extension to have the more expensive feature telephone.

Computer-telephone integrated systems allow an interface between computer and telephone systems and the sharing of information between them. At present, this technology is new and used only in limited situations.

Telephone Lines

Every practice should designate phone lines and numbers for both incoming and outgoing calls. For incoming calls, one line should be designated as the main number, and additional lines should roll over from the main number. In larger practices there may also be separate lines for each department. This allows callers to either dial directly to the department or dial the main number first and then request the department. These features of incoming telephone lines are shown schematically in Figure 9–6. Lines for outgoing calls should have unpublished numbers to assure adequate open lines for outgoing calls.

Telephone System Features

There are many different features available for telephone systems. These features should be reviewed when selecting a new system or upgrading an old system to be sure that the features selected are right for the practice. Some practices are not aware of and do not use all the operational and cost-saving features available with their telephone systems. The following features may be helpful in increasing productivity and processing calls more efficiently (Matherly & Hodges, 1992; "Phone Systems," 1994):

- The hands-free feature allows a person to hear the dial tone, ringing, and busy signal and to hold a conversation without lifting the receiver; must be used selectively to avoid problems with confidentiality and background noise
- The speed dial feature allows frequently called numbers to be preprogrammed into the unit or system so they can be dialed automatically by entering a short code number or pushing one button; beneficial for frequently called numbers, such as physician pagers, physicians' homes, hospitals, pharmacies, and referral physicians
- The conference call feature allows more than two parties at different locations to participate in a call; useful in an variety of situations
- The call pick-up feature allows other telephone lines to be answered from a nearby location; provides back-up answering capability

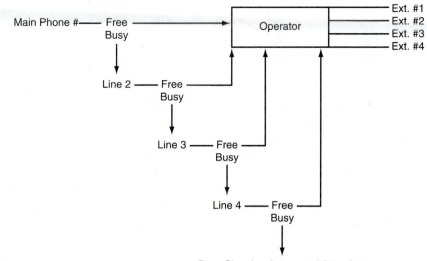

Callers dial main published telephone number; incoming calls roll over to free lines, are attended by operator, then routed to internal extensions by operator.

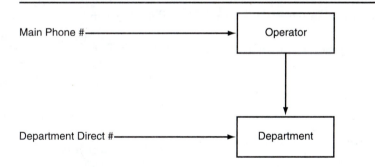

Callers may connect with a department by dialing the main published number or the department's direct number.

FIGURE 9–6 Features of Incoming Telephone Lines

• The call forwarding feature allows calls to one telephone number to be forwarded automatically to another location; used by practices to transfer calls to the main number to the answering service or to transfer calls from one extension to another internally

• The call hold feature allows calls to be placed on hold and then picked up again at the same location or from another telephone extension

• The call transfer feature allows calls to be transferred to another line or extension by entering the target number

• The voice paging feature allows paging to be done from phone units; serves as an intercom through the office so may risk confidentiality

• The busy lampfield feature allows the operator to identify which lines and extensions are in use and to offer alternatives to incoming callers

- The automatic privacy feature assures that calls cannot be picked up by another extension
- The distinctive ringing feature allows for distinctive rings to distinguish between internal calls and external calls
- The automated voice messaging feature allows recorded messages to be sent automatically by telephone; often used for reminding patients of appointments
- The automatic call distribution feature allows the caller to hear a recorded message and then press a number to send the call to the appropriate extension; helps keep callers from being placed on hold and reduces staff costs
- The music or messages on hold feature plays music or messages to callers on hold and allows callers to know the line has not been disconnected and they are still on hold; may make hold time more pleasurable and beneficial
- The long-distance lockout feature allows long-distance calling only from designated phones; valuable when courtesy telephones are placed in patient waiting areas
- The queuing feature holds calls in the order in which they are received; allows calls to be answered in order and reduces hold time
- The voice mail feature allows calls to be received and messages stored when no one is available to take them

Some of these features are described in greater detail below.

Automated Voice Messaging

Appointment reminder calls decrease the no-show rate for appointments. This can improve practice productivity and also reduce the risk of liability for lack of follow-up care. Manual reminder telephone calls are labor intensive. Through the use of an automated voice messaging system, a large volume of calls can be made with minimal staff. Thus, primary advantages of automated message systems are reduced no-show rates for appointments and decreased staff time needed for appointment reminder calls.

An automated message system can also be used to remind patients to bring the necessary insurance information with them to their appointments. This is an important feature for the confirmation of insurance eligibility or the authorization of incoming referrals. In addition, automated messaging systems can be used to convey preventive care reminders and information. It should be noted that patient satisfaction increases with thoughtful, well-designed, and timely messages.

The cost of an automated message system includes the cost of the system itself plus the costs of maintenance, local phone charges, and staff time. Cost recovery for an automated message system can be estimated by measuring lost revenue or loss of physician clinical time because of missed appointments. Patient volume determines the cost recovery time.

The following features should be evaluated when selecting an automated voice messaging system (Von Tanke & Morrow, 1994):

- Ease of use and learning (initial and ongoing training support should be provided)
- Flexibility of system (system should be able to change messages and create new messages quickly)
- Costs of expanding and upgrading the system (costs should be relatively inexpensive)
- Upgradability (vendor should guarantee upgrades for several years)
- Integration with existing information systems (electronic record transfer to and from the messaging system should be automated)
- Voice quality (speech quality should be high)
- Control of call processing (system should be able to control different answering options such as answering machines)
- Call log reports of calls generated and their outcome (these should be available)

Voice Mail

In a medical office it is advantageous to have an operator/receptionist answering calls during office hours. This provides the personal contact patients want and need for answering their questions or receiving necessary information. A receptionist who is caring, informed, and competent can direct the patient to the

---

CASE STUDY 9-2

UPDATING TELEPHONE SYSTEMS

Over the past two years, a busy family practice has recruited three new physicians who have an excellent reputation in the community, the practice continues to grow, and the volume of telephone calls has increased. Patients have started complaining about the constant busy signals they receive and the number of times they are placed on hold. Frustration continues to increase for the patients, staff, and physicians. The telephone system was upgraded five years ago. Features of the present system that the staff uses include calls on hold, call transfer, and intercom paging. The front desk has three telephones for five staff members. The nursing staff must use the telephone in the laboratory. Business office personnel feel they could use another telephone, and the physicians are worried about the increasing level of patient complaints.

Case Discussion Questions

1. What steps should be taken to identify specific problems in this practice's telephone system?
2. What recommendations should be made for a more effective and efficient system?

---

proper person to resolve the issues. Unfortunately, it is not always feasible to have the operator/receptionist spend adequate time with every caller. Voice mail, which receives and stores a message from the caller, can enhance the ability of the operator/receptionist to respond to individual callers and significantly reduce the time necessary to process each call. If the appropriate staff member is not available, the caller can be transferred into voice mail to leave a message. Thus, voice mail allows the receptionist to answer more calls, leading to greater satisfaction, efficiency, and a balance between cost and service.

The long-term benefit of processing a higher volume of calls can offset the initial expense of a voice mail system. A cost-benefit analysis shows the length of time necessary to cover the initial investment. As with any decision to purchase equipment, it is important to choose a reputable vendor. Reliability of the equipment, maintenance of the system, and training of staff also should be factors in the decision-making process.

Systems vary in options and limitations, but several features are considered standard in most systems. These features should be considered in the selection of a voice mail system. Mailboxes, for example, can be used as storage units for individual extensions to receive messages. Mailboxes might be established for designated people within the organization, pharmacy calls, business office calls, or other special designations. A password or code for each mailbox ensures confidentiality for the caller. Primary/secondary call handling allows the choice of having calls answered first by the mailbox or having the mailbox answer calls only if the operator is not available. Call storage allows messages to be saved on request of the owner of the mailbox.

Voice mail provides cost-effectiveness, accuracy, and reliability. Cost savings occur when fewer people process more calls. Accuracy occurs in retrieval of the actual message of the caller, and reliability occurs in the consistency of handling every call. Voice mail also can be convenient to the caller by allowing messages to be left day or night from any location. Staff time can be saved by not taking messages but transferring the caller directly into the voice mail of the person receiving the call.

When the decision has been made to install a voice mail system, the process of informing employees and patients is important. The system's advantages as well as its potential problems should be discussed and explored. Advantages of the system, specified above, should be explained to build enthusiasm for everyone using the voice mail system. Possible disadvantages, including equipment failure, patient dissatisfaction, and training time, should be reviewed and plans should be made to address each issue. Training sessions for staff provide the opportunity to test the advantages of the system and to address its disadvantages. Training also allows staff to be in a better position to explain the system to patients. Despite its advantages, some patients are not comfortable using voice mail. Therefore, callers should have the option to transfer out of voice mail to the operator.

Message on Hold

The goal of practices should be to minimize the hold time for their patients. Despite the best intentions of staff, patients are sometimes left on hold longer than the practice realizes, and the time on hold can be a source of frustration for patients. This can be mitigated by providing patients with information while they are holding. The information may be beneficial to them, and it also reassures them that they have not been disconnected.

Message-on-hold systems can provide an audio cassette or digital voice communication setup that is linked with the telephone system. Common messages include educational information, information on featured services or personnel, practice information, public relations announcements, and entertainment. Professional studios can produce a set of messages that features the information the practice wants its patients to receive. These messages provide an opportunity to create interest in a new provider or new service, provide information on the practice location and hours, create an understanding of the services provided, and furnish medical information and education.

Answering Service

Traditionally, medical practices have used answering services to answer calls after hours and on weekends when the office is closed. The answering service is instructed to answer calls with a given set of protocols. The primary advantage of an answering service is that it is a personal service. The answering service also has the responsibility of following up with the physician. If the physician does not return the page, then the service pages the physician again. If there is no response after the second page, the service may be instructed to page another physician. The personal contact and follow-up are critical components of the answering service.

An answering service must be able to provide reports logging the name of the caller, the telephone number, and the initial complaint. The time the physician was paged and the time the physician answered the page also should be logged. In addition to providing management information, these reports provide the required documentation for liability protection for the physician.

The primary disadvantage of an answering service is its cost. Answering services use various methods to charge their clients for the service. Some charge an all-inclusive flat fee, and others charge per call. A management reporting feature, which assesses call activity, may be charged separately or as part of the overall fee. The fee structure may affect practices differently, depending on the volume of their after-hour calls. Other disadvantages of an answering service include operators who occasionally take incorrect information, deliver inaccurate messages, fail to follow protocols, or treat patients rudely. If the service is understaffed or experiencing a high volume of telephone calls, callers may be placed on hold for long periods of time.

In selecting an answering service, references from other physician offices should be checked. The interaction the service has with the physician is extremely important in the exchange of information. The ability of the service to update and maintain equipment directly affects the service's ability to respond to the needs of the practice and provide the telephone coverage necessary for continuity in and availability of patient care.

An answering service provides an important and necessary service to a medical practice. The advantages and disadvantages of this service should be reviewed in the overall context of the telephone communication system. The use of an answering service in conjunction

---

CASE STUDY 9-3

AUTOMATED SYSTEMS

Changes in the delivery of health care are increasing the need for more support for home care and instruction to the patient. In addition, patients are being discharged from the hospital sooner with more medical care needs at home. This creates a need for greater monitoring to assure continued improvement and compliance with medical care.

An internal medicine practice, which has a patient base consisting primarily of elderly people, has experienced an increase in the volume of telephone calls and is considering adding an automated attendant to help with patient phone calls. The practice also feels that voice mail would help relieve the receptionist and operators of some of the labor-intensive message taking. However, the practice is concerned with patient reaction and satisfaction, because the elderly are more likely to resist automation.

Case Discussion Questions

1. Would you recommend an automated system for this practice? Why or why not?
2. How would you go about instituting automated features within this practice, considering its high elderly population.

---

with other telephone features may provide the most reliable, cost-effective solution.

System Management Reports

For the initial assessment of the telephone communication system, the telephone company can provide reports on utilization. The telephone company can also interpret the reports and make recommendations regarding the number of lines needed and the type of equipment necessary.

Many internal phone systems also have the ability to generate reports. Management reports generated as a function of the telephone system are helpful in determining the effectiveness and efficiency of the system. The reports provide data regarding the volume of calls, peak calling times, employee productivity, and market distribution, and they are extremely important in accessing the efficiency and adequacy of the system's equipment and staffing. Monitoring the volume of calls by time of day as well as by day of week helps practices maintain the ap-

propriate levels of staffing and assures adequate incoming line availability. Equipment enhancement or expansion may be necessary to meet the demands of increased patient volumes so it is extremely important to continually monitor the calls of the practice.

The reports described below are a sample of the information necessary to monitor the operation. Different systems may have additional standard reports and may be able to provide customized reports.

Busy Signal Reports

This report measures the number of incoming calls that receive busy signals. Callers who continually receive busy signals may become frustrated, and this can lead to loss of business for the practice. Frequent busy signals can also pose a liability in emergency situations, because open lines must be available for emergencies. Information from a busy signal report can help identify when and where additional staffing and/or equipment may be required.

Time on Hold Report

This report measures the length of time callers spend on hold. Most practices are aware that callers spend time on hold, but they are usually surprised by the frequency of holds and the length of time on hold. Time on hold is a major frustration for the caller and may be perceived as poor customer service. Excessive hold times can be a sign of inadequate staffing or equipment.

Time of Day Report

This report measures the number of incoming calls at designated intervals of the day. Physician practices usually experience peak calling times, and it is important to provide adequate staffing for them. Calls should be processed efficiently to minimize frustration for staff, physicians, and patients.

Calls per Day Report

This report measures the volume of calls for each day of the week. This allows management to adequately staff for peak days as well as peak times of day.

Number of Calls Processed

This report measures the number of calls processed by each extension. The ability to process a large volume of calls is dependent upon equipment, adequate training, and established protocols for staff.

Amount of Time on Each Call

This report measures the time employees spend on each call. The report can also be used in conjunction with telephone logs to identify the issues callers present to staff. Protocols that specify actions for different types of calls improve staff efficiency.

Market Analysis

Market analysis allows the practice to know where calls are initiated. It can provide information needed to identify locations that could be future service areas for the practice.

PATIENT SCHEDULING SYSTEM

A major part of a medical practice communication system is the patient scheduling system. The scheduling system is critical to the successful operation of the practice, because it allows patients access to the practice and contributes to the most efficient use of provider time and resources (Joshi, 1994). The process of making an appointment is generally the patient's initial communication with the practice, and this first impression may have a significant impact on the patient's perception of the quality of care received. This, in turn, may influence patient satisfaction, repeat visits, and referrals. In addition, the scheduling of patients has a significant impact on operational and financial issues within the practice. An effective patient scheduling system translates into smooth operations and financial solvency.

Effective patient scheduling optimizes the resource management equation, which involves the interaction of patient demand time, staff, equipment, and space (Matthier, 1995). All of these factors are related and dependent upon effective patient scheduling to assure smooth operations. If any one factor is out of balance, then practice efficiency is not optimized. The telephone communication system and the staffing priorities described earlier in this chapter are essential components of an effective scheduling system. Without this basic foundation, the scheduling system, no matter how well planned, cannot support the practice.

The purpose of this section of the chapter is to provide an overview of the patient scheduling function. The section includes the objectives of a well-functioning system, methods of analyzing the effectiveness of a system, and the various types of scheduling systems.

Scheduling System Objectives

As noted above, patient scheduling is a critical component of practice operations, patient satisfaction, and provider efficiency. The system must support the patient's needs and interactions with the medical practice, as well as complement the operational functioning of the practice.

The patient's initial contact with the practice is usually through the telephone system at the time an appointment is made. This process should be as easy as possible for the patient. Numerous rings before a phone line is answered, long hold times, repeated transfers, and an inability of staff to answer questions or provide service make it difficult for patients to access quality medical care. If the problem is compounded by difficult check-in, long waiting room waits, and a perception that a physician is overbooked, the patient may eventually look elsewhere for medical care. Patient satisfaction is a critical component in establishing long-term relationships with patients and payers who are concerned about quality. This makes it imperative to review and monitor patient care systems on a continuous basis.

Scheduling should balance patient demand to be seen with the available resources of time, staff, and facility capacity. A scheduling system that maintains this balance helps keep patients satisfied with the service. It also helps keep the staff operating in the most productive manner. The scheduling system also should allow for unanticipated or extraordinary events, such as no-shows, walk-ins, emergencies, and new patient registration. In addition, the scheduling system should enhance the functioning of the practice's operations by interacting automatically wherever possible with other relevant systems in the practice. Examples of these other systems include chart ordering and tracking, patient registration, and patient recall. All should be aligned with the appointment scheduling system.

A good scheduling system accommodates both providers and patients. It adjusts, to a reasonable degree, to different providers with individual schedules and practice styles, patients with different needs, and other variables, such as availability of resources. Simplicity and user friendliness for staff are also necessary for a truly effective and efficient scheduling system.

Scheduling System Analysis

The analysis of an existing or proposed patient scheduling system should be based on as much statistical data as possible but also must consider the multitude of subjective factors that always influence a practice. The analysis involves determining both patient demand and the practice's ability to meet that demand. A balance must be struck between patient needs and practice resources.

A medical practice needs to identify who the patients (customers) are and what their needs are. This is the demand side of the equation. To properly assess demand, data are needed on the number of patients that must be seen per hour, day, and week; peak demand periods each day, week, and year; and the amount of time per patient usually required for making appointments, check-in, waiting in both the waiting room and the exam room, provider visit, and check-out. All of these data are or can be available from prior scheduling records and/or time study surveys. Staff input is critical to the accuracy of the information. It is important to allow for the time it takes to prepare the patient for procedures and the time it takes the patient to undress and dress again. Keep in mind that some patients, including the disabled or elderly, may need more time than others.

The resource side of the equation includes staff and other resources. Data are needed on the number of patients physician(s) can (or will) see per hour. It should be assessed whether they see more or fewer patients, and whether this can be supported by staff. It also must be determined whether the number of staff is adequate and whether they are appropriately trained; and whether there is enough parking and waiting room and exam room space available to accommodate the patient visit load. Finally, it is important to know whether demand and/or capacity are fairly predictable. Again, staff input is valuable in assembling information.

The analysis should include a financial impact study of potential changes to determine whether the practice should continue with the current system. A practice analysis sometimes reveals how the physicians and practice can see more patients and produce more income. This may involve a cost in terms of staffing, equipment, or other additional resources. One way to measure the financial impact of a potential change is to determine the practice's patient-per-hour rate and convert this rate into dollars. The additional income expected, relative to any changes in costs, can then be determined. Not all system changes must lead to additional income or cost savings; sometimes a significant improvement in quality of care more than justifies a scheduling change.

To illustrate this method, assume a practice has one primary care physician with minimal hospital or surgical practice. The annual practice profit (physician income) equals $115,000. Annual practice hours are 1,296, and annual visits are 3,888. The profit per hour can be calculated as:

$$\frac{\text{Annual profit}}{\text{Annual hours}} = \frac{\$115,000}{1,296} = \$88.73$$

The number of visits per hour can be calculated as:

$$\frac{\text{Annual visits}}{\text{Annual hours}} = \frac{3,888}{1,296} = 3$$

The primary variables here (excluding patient fees) are the number of patients seen per hour, hours worked per day, or hours worked per year. Assume the analysis shows that the reason only three visits per hour are scheduled is that the number of exam rooms (two) is a constraining factor, and the physician frequently has to wait while a patient finishes dressing before the next patient can be put into the room. The administrator recommends that the physician's office be used as a combination office/exam room. This will increase the number of patients that can be seen per hour from three to four. This has a significant impact on physician annual income, or profit, with minimal increase in costs (primarily supplies) and no change in practice hours. The hourly profit increases from less than $90 per hour to $118 per hour, or 33 percent, and the annual profit increases from $115,000 to $152,000. This example shows how an analysis of patient scheduling, financial information, and resources can lead to a recommended operational change that results in a significant increase in practice profits.

Centralized and Decentralized Scheduling

The question of using centralized or decentralized scheduling has been debated since the formation of larger groups. Both methods have their pros and cons, and neither method is right for all practices. In some cases a practice may elect to use a combination of both systems.

In decentralized scheduling, the scheduler or receptionist works closely, usually at the location, with the physician and immediate support staff. This system is usually supported by a manual scheduling book, but it can function easily with a computerized system. The primary advantage of this type of scheduling is the close working relationship between the scheduler and provider unit. This allows providers to have total hands-on control of their scheduling activities, which some providers prefer. In decentralized scheduling, the scheduler also develops familiarity with the physician's patients and practice style. In some cases, the scheduler also performs other office duties at the point of patient service.

Centralized scheduling tends to be found in larger groups. In centralized scheduling, a small number of schedulers set appointments for all or most of the providers in the practice. These schedulers may be remote from the providers' locations and function essentially as telephone operators. Although not mandatory, a computerized scheduling system makes centralized scheduling much easier and more efficient. The primary benefit of centralized scheduling is its efficiency and lower cost. Presumably, a few schedulers taking calls in the order they are received for the entire group can handle more calls per hour than can schedulers working under the decentralized method. Analysis or actual experience is needed to confirm whether or not this is the case in specific practice situations.

A potential disadvantage of centralized scheduling is loss, to some degree, of the close working relationship between the scheduler and the provider unit and its patients. In practice, scheduling efficiency may be improved with centralized scheduling, but cost reductions may not be realized because receptionists are still needed at the point of patient service. On the other hand, relieving receptionists of scheduling duties may allow paperwork from the back office to be reassigned to the front office, thereby making the provider and nurse more effective.

There are many variables involved in deciding whether to choose centralized scheduling or decentralized scheduling, and the final decision should rest on an evaluation of both objective and subjective factors. It is important to remember that the individual

CASE STUDY 9–4

PHYSICIAN SCHEDULING AND WORKLOADS

A small family practice with three physicians in North Dakota recently hired a new manager, Beatrice Lane. The physicians want to know whether the three-way split of internal expenses and temporary help costs (to provide coverage when nursing and reception staff go on vacation throughout the year) is equitable. Beatrice has obtained the graph shown in Figure 9–7 from the patient scheduling system. The graph shows that one provider sees significantly more patients than the others and that the physicians see significantly fewer patients in the summer.

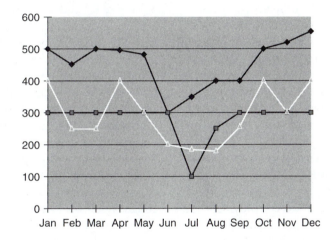

Figure 9–7 Patient Visits per Month, by Physician

Case Discussion Questions

1. Is it fair for the physicians to split all costs equally? If not, which costs should not be split equally? How should they be split?
2. If physician vacation plans don't coincide with staff plans, what are some options to consider? How does this impact patient needs? What are some questions you need to ask to obtain more information?

practice situation must again be considered in determining the feasibility of either system or a combination of the two systems.

Manual and Automated Systems

A manual scheduling system uses an appointment book to schedule patients for the provider. Staff members access the book and make entries manually. The system is fairly easy to operate and inexpensive, and it works well in relatively simple practice situations. Combined with the appropriate scheduling method, a manual system may be completely adequate for many practices.

Advantages of a manual appointment system include the ability to easily review previous or upcoming appointments which requires no added cost. Disadvantages include the ability of only one staff person to access the appointment book at any given time, the need to prepare management reports manually, illegible handwriting, and lack of interaction with other practice systems that are automated.

An automated, or computerized, system is more complicated and expensive initially, but it has considerably greater capacity and more features. This is important for practices growing in numbers of providers and locations. An automated scheduling system also allows multiple users to access the patient schedule at the same time, and it decreases the time needed to make an appointment. It can be used to schedule other facility resources as well as to manage complex, multiprovider scheduling system requirements.

An automated system can also be integrated with the patient demographic data bank so that each patient's medical record number, date of birth, address, phone number, and insurance information can be retrieved easily. This information is valuable for ordering patient charts, creating charge tickets, and printing appointment lists. In addition, an automated scheduling system can be tied to the patient billing system so that necessary insurance information, referral authorizations, or payment arrangements can be obtained.

Other benefits of an automated system include a diversity of features that can be set up to accommodate a wide variety of practice needs. Individual physician time schedules, practice styles, patient appointment types, procedures, and locations can all be managed with an automated system. A good system allows appointments to be made at remote locations with other providers and ancillary services. Also, linked appointments can be programmed for certain procedures that require a provider visit tied to other ancillary services. In addition, schedule changes, either provider- or patient-initiated, can be handled relatively easily.

The choice of an automated scheduling system, like the choice of a telephone system, requires adequate research. The system must be proven and references must be checked. Vendor reliability and ongoing support are critical. A good scheduling system should be user friendly, allowing for easy training and ongoing support. It should have the flexibility to interface with existing practice systems while allowing for different provider schedules and different appointment types. It should allow patient calls to be processed quickly. Computer screen design, screen step sequences, variable programming, and security are all factors that impact the function of a scheduling system.

As stated earlier, the practice setting helps determine the need for a manual or an automated system. An adequate system is critical to practice operations, so it is important to obtain the functional capacity that is needed and can be afforded.

Automated System Report Features

Health care is changing rapidly in terms of how standards and quality of care are defined. Medical legal responsibility is placing an ever-increasing burden on the practice to manage patient care, and patient follow-up is often the provider's responsibility. Reducing the numbers of canceled and missed appointments is important for follow-up and to prevent liability. An automated appointment system can be tied to the recall system to help providers track continuity of care and assure quality medical care for patients.

Health care changes have also increased the need for greater practice efficiency. If practice revenue is stagnant or declining, then operational efficiency is one place to look for additional profits. Adequate information is critical to the analysis of operational efficiency, and financial information is only part of the picture. How patients are scheduled is also likely to be important. An automated system can produce the management reports necessary for both quality of care and analysis of the production and efficiency of the practice. Some reports that an automated scheduling system might be able to provide include number of patient visits, type of patient visits, number of no-shows and cancellations, and appointment availability.

The number of patient visits report tracks the frequency of visits by practice, provider, or service, per hour, day, month, and year. This is done for analysis purposes, such as comparing productivity of providers or practices or tracking trends in patient volume to determine times at which more practice resources are needed.

The type of patient visits report can track scheduled visit type, diagnosis, and visit length. This information can be used to fine-tune a provider's individual schedule. Appointment slots can be established for specific types of patient visits in order to reduce unproductive waiting times for both physicians and patients.

The number of no-shows and cancellations often can be tracked by frequency and even by name. Patients who routinely do not show up for scheduled appointments can be counseled and eventually dismissed from the practice for noncompliance if necessary. A high number of no-shows may point to the need for an appointment reminder system.

The appointment availability report tracks the average length of time before patients can be seen by the different providers for various procedures. This information can be important for marketing and resource allocation purposes. Excessive waits for a nonurgent physician visit may drive away both new and long-term patients. Excessive waits for routine exams, such as ultrasound or mammography, may point to the need for additional equipment, alternate sources of care, or extended hours.

Scheduling Policies and Procedures

The number one complaint of patients is long waits to see physicians. Effective and efficient scheduling policies and procedures can help the practice plan for late patient arrivals, emergencies, walk-in patients, and urgent same-day care. In establishing an effective scheduling system, it is important to develop specific policies and procedures that are tailored to the practice situation. Other issues to include in establishing policies and procedures are individual physician hours and practice habits. A list of issues and situations that should be addressed by scheduling policies and procedures is given in Table 9–2.

Most efficient scheduling systems allot extra time for unexpected walk-ins; patients needing emergency, urgent, and same-day care; new patients; and other interruptions. Same-day appointment slots should be filled with the first request for an appointment to assure adequate availability throughout the day. This allows time for the provider to see all the patients who need to be seen that day and to fill up open slots later in the day. Excessive free time is very costly, but it is necessary to have some open slots for same-day care and emergencies. Previous experience is the best guide for establishing these openings. Typically, most medical practices have a high patient volume in the morning, a drop at lunch time, a slightly higher volume after 1 P.M., and another drop at 4 P.M. Increasingly, practices are experiencing patient demand for evening and Saturday appointments for both sick and routine care. This request

TABLE 9–2 Scheduling Policies and Procedures

Scheduling Policies and Procedures Should Address:
1. Confirming established appointments
2. Emergencies and walk-in patients
3. Urgent and same-day care
4. Answering patient questions, both medical and business
5. Obtaining insurance information
6. Obtaining referral information
7. Filling the earliest open slots
8. Changing appointments
9. Late arrivals
10. No-shows
11. Cancellations
12. Handling interruptions, both routine and nonroutine

should be explored by every practice to assess the needs of each particular patient population.

Finally, one part of the policy and procedure statement that is often neglected is the need for the scheduler to constantly keep the needs of the patient as top priority. The scheduler is often the first person to whom the patient talks; it is therefore imperative that the scheduler maintain and project a professional image. A scheduler with strong communication skills is necessary when interacting with people who are not feeling well and need to be treated courteously and efficiently. Patients always should be informed of any delays and the estimated length of the delay. When delays occur, an offer to reschedule the appointment should be extended.

Schedule Types

There is a variety of methods for scheduling patients. Individual scheduling, a traditional and easily managed system, allows a designated time slot for each individual patient. It is designed for minimal waiting time for the patient and allows for the appropriate length of time to address the patient's health concerns. Specific time slots by type of visit can be established, and the scheduler can be allowed to use judgment in filling these slots. For example, a physician may schedule the first 30 minutes of each hour for routine physicals or multiple-problem patients, the second 20 minutes for moderate or routine problems, and the final 10 minutes for one or two follow-up visits. This system is good for the patient because, when it is operating well, it reduces waiting time. However, it allows little flexibility for emergencies or visits that extend beyond the scheduled time. For these situations to be addressed in an individual scheduling system, open time for the provider must be included in the day's schedule.

In block scheduling, multiple patients are scheduled for the same time. Block scheduling reduces the risk of a provider waiting for a patient, but it usually results in longer wait times for patients. An example of block scheduling would be to have all morning patients scheduled at 9 A.M. The patients would be seen in the order of arrival. This type of scheduling can lead to patient dissatisfaction due to extended wait times.

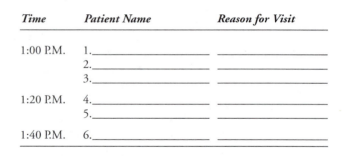

Time	Patient Name	Reason for Visit
1:00 P.M.	1._____	_____
	2._____	_____
	3._____	_____
1:20 P.M.	4._____	_____
	5._____	_____
1:40 P.M.	6._____	_____

FIGURE 9–8 Sample Modified Wave Schedule

A wave scheduling system counters this problem with a small built-in wait time for the patient—never more than 30 or 40 minutes. In wave scheduling, all visits are scheduled on the hour, and patients are seen in the order of check-in. This allows for the late arrival of a patient without it delaying the provider. A modified wave schedule might schedule three patients on the hour, two patients at 20 minutes after the hour, and one patient at 40 minutes after the hour, as shown in Figure 9–8. It is assumed that at least one of the patients scheduled for on the hour will arrive early or on time. It allows a small amount of flexibility for delays for some patients without inconveniencing other patients.

Some physicians establish certain days or blocks of time in a day to handle specific types of visits or procedures. One surgeon may establish Mondays for all surgical follow-up visits for procedures completed the preceding week. Another surgeon may schedule all of one type of office-based procedure for a specific day of the month so that the office staff needs to prepare for that procedure just one day a month.

COMMUNICATION SYSTEMS AND EFFICIENT PRACTICES

Communication systems within a medical practice are integral components of successful operations and efficient use of resources. Effective communication systems maintain patient, staff, and provider satisfaction. Telephone and scheduling systems provide the support necessary to access the practice and the care needed.

A telephone system operating at the optimal level assures proper communication between providers and patients. The successful combination of a telephone system's staff and equipment provides for smooth operational flow of communication. Adequate telephone system analysis is critical to system selection and ongoing monitoring of system effectiveness.

An effective patient scheduling system optimizes provider and staff efficiency as well as providing patient satisfaction. Balancing patient demand with practice resources assures the viability and success of the practice. Scheduling decisions concerning policies, schedule types, and the scheduling system should be made by each practice to balance the needs of patients with practice resources. An efficient scheduling system has significant impact on patients' perceptions of the quality of care that is provided.

Communications systems can be designed to perform only the basic tasks, or they can be enhanced to provide sophisticated management-reporting and analytical tools. Systems can be as simple or complex as the practice's situation demands, as long as they work efficiently and effectively and are managed appropriately. Successful systems are the result of careful planning, ongoing maintenance, and frequent fine-tuning to keep up with changing practice conditions. Adequate financial and planning resources are needed to assure that a practice's communication systems meet practice needs.

REFERENCES

The phone systems & voice processing. (1994). *What to buy for Business Series,* (Issue 9). Rye, NY: What to Buy, Inc.

Barnett, A.E. (Ed.) (1992). The telephone challenge: From costly nuisance to profitable tool. In *Ambulatory care management and practice.* Gaithersburg, MD: Aspen Publishing.

Conklin, M. (1994). Phone services help control patient demand, reducing unnecessary utilization. *Healthcare Strategic Management, 12*(6), 13–14.

Jones, C. (1990). Telephone etiquette. *Group Practice Journal, 39*(2), 51–53.

Joshi, M.S. (1994). Improving the appointment scheduling process: A national, multi-HMO benchmark initiative. *HMO Practice, 8*(4), 180–83.

Matherly, S. & Hodges, S. (1992). *Telephone nursing: The process.* Englewood, CO: Center for Research in Ambulatory Health Care Administration.

Matthier, F. (1995). A checklist for scheduling success. *Family Practice Management, 2*(1), 68, 71.

Von Tanke, E.L. & Morrow, D. (1994). Cost saving through automated voice messaging. *Group Practice Journal, 43*(2), 56–60.

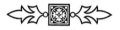

CHAPTER

10

Management Support Systems and Medical Records System Management

Bette A. Waddington

LEARNING OBJECTIVES

Upon completing this chapter, the reader should be able to:

- Discuss the processes basic to effective human resource staffing and management
- Explain the importance of developing practice standards by adapting policies and procedures to medical record information management systems
- Describe how to implement organized processes that deliver an efficient system for the appropriate management of the medical health information of the practice's patients
- Describe and discuss the significance of good customer service as it relates to health information management

A well organized medical records department of a group practice can efficiently manage patient flow, reduce malpractice risks, and provide accessible data to satisfy the information needs of the authorized medical records customer. The internal benefits of a well organized and managed medical records system include efficiencies in patient flow and staff and physician productivity, which result in patient satisfaction with the level of service and the response of staff and physicians to patient needs and wants. The practice also benefits financially through the appropriate use of human resources, especially given that personnel costs comprise the greatest expense for a medical group. Inefficiencies are often compensated for by overstaffing in medical records departments. Therefore, appropriate staffing and assignment of work functions, as well as the provision of tools needed for staff members to accomplish their assignments, can significantly reduce the costs of medical records departments.

Meeting the requirements for medical information from hospitals, patients, third-party payers, ancillary facilities, pharmacies, and consultants significantly improves the relationship between these customers and the practice and demonstrates the quality of the practice to those the practice serves.

This chapter presents criteria necessary for implementing efficient systems in a practice's medical records department. A case study that incorporates common problems in medical records departments is provided. It illustrates how to proceed with the reorganization of a medical records department.

PERSONNEL IN MEDICAL RECORDS

The personnel of the medical records department are key to the success of the department. Appropriate staffing and distribution of work, adequate policies and procedures for managing the record flow, and maintenance of positive morale are necessary for the overall success of the department. Distribution of work contributes to the efficient flow of medical records throughout the clinic. It also contributes to the most effective use of staff. Training and orientation are also important for employee success. How employees are developed, managed, and given incentives to perform to their maximum potential determines the success of the medical records department in providing medical information to physicians, nurses, receptionists, the business office, transcriptionists, patients, and outside entities requiring medical information.

Utilizing a certified medical records technician (with an associate degree in records technology or with a registered records technician certification) to manage the department establishes the foundation for monitoring and managing the department with professional and sociolegal influences that assure a well organized and efficiently run department. This person should have the knowledge and expertise to facilitate the development of a written set of guidelines for the management of medical records, to accommodate legal and ethical issues related to medical records, and to provide appropriate ongoing management of the department in an efficient, cost-effective manner. The guidelines will be implemented and applied most effectively when the medical records committee establishes, monitors, and maintains the guidelines and compliance with them.

Recruiting and Evaluating Staff

To begin the process of organizing the staff within the department, written job descriptions for all department employees should be prepared, identifying specific tasks and responsibilities. The job descriptions provide the basis for performance evaluations and the setting of performance objectives for each employee (Price, 1995). Job descriptions are also used when recruiting and hiring in order to attract individuals who meet the qualifications necessary to fill the positions successfully. Skill levels should be assessed through testing in spelling, penmanship, alphabetizing, numerical filing, and legal and ethical knowledge. Job recruits should be asked to demonstrate their skill levels during the interview by actually performing some of the required tasks, such as filing, typing, or spelling. If these guidelines are followed when recruiting and hiring, new employees will be more likely to be qualified, and whatever training they need will already have been assessed.

A formal, written evaluation should be used for all staff, and their input should be obtained in the establishment of performance objectives. Performance objectives should include but need not be limited to:

- Knowledge of legal and ethical issues, including records release
- Knowledge of transfer and release guidelines
- Knowledge of documentation requirements
- Knowledge of retention and termination laws and policies
- Possession of relevant skills, including ability to alphabetize, organizational skills, low error rate, optimal volume of work output, and careful attention to details

When employees are involved in establishing job performance objectives, they have more incentive to maintain quality performance. Using performance objectives also encourages consistency and excellence in performance. A sample performance evaluation tool is provided in the Appendix to this chapter.

Customers requiring medical records can provide valuable information to assist management with the decisions necessary to maintain quality in the management of medical records. Conducting periodic surveys of the department's customers regarding the department's efficiency, availability, and similar factors provides a tool for measuring the department's performance and for identifying deficiencies proactively, so they can be corrected before they cause problems. Customer surveys can also provide additional information for employee performance evaluations. Customer surveys should be conducted by the department supervisor regularly and consistently.

Orientation and Training

The orientation and training process should be put in writing, specifying who is responsible for training, how long training will last, and which functions will be part of the training program. It should be kept in mind that staff members with deficient performance are likely to pass on bad habits and inefficient methods to new employees if chosen to provide the training. The manual,

Medical Records: Policies and Guidelines (Liebler, 1990), can be used in developing an orientation and training program by providing topics for training. Another resource for training materials is the American Health Information Management Association.

Employees should be kept current through continuous medical record issues updates and through other means, including in-service training in the practice, provision of a library of resource information on medical records management, and outside educational programs. Often hospital medical records departments have training and educational seminars available to the staffs of affiliated practices.

Some topics bear repeating periodically, whereas others need to be reviewed only occasionally. In-house training on legal and ethical issues, documentation, patient rights, care planning, policy changes, regulation changes, and procedures and protocols for efficient management of the medical records improves the effectiveness of staff members and eliminates some of the frustrations that occur when employees want to perform well but fall short of customer expectations.

Employee Morale

Employee morale in medical records departments is often jeopardized by the actions and attitudes of physicians and employees outside the department. Often, frustration caused by the lack of immediate availability of records is directed at department employees, even though other systems in the practice may be responsible for the department's inability to respond to record requests. The facilitation of communication with other departments and with physicians can foster mutual understanding of one another's needs and limitations and lead to support, rather than criticism of department staff.

Department director meetings can be used as a forum in which to significantly influence the attitudes of employees of other departments toward the medical records staff. Department directors can, in turn, influence their employees' attitudes and behaviors toward medical record staff members by their own attitudes and their participation in cooperative management strategies with other department supervisors. Problem solving at the department director level is most effective in changing attitudes and establishing cooperation between departments. Involving key staff members in problem-solving meetings using a continuous quality improvement (CQI) approach provides the most effective mechanism for accomplishing this goal.

All clinic employees should be informed of the procedures and policies of the medical records department to facilitate better understanding of expectations in the management of medical records. This can be accomplished by preparing a list of general policies and reviewing them at a staff meeting. Items that should be addressed include patient information confidentiality, policies restricting access to the records room and records, and information transfer policies.

Numbers of Staff

Frequently, medical records departments are overstaffed due to their own inefficiency. Typically, more people are added to a department in response to demands and complaints regarding access to and availability of records. This overstaffing is necessary usually due to lack of effective policies regarding the use and movement of records and to lack of resources necessary to perform work functions effectively. Necessary resources include well-designed charts, appropriate filing systems, and use of the computer to monitor and track records or even to digitize the records.

Calculating a staffing ratio, by comparing one practice's department to departments in other practices, can provide a picture of a department's level of efficiency in work performance as well as justify the need for additional staff if inefficiencies are found to be due to understaffing. The MGMA *Cost Survey* and the *PEER* report from the Center for Research in Ambulatory Health Care (CRAHCA) can provide comparative data for this purpose.

Work Distribution

How work is distributed, responsibility delegated, and authority assigned significantly impact the efficient use of staff and contribute to the quality of staff performance. Work processes for the employees in the department should be organized according to primary work functions. Primary responsibilities should be assigned to individuals, with secondary tasks assigned as needed to help or fill in for absent or deluged employees. This helps assure continuity and improves the quality of job performance because the scope of responsibilities is narrowed,

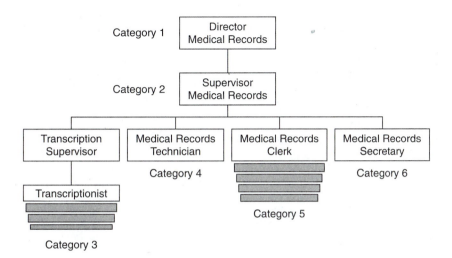

FIGURE 10–1 Organization Chart for a Medical Records Department: Job Categories

and this increases the likelihood of job success. Primary responsibilities to be assigned to the staff members in each of the job categories shown in Figure 10–1 include:

Category 1.   Managing the department, including planning, monitoring, and controlling department functions to assure compliance with policies, procedures, and regulations affecting medical records

Category 2.   Managing daily operations of the department, including managing staff and systems and processes management

Category 3.   Managing work functions of transcriptionists and assuring their compliance with all department policies and procedures

Category 4.   Managing mail handling and distribution and original chart requests; providing chart audits, abstracts, and reports; and managing the organization of information in medical records

Category 5.   Pulling, filing, locating, retrieving, and deleting records; logging requests; and maintaining an accurate filing system

Category 6.   Transferring clients, maintaining logs, managing and responding to information requests, typing, answering phones, and duplicating

POLICIES AND PROCEDURES

This section addresses the issues of documentation completeness, form, legibility, and uniformity. It also covers such areas as records transfer and release; information organization within the medical record; construction and assembly of the medical record; storage, retention, destruction, and purging of medical records; and legal and ethical issues.

Medical Records Committee

Each practice should establish a formal medical records committee that is responsible for the development of policies and procedures; management decisions related to the department; and ongoing monitoring, planning, and development. The committee will be most effective if there is representation from each department that has significant interactions with the medical records department. The medical records committee for a typical practice might consist of the following members:

- Two physicians
- Director of nursing
- Medical records supervisor
- Front office supervisor
- Assistant administrator

These individuals would be responsible for establishing policies and procedures for the department, directing decisions for reorganization, and acting as ongoing policy makers and advisors for the department. If a practice has not had a medical records committee previously, then the committee will need to meet more often at first to establish and implement policies. After the department begins to function efficiently, the number of meetings can be reduced.

Typical issues that require the committee's immediate attention might include:

- Removal of medical records from the clinic
- Individuals other than medical records staff pulling charts
- Dictation to be returned within 24 hours
- Mandatory dictation of all progress notes
- Standard and uniform organization of the information within the chart
- Holding of medical records in clinical areas
- Flow of ancillary test reports (these should go to the physician and then to medical records for filing)

Policies and Procedures Manual

A policies and procedures manual for the medical records department should be developed that specifies policies and procedures for managing patient records. Development of the manual provides an opportunity to scrutinize department processes and clarify the management process. The development of sound professional practice, conveyed through well written and enforced policies and procedures, contributes directly to high-quality patient care. *Medical Records: Policies and Guidelines* (Liebler, 1990) is an excellent resource for developing a department's unique set of policies. As the committee prepares written policies and procedures for the management of medical records and related department functions, the following items should be addressed:

- Records release guidelines based on state laws
- What information is subject to confidentiality compliance
- Who is responsible for legal implications
- Confidentiality statement signed by all employees (see sample in the Appendix of this chapter)
- Who is authorized to release records and how (for example, workers compensation, state health department, attorneys, family members)
- Who gives consent for treatment and how
- Court orders, subpoenas
- No financial information to be recorded on the chart
- Records transfer charge
- Time requirements to retrieve and return charts to filed status
- Where charts are stored for active/inactive status
- When charts are moved to inactive status, purged, terminated
- When and how charts are remade and who is responsible
- Definition of the format for information organization within the chart

Test Results

After the policy for releasing test results to patients has been defined, consistent procedure for communicating test results to patients should be implemented. One very efficient procedure is to place the results on voice mail and to provide each patient with a unique security code that allows access to test results. There are several computerized phone applications that accomplish this end and reduce the effort necessary to accomplish this function manually. As an alternative to the electronic notification of patients, a preprinted letter or postcard, listing common tests, can be completed and mailed to the patient. This eliminates the telephone tag that occurs when nurses and patients try to reach each other (see the ancil-

lary test report response form in the Appendix to this chapter). When an automated lab and X-ray requisition and response application is not available, nurses should be assigned to maintain a lab log when tests are ordered. This provides an audit trail of the returned results.

Records Control and Responsibility

Many times medical records departments yield to the demands of the most insistent personnel in the practice. When this occurs, efficient management of chart flow is jeopardized. Responsibility for the control and management of medical records must be placed entirely within the medical records department. To accomplish this, all reports must be filed in the patient chart in the medical records department after it comes back from the physician's office and has been signed off. This provides a mechanism for consistent management of the information within the chart and control of the location of charts to assure accessibility to all customers. Thus, all records should be sent back to the medical records department after the patient is seen, and they should no longer be held in clinical areas. Dictation, reports, consult letters, and similar communications should go to the physician. If the reports are positive or a medication has to be adjusted, a chart should be requested. If reports are negative, they are signed off and returned to the medical records department where they are filed in the patient's chart. This procedure greatly enhances the accessibility of records and eliminates massive redundancy in the record clerks' work efforts, as they spend significant amounts of their time searching for records.

All paper filing in the medical record should occur within the medical records department. This assures consistency and uniformity in a neat and orderly record, where information can be accessed quickly and easily by physicians.

All physicians should be required to dictate chart notes according to National Committee on Quality Assurance (NCQA) documentation standards. (A copy of the standards titled Chart Audit and Review Form is contained in the Appendix to this chapter.) Some physicians' chart notes place the practice and the physicians at high legal risk due to their illegibility. Contracts also depend on records quality. Managed care organizations and Medicare audit the records of participating providers. This audit is used as part of the decision process to allow physicians to remain on their panels; it also affects reimbursement if documentation does not support coding levels. Documentation can be simplified by the use of forced-choice forms and flow sheets when dictation is not used in the clinic. However, transcribing produces the most efficient and highest quality of documentation.

No personnel other than medical records department staff should be allowed to enter the medical records room and remove charts. Billing staff, nurses, and physicians must place requests for charts through the normal channel. Otherwise, charts are likely to be misplaced, which again leads to redundant work effort for record searches as well as frustration on the part of customers of the medical records department. Unauthorized access also provides the potential for breach of confidentiality of patient medical information.

Many practices overlook the importance of documenting educational materials given to patients. Providing educational and health care directives can be a significant risk management tool. A flow sheet in each chart can be used by the nurse to record information. A master list of all patient education materials should be kept on file for future reference. This list should be updated with new materials, although the original list should also be kept on file.

Most groups have a policy prohibiting removal of charts from the facility, although the policy may not be adhered to consistently. If charts are lost or not available to providers when patients present for treatment, it becomes a high-risk management issue. The extra effort on the part of staff members to search for missing charts is not efficient use of their time, and the inconvenience to patients when their charts are not available is poor customer service. The medical records committee should enforce the policy when physicians fail to comply. Some practices impose financial penalties or even withhold compensation checks to enforce compliance.

ASAP requests for medical records should be used only when records truly are needed within 30 minutes.

Repeated unnecessary ASAP requests can lead to slower response time as abuse of the requests is recognized. Ideally, there should be a 30-minute turnaround on ASAP chart requests. This may not be possible with all charts, but at least 85–90 percent of ASAP chart requests should have a 30-minute turnaround rate. With proper organization of work functions and appropriate policies and procedures, records will be delivered promptly, and overuse of ASAP requests will not be necessary to assure that charts are found in a reasonable amount of time.

A policy should be established that requires the chart to be pulled for abnormal results to evaluate previous conditions. This requires that all records be returned to the medical records room to be refiled and test results and transcription be sent to the physician to be reviewed and signed. Normal results should be returned to the medical records room to be filed in the patient's record. One or two individuals in the department should be assigned the responsibility of filing materials in the chart in the order set by the medical records committee for the standard organization of information in the chart.

There should also be a policy for chart termination, reconstruction, and purging of data. Accountability for these functions should be assigned to specific individuals to assure consistent, ongoing management of records. All medical records should be purged at three years to open space in the medical records room and to most effectively utilize storage space.

To assure consistency in the management of patient confidentiality, a confidentiality statement should be developed and signed by all employees. It should be signed annually and placed in each employee's personnel file. Infraction of the policy should result in immediate dismissal, and this should be stated in the personnel policy manual. A sample confidentiality statement is included in the Appendix. It could be expanded at the discretion of the medical records committee.

Compliance with all policies set for the medical records department will help assure the success of the records management system. To encourage compliance with policies, when charts are transferred without appropriate record-keeping, for example, the responsible individual must be held accountable.

RECORD AND INFORMATION MANAGEMENT

This section explains how the computer system can contribute to the efficient management of medical records. The purpose and use of forms, the management of information that goes into the patient's chart from outside sources, and the management of information within the medical record are also covered in this section.

Computer Tracking of Medical Records

A computerized chart-tracking system with bar-coding capabilities should be implemented. This provides concurrent location recording and tracking, which expedites the pulling and filing of charts and also provides a mechanism for interdepartmental transfer recording. In addition, it eliminates the redundant handwritten out-guides required in a manual system. The necessity of having requests taken by clerks is eliminated, because the requests are received electronically and printed out in the medical records department. These printed requests are then inserted into the out-guides when the chart is pulled and serve as documentation of the location of the chart in the chart rack. The chart-tracking system can be used to generate a report of record release requests. This monitors where patients are going who are leaving the practice and provides documentation of information released. Upon implementation of the chart-tracking system, in-service training for staff and physicians should be provided to facilitate the smooth transition to the new system and assure its success.

All medical records requests should come into the department via the electronic tracking system, which eliminates multiple locations and constitutes a record of requests, because requests are printed in the department. The file format of this system should include the name of the requesting physician as well as the name of the individual entering the request. Nurses need computer terminals at their stations in order to have access to the chart-requesting process.

Implementing an electronic appointment scheduler on the computer system is necessary to accommodate a chart-tracking system. The scheduler allows the track-

ing system to pull record requests from the scheduler, and this eliminates handwritten requests. An electronic scheduler also allows nurses to use terminals at their stations to schedule patients. Security levels can be placed on the scheduler to prevent inappropriate scheduling. Electronic scheduling allows anyone from any location in the practice to schedule patients, look up patient arrival status, and review changes in the day's schedule at a glance. It also allows the medical records clerks access to new patients so they can make up new charts ahead of the scheduled arrival, and it eliminates the need to search for records of patients who are not marked in the appointment book. Walk-in or same-day patients can be registered on the electronic scheduler, and their charts will be requested automatically in the medical records room, thus expediting the retrieval of the records for immediate care.

Purged Records Storage

CD ROM storage of purged medical records is one of the latest technologies that can decrease storage costs and provide immediate access to patient histories. This technology reduces the amount of space needed for storage and the cost of storage and retrieval. A data reader to scan records onto the disk can be leased rather than purchased. After the initial purge of records, the scanner can be rented once a year for two or three months to keep the purging current.

A consistent audit trail for purged charts can be established through the use of chart tracking on the system report generator. Purged charts should be logged consistently with the chart-tracking report generator. This eliminates the manual log.

Records Filing and Organizational Systems and Concerns

Terminal-digit labeling for medical charts is the best filing system in terms of accuracy, even work distribution, even distribution of charts in the filing racks, and ease in purging charts from the tracking system. In a terminal-digit filing system, a unique six-digit number is assigned to each patient. This number is then divided into three sets of two-digit numbers ranging from 00 to

99. The last two digits, or primary digits, are the first to be considered by the clerk when filing. Once the corresponding primary section is located, the middle two (secondary) digits are considered, followed by the first two (tertiary) digits. An example of terminal-digit sequencing is as follows:

17-10-52	05-20-52	47-00-53
47-10-52	77-20-52	02-13-53
62-10-52	40-00-53	02-14-53

It is necessary to implement electronic chart tracking in order to succeed with a terminal-digit filing system, because the filing system is needed to cross-check patients' names and their chart numbers. Chart vendors can supply charts with some of the digits preprinted on them, which helps to reduce the amount of time necessary to prepare new charts and to assure correct numbering.

During the conversion to terminal-digit labeling is an excellent time to convert the entire chart jacket to a heavier weight of paper, insert fasteners to secure the loose papers, and add information dividers. Vendors can supply jackets with preprinted numbering to reduce the amount of time required by staff to label them. Using the computer to print name and date-of-birth labels for medical records further reduces the labor needed to complete the chart by eliminating the need to hand type patient record labels. All papers in medical records should be secured with binder tabs. Loose papers increase the risk of losing important patient medical information. Binder tabs can also be placed by the vendor to eliminate manual effort in the practice.

A single chart should be maintained for each patient in the clinic to assure continuity and consistency in filing. A single chart also assures that physicians have access to all the medical information for each patient. All pieces of paper in the medical record must have patient identification on them, either name or account number, and date of birth. Some practices have a second chart for patients scheduled for executive physical or workmen's compensation. Duplicate records increase the risk of losing pertinent patient data.

Providing the appropriate number of computer terminals in the department is essential for efficient and effective use of staff work efforts. When staff have to wait in line to look up patients' record numbers, congestion occurs at the terminal and there is down time for staff. Waiting to use a computer terminal decreases efficiency and productivity.

Formatting the information in the chart in an organized system makes accessing the information easier. Formatting also helps prepare the clinic for future efficient management of information related to quality of care. In addition, it facilitates chart audits by managed-care organizations and Medicare. Using preprinted flow sheets on the internal chart dividers helps in the documentation and location of information related to medications, history, surgeries, immunizations, chronic problems, and/or other categories determined by the practice's medical records committee. Chronological filing of information within each divider category in the chart is the most efficient system for retrieving information and for purging data. The use of brightly colored allergy stickers on the outside of the medical record alert providers to potential medication problems. A list of specific allergies should be put in a prominent place in the chart where all providers can access the information quickly.

When converting to a chart system, it is useful to establish a conversion schedule. A predetermined number of established and current patients' charts should be converted each month by designated staff during a specified period of time each day. Purging of old data (as determined by the medical records committee) could also be done at this time. New patient charts could be added to the chart system as they present for their appointments.

With the advent of managed care and the establishment of documentation standards to meet NCQA standards, many practices now conduct regular random internal chart audits by qualified clinical staff (RNs) who are capable of reviewing quality assurance and utilization issues. They use a chart audit form and documentation standards from the NCQA, which are included in the chapter Appendix.

Integrating with the hospital's computer system—to provide electronic access to patient ancillary test results, write orders from the clinic, and review patient hospital records—leads to more efficient use of providers' time and satisfaction of patients' needs. There may be some computer system integration barriers, but these can usually be overcome with a little perseverance.

As previously indicated, it is essential to develop uniform policy on how and what is documented in the medical record. The use of forced-choice forms, flow charts, medication lists, problem lists, preprinted history/physical forms, and preprinted charts and graphs greatly reduces the amount of dictation required and provides convenient and immediate access to clinical information in the chart. Many chart vendors offer a variety of unique forms to fit every specialty. A consistent documentation format, when it is followed by all providers, provides good risk management as well as convenient access to information. Guidelines for documentation must be set by the medical records committee, with monitoring and control of the documentation process the responsibility of physicians on the committee. These steps are necessary to reach a practice-wide standard.

Telephone messages should be filed consistently in the chart, always using the same location and format. The Bibbero System has an excellent telephone message pad that is unique to medical practices. It can be hung on a note page or attached to the chart note with a sticky backing. Again, only one method should be selected and used consistently. The notes should be filed by medical assistants or nurses to eliminate the possibility of misplacing them and to reduce the time required to write in the chart.

Records Responsibility

A master list, with signature and initial lines and dates of implementation and termination should be created and used by all providers in the practice who document in the medical chart. The list can be used by the medical records department to assist in the recognition and verification of provider signatures. This provides a risk management tool for provider identification in the future, which is especially necessary when initials only are used to sign off on notes and orders and when the handwriting is illegible.

The authorization to release information should include all information, even sensitive information, that patients may not want to have transferred, such as HIV test results, substance abuse information, and psychi-

atric treatment notes. State laws regarding guidelines for the retention and transfer of HIV information must be consulted, because the regulations are state-specific. It may be necessary to store this information, including lab reports and other information related to HIV, in a location other than patients' charts.

Individuals responsible for acquiring medical record release forms, including receptionist, registration clerks, and nurses, must assure that all information is gathered on the form before transferring the request to the medical records department. The lack of proper information interrupts the transfer process and causes extra work for the medical records department staff.

Responsibility should be established in the medical records department for chart information management, including the purging of old information in charts and the organization of data in charts according to guidelines established by the medical records committee. This responsibility should be assigned to just one or two people to reduce the error rate caused by incorrect filing of data in patients' charts and to help achieve consistency in the management of the information in the records.

Electronic Systems Implementation

Implementation of an electronic medical record should be considered. This provides the most effective access to patient medical histories and improves efficiency in treating patients. The electronic record provides concurrent access to more clinical data for multiple providers. It also allows for data retrieval for clinical applications. For example, it can generate a report on all patients with a particular medical problem. As the industry moves toward implementation of requirements to report clinical outcomes, practices must be prepared to address information retrieval requirements. The *Directory of Software Vendors for Group Practice* (1994), which can be purchased from the MGMA Library Resource Center, provides a list of vendors with electronic medical records.

If a practice is not in a position to adopt electronic medical records, during the interim a bridge from transcription that is placed on WordPerfect can be achieved to allow nurses and physicians access to the transcribed notes. Security levels can be assigned by employee to assure confidentiality, and current chart notes can be accessed when the record is not immediately available.

A system for collecting prescription refill requests should also be implemented. This can be accomplished by installing a tape recorder on a dedicated phone line that the pharmacist uses to place refill requests, and instructing patients to call the pharmacy. This method leads to more efficient work efforts by receptionists, nurses, and medical records clerks. However, it may take time to retrain personnel.

Financial information about patients should not be kept in medical records. This includes superbills, financial agreements, and notes regarding payment plans on the patient's account. Financial data can be accessed easily from the computer and should not need to be recorded in the chart. Malpractice liability companies discourage the recording or storing of any financial information in the chart, because prosecuting attorneys have used this information to imply that physicians are interested only in money and not in patient care.

Each department or clinical area should have the same location for its in and out bins for medical records. Using different locations in each area makes inefficient use of medical records staff time in picking up and delivering records, especially for temporary staff members, who must learn the many different locations that charts are placed.

Implementing a policy that requires the return of medical records to the medical records department within 24 hours of the record request or patient visit helps the department manage availability consistently. Some practices even lock up records to maintain control over them. This is not recommended because it creates frustration and additional work on the part of the medical record staff when charts are unavailable.

The medical records department should be required to deliver all scheduled patients' charts to the appropriate departments 24 hours prior to patient visits. This gives nurses an opportunity to review charts prior to patients' being seen. This review does not need to be comprehensive when the chart is well organized and consistently maintained in the medical records depart-

ment. However, a few months may be needed to reach a level of organization that assures efficiency.

SPACE FACILITY UTILIZATION

Providing a centralized system for the storage and retrieval of medical records is important for properly managing patient health histories. The processes and procedures of a centralized system should meet the following objectives:

- Promote continuity of care through ready accessibility and prompt retrieval of medical information
- Comply with guidelines for use of medical records that are set down in the department policies and procedures
- Comply with all legal, regulatory, and accrediting agency standards that are summarized in the department policies and procedures
- Protect records from loss, tampering, and inadvertent destruction
- Restrict access of unauthorized individuals to protect patient confidentiality

Support systems of the medical records department should assure availability of records even when the chart room is distant from patient care. These support systems include chart tracking, electronic scheduling, terminal-digit filing, and distribution of work functions appropriately to the medical records staff, all of which were described above.

Providing the appropriate amount of work space and equipment for clerks to manage their tasks efficiently as they are organizing, sorting, and transferring records is key to record availability and efficient employee work effort. Adequate counter space, sufficient telephones and computer terminals, rolling carts, and adequate shelving are resources that can have a significant impact on department efficiency. The shelving must permit easy access to records by numerous people concurrently. It also must be able to hold large numbers of charts per square inch without overcrowding and have appropriate safety features to provide a hazard-free environment for employees. Proper support equipment such as ladders, step stools, telephone headsets, and ergonomically correct chairs must be selected and maintained with consideration for employee safety and comfort. The storage space also must provide adequate lighting, a controlled environment (60° to 80° F with 50 percent humidity) that is devoid of dust, and protection from hazards such as fire or flooding and from damage due to broken water pipes or leaking ceilings.

Special filing areas should be designated for some types of records, such as records of employees who are treated as patients of the facility, records containing HIV status or other sensitive information, records of individuals of unusual fame or notoriety, or records relating to cases under active litigation.

Storage of inactive records must be managed with the same care as the storage of active records. To minimize space, records can be stored on microfilm or CD ROM. These storage media require a minimal amount of physical storage space and provide easy access to medical information.

Planned destruction of medical records can be accomplished systematically as part of the normal routine of operations in the department. Destroying unneeded records contributes to effective use of space in chart storage. The method, schedule, and documentation of record destruction should be set out in the policies and procedures of the department and overseen by the department director to assure that the guidelines are carried out appropriately. In general, the policies relating to the use, retention, and destruction of records should be reviewed and approved by the medical records committee, legal counsel, and chief executive officer. Distribution of policies and procedures to all patient care services and providers promotes compliance and results in the most efficient and effective management of the medical records facility.

TRANSCRIPTION

The purpose of the dictation/transcription system is to support the documentation associated with quality patient care and continuity of care. The processes and procedures to accomplish this purpose must meet the following objectives of the medical records department:

- Expedite the transmittal of information on a priority basis
- Encourage timely and accurate documentation in medical records
- Facilitate compliance with standards of documentation
- Promote legible, uniform, and complete medical records documentation

To achieve these objectives, dictation must be standardized and include the following information:

- Name of facility
- Type of report
- Patient identification
- Dates of admission and discharge
- Date dictated
- Date transcribed
- Initials of transcriptionist
- Signature of authenticator

Quality control should be built into the policy manuals including the requirement for routine and periodic audits of dictated/transcribed reports. Audits should include a review of the following aspects of the dictation/transcription system:

- Proper patient/client identification
- Adherence to standard format
- Proper use of abbreviations and symbols
- Correction of typographic errors, spelling errors, and mistakes in medical terminology
- Overall appearance
- Adherence to processing times and priorities
- Updates to abbreviations and symbols
- Adherence to distribution policies
- Down time and equipment malfunction

Setting processing times and designating priorities for transcribed materials greatly facilitates access to medical information and promotes efficient use of staff work efforts. This requires determining the amount of time it should take to process routine dictation for specific summaries, reports, consultations, histories, and physicals. Most routine transcription can be turned around in 24 hours, although some offsite reports, such as autopsies, may take 7 to 21 days. STAT reports usually are

CASE STUDY 10–1

DETERMINING FILE MANAGEMENT POLICY

A 35-physician multispecialty group has a staffing ratio of medical records department full-time-equivalent employees to full-time-equivalent physicians that is significantly higher than that of similar practices. The entire staff of the practice is exasperated with the employees of the medical records department, believing they are the sole cause of the slow response time to chart requests and the lack of availability of medical records.

Each department of the clinic has its own storage area for charts to which it must have immediate access. The information in these charts is not recorded in the main medical record room. Some departments go to the extent of locking up their charts to assure they are available when the physician needs them. Nurses from these departments regularly request charts from the medical record room, when the charts are already located in their own department's storage area. This causes medical records clerks to waste time searching other areas of the practice for "missing" charts.

The end results are frustrated physicians, embarrassed nurses, and angry clerks who feel they must waste valuable time and be blamed for the mismanagement of the medical records. Clearly, policies and procedures are needed in this practice to control the flow of records more efficiently.

Case Discussion Question

1. What policies and procedures should be established by this practice? Specifically, where, when, how, and who should file charts, track audits, and follow up with reports and data filing in the medical records?

processed within three hours, or immediately the next morning if dictated at night, but this may depend on what is being dictated, when it is dictated, and what mechanism is used for dictating.

THE IMPORTANCE OF INFORMATION

Today there is a significantly higher demand for information from patients' medical records than in the past. Requests for information come from consulting physicians, third-party payers, patients, attorneys, hospitals, ancillary providers, and state and federal agencies. These requests for information require medical groups to organize and manage information more efficiently and effectively in order to provide complete and accurate information in a timely fashion. Implementing systems, processes, protocols, consistency,

and uniformity greatly improves availability of medical information to all authorized customers. This better serves patients, the practice, and all providers of medical services.

REFERENCES

(1994). *Directory of software vendors for group practice.* Denver, CO: Medical Group Management Association.

Liebler, J.G. (1990). *Medical records: Policies and guidelines.* Gaithersburg, MD: Aspen Publishers.

Price, C. (1995). *The group practice job description handbook.* Denver, CO: Medical Group Management Association.

APPENDIX: SAMPLE FORMS

PERFORMANCE EVALUATION

Employee: _____ Scheduled Review Date:

All [NAME OF PRACTICE] employees must have a written evaluation at the completion of their probationary period and at least annually thereafter to assess their job performance. The results of these evaluations must be discussed with the employee and a copy of the evaluation must be placed in the employee's personnel file.

The performance review should:

- Build upon positive elements of the supervisor/employee relationship and improve two-way communications
- Accomplish a fair appraisal of the job performance in the previous work period
- Identify the employee's strengths and weaknesses and specify clear recommendations
- Serve as a guide to equitable salary administration when applicable

Reviewer's responsibilities:

1. Review the major job functions and factors you will rate with the employee.
2. Review the employee worksheet with your subordinate. Ask him/her to rate his/her performance on the major job functions and job factors.
3. Enter positive and/or negative comments under each factor. Your comments should substantiate the performance level that you assign.
4. Enter a summary of the employee's strengths and weaknesses in the designated area.
5. Consider specific objectives for the next review period.
6. Determine overall performance level
7. Conduct a review session with the employee as follows:
   a. Review major job functions and job factors, adding comments to substantiate the performance level assigned; discuss employee's self-ratings as they relate to yours.
   b. Review summary of strengths and weaknesses.
   c. Determine with employee specific objectives to improve or develop job performance; specify timetable for reviewing objectives and/or areas for improvement.
   d. Give employee an opportunity to complete the section for employee's comments.
8. Give the employee his/her copy of the form and send self-appraisal and supervisory appraisal copy to Human Resources for employee's file.

Major job functions: Functions rated as *Exceeds Standards* or *Below Standards* must be substantiated with specific examples.

1. _____

_____

☐ Exceeds standards   ☐ Meets standards consistently
☐ Usually meets standards   ☐ Below standards
Comments:

2. _____

_____

☐ Exceeds standards   ☐ Meets standards consistently
☐ Usually meets standards   ☐ Below standards
Comments:

3. _____

_____

☐ Exceeds standards   ☐ Meets standards consistently
☐ Usually meets standards   ☐ Below standards
Comments:

4. _____

_____

☐ Exceeds standards   ☐ Meets standards consistently
☐ Usually meets standards   ☐ Below standards
Comments:

5. _____

_____

☐ Exceeds standards   ☐ Meets standards consistently
☐ Usually meets standards   ☐ Below standards
Comments:

6. _____

_____

☐ Exceeds standards   ☐ Meets standards consistently
☐ Usually meets standards   ☐ Below standards
Comments:

7. _____

_____

☐ Exceeds standards   ☐ Meets standards consistently
☐ Usually meets standards   ☐ Below standards
Comments:

8. _____

_____

☐ Exceeds standards   ☐ Meets standards consistently
☐ Usually meets standards   ☐ Below standards
Comments:

9. _____

_____

☐ Exceeds standards   ☐ Meets standards consistently
☐ Usually meets standards   ☐ Below standards
Comments:

10. _____

_____

☐ Exceeds standards   ☐ Meets standards consistently
☐ Usually meets standards   ☐ Below standards
Comments:

JOB KNOWLEDGE considers employee's understanding of duties and what is expected of the position.

☐ Exceptional knowledge of job trends and resources; consistently endeavors to learn more.
☐ Complete knowledge of job responsibilities and resources; efficient and thorough.
☐ Job knowledge adequate to complete assignments.
☐ Job knowledge adequate for only simple tasks; should improve.
☐ Poor job knowledge; does not understand job duties.

SUPERVISION REQUIRED considers employee's ability to work independently with minimal supervision by making routine decisions, completing assignments, displaying adequate knowledge of equipment used, correctly using relevant forms, and following departmental policies and procedures.

☐ Works independently; requires minimal supervision.
☐ Regularly follows instructions; requires little follow-up.
☐ Requires regular checking to be sure work is done on time and in accordance with instructions.
☐ Requires very close supervision.

Comments:

During the past review period, the performance with respect to this job factor has:
☐ Improved   ☐ Remained the same   ☐ Declined

QUANTITY OF WORK considers volume of work completed as compared to desired objective.

☐ Output of work is ordinarily high; regularly produces above and beyond established requirements.
☐ Output of work occasionally exceeds amount deemed necessary for normal operations.
☐ Turns out normal amount of work but seldom more than required.
☐ Work output is below established requirements.

Comments:

During the past review period, the performance with respect to this job factor has:
☐ Improved   ☐ Remained the same   ☐ Declined

QUALITY OF WORK considers accuracy, thoroughness, and neatness of work.

☐ Work consistently exceeds standards.
☐ Work consistently meets standards.
☐ Quality of work inconsistent, ranging from acceptable to unacceptable.
☐ Work often unacceptable; quality is poor.

Comments:

During the past review period, the performance with respect to this job factor has:
☐ Improved   ☐ Remained the same   ☐ Declined

ATTENDANCE considers punctuality, absenteeism, and use of sick leave.

☐ Very prompt.   ☐ Regularly in attendance.
☐ Usually on time.   ☐ Usually in attendance.
☐ Lax in reporting to work.   ☐ Lax in attendance.
☐ Shows disregard for policies regarding punctuality.
☐ Shows disregard for attendance policies.

Comments:

During the past review period, the performance with respect to this job factor has:
☐ Improved ☐ Remained the same ☐ Declined

CUSTOMER RELATIONS considers the attitude of the employee toward visitors and outside agencies.

☐ Always cooperative, helpful, and polite.
☐ Usually cooperative, helpful, and polite.
☐ Usually cooperative, but occasionally abrupt in dealing with others.
☐ Frequently blunt and discourteous.

Comments:

During the past review period, the performance with respect to this job factor has:
☐ Improved   ☐ Remained the same   ☐ Declined

CO-WORKER CONTACT considers aspects of interaction with co-workers, such as seeking to improve relationships with co-workers, sincerity, and courtesy.
☐ Always cooperative, helpful, and polite.
☐ Usually cooperative, helpful, and polite.
☐ Usually cooperative, but occasionally abrupt when dealing with others.
☐ Frequently blunt and discourteous.

Comments:

During the past review period, the performance with respect to this job factor has:
☐ Improved   ☐ Remained the same   ☐ Declined

EMPLOYEE PERFORMANCE APPRAISAL, Employee comments:

_____
_____
_____
_____
_____
_____
_____
_____

SUPERVISOR COMMENTS:

_____
_____
_____
_____
_____
_____
_____
_____
_____
_____

SIGNATURE OF
RATING SUPERVISOR: _____

DATE OF REVIEW: _____

EMPLOYEE SIGNATURE: _____

CONFIDENTIALITY STATEMENT

I, (NAME), understand that in the performance of my duties as an employee of (NAME OF HEALTH CARE FACILITY) I am required to have access to, and am involved in the processing of, patient care data. I understand that I am obliged to maintain the confidentiality of these data at all times, both at work and off duty. I understand that a violation of these confidentiality considerations may result in disciplinary action, including termination. I further understand that I could be subject to legal action. I certify by my signature that I have participated in the orientation and training session given on (DATE) concerning the privacy and confidentiality considerations of patient care.

_____   _____
DATE   SIGNATURE

Original to be placed in the employee's permanent personnel file.
Copy to be placed in orientation and training session file.

ANCILLARY TEST REPORT RESPONSE

PRACTICE NAME
PHYSICIAN NAME
ADDRESS
CITY, STATE, ZIP
TELEPHONE NUMBER

TODAY'S DATE

Dear _____ ,

(Use the patient's full name)

The following tests were conducted (or ordered) on _____

☐ Urinalysis ☐ Pap Smear
☐ Hematocrit ☐ Lipid Profile
☐ CBC ☐ _____ Culture
☐ Biochemical Survey ☐ Mammogram
☐ X-ray _____
☐ _____ Cholesterol ☐ _____ LDL
☐ _____ HDL

Comments:

_____

_____

_____

_____

_____

Please call if you have any questions.

Sincerely,

PHYSICIAN NAME
PHYSICIAN SIGNATURE

Format with three-fold structure and print your return address in upper left corner.

CHART AUDIT AND REVIEW FORM

Chart Number/Name:
Date:
Comments:

Appearance of chart (overall)	good/fair/poor	
Chart organization	good/fair/poor	
Chart Contents	**Y/N:mark Yes when present; if No, give reason**	
Date entry documented		
Patient's initial complete exam		
Chief complaint/initial assessment		
Medical history (current & past)		
Family history (current & past)		
Physical exam		
Screening for problems		
Allergies/alerts (up-to-date?)		
Medications and dosage (dates)		
Progress notes		
Physician/provider signature		
Date/vital signs		
Medications		
Problem management		
Abnormal findings		
Continuity of physician		
Referrals		
Special documentation		
Procedure		
Consent for in-office services		
Consent for out-of-office services		
Consultant notes		
Hospital documentation		
Other		
Assignment of benefits		
Release of information		
Medical necessity (waiver form)		
Surgical office ($500 waiver)		

MEDICAL RECORD DOCUMENTATION

Principles of Documentation:

1. The medical record should be complete and legible.

2. The documentation of each patient encounter should include: the date; the reason for the encounter; appropriate history and physical exam; review of lab and X-ray data and other ancillary services, where appropriate; assessment; and plan for care (including discharge plan, if appropriate).

3. Past and present diagnoses should be accessible to the treating and/or consulting physician.

4. The reasons for and results of X-rays, lab tests, and other ancillary services should be documented or included in the medical record.

5. Relevant health risk factors should be identified.

6. The patient's progress, including response to treatment, change in treatment, change in diagnosis, and patient noncompliance, should be documented.

7. The written plan for care should include, when appropriate; treatments and medications, specifying frequency and dosage; any referrals and consultations; patient/family education; and specific instructions for follow-up.

8. The documentation should support the intensity of the patient evaluation and/or the treatment, including thought processes and the complexity of medical decision making.

9. All entries to the medical record should be dated and authenticated.

10. The CPT/ICD–9 codes reported on the health insurance claim form or billing statement should reflect the documentation in the medical record.

What Is Documentation and Why Is It Important?

Documentation is the recording of pertinent facts and observations about an individual's health history including past and present illnesses, tests, treatments, and outcomes. The medical record chronologically documents the care of the patient in order to:

- Enable the physician and other health care professionals to plan and evaluate the patient's treatment.

- Enhance communications and promote continuity of care among physicians and other health care professionals involved in the patient's care.

- Facilitate claims review and payment.

- Assist in utilization review and quality-of-care evaluations.

- Reduce hassles related to medical review.

- Provide clinical data for research and education.

- Serve as a legal document to verify the care provided (for example, in defense of an alleged professional liability claim).

What Do Payers Want and Why?

Payers want to know that they are getting value for their health care dollars.

Because payers have a contractual obligation to enrollees, they may request additional documentation to validate that services provided were:

- Appropriate to the treatment of the patient's condition
- Medically necessary for the diagnosis and/or treatment of an illness or injury
- Coded correctly

What Are Covered Services?

Covered services are those services that are payable in accordance with the terms of the benefit plan contract by the insurer. Such services must be documented and medically necessary in order for payment to be made.

What Are Medically Necessary Services?

Typically, payers define medically necessary services as those services or supplies that are:

- In accordance with standards of good medical practice
- Consistent with the diagnosis
- The most appropriate level of care provided in the most appropriate setting

Note that the definition of medical necessity may differ among insurers. Medically necessary services may or may not be covered services depending on the benefit plan.

How Does the Documentation in Your Medical Record Measure Up?

1. Is the reason for the patient encounter documented in the medical record?
2. Are all services that were provided documented?
3. Does the medical record clearly explain why support services, procedures, and supplies were provided?
4. Is the assessment of the patient's condition apparent in the medical record?
5. Does the medical record contain information on the patient's progress and on the results of treatment?
6. Does the medical record include the patient's plan for care?
7. Does the information in the medical record describing the patient's condition provide reasonable medical rationale for the services and the choice of setting that are to be billed?
8. Does the information in the medical record support the care given in the instance that another health care professional must assume care or perform medical review?

ADDITIONAL RESOURCES

MGMA Resources (303-397-7887):

The Group Practice Personnel Policy Manual (Courtney Price, Ph.D.)
Directory of Software Vendors for Group Practice, 1994 Edition
Performance Efficiency Evaluation Report
Cost Survey

Other Sources:

Bibbero Systems (800-358-8240)
American Health Information Management Association (312-787-2672)
Medical Records Policies & Guidelines (Joan Gratto Liebler, Aspen Publishers, 800-638-8437 or 800-621-6828)

CHAPTER

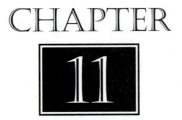

11

Information Management Technology

Doran A. Dunaway and Steven P. Nohe, Sr.

LEARNING OBJECTIVES

Upon completing this chapter, the reader should be able to:

- Explain current needs for information technology
- Identify future trends in information systems
- Explain the benefits of new information technology
- Demonstrate the application of information technology

The health care industry faces increasingly challenging objectives in the future. Information is more important than ever before in addressing goals such as improved quality of health care and greater cost efficiency. Simultaneously, the industry must search for ways to provide health care to larger and older patient populations. To meet these challenges, new technology in information systems and communications is rapidly being developed and adapted to all aspects of health care. Computer-based patient record (CPR) systems are emerging as the unifying foundation of health care information (Ball & Collen, 1992). An effective understanding of the new technology is a critical component of success in the health care industry today.

The purpose of this chapter is to demonstrate the future direction in technology trends, reviewing today's health information systems environment, assess the technology employed in that environment, and explain the key applications and challenges of CPR systems. Trends in health care information systems are listed in Table 11–1.

TABLE 11–1 Trends in Health Care Information Systems

Focusing on next-generation clinical systems
Taking advantage of graphical user interfaces (GUI)
Shifting from proprietary to open systems
Developing strong interface engines to allow free manipulation of data
Designing enterprise networks
Creating multiple paths to the patient data repository

THE VISION

In the future, when a patient arrives at a physician's office or other health care setting, he or she will be identified quickly as either a new or existing patient. Patients who have been seen by the practice before will have records that can be viewed quickly at a computer station. These records will include payer information, laboratory test results, imaging results, demographic and financial data, and historical clinical care data. Patient records will also contain highlighted information to warn physicians about special concerns, including drug allergies, drug contraindications, and other patient-specific information that will enhance clinical care.

When needed, information will be transmitted over a network to a specialists for consultation and immediate feedback. The referring physician and the specialist will examine the data on the screen while conferring online or by telephone. New treatment will be documented and added automatically to a central repository accessible by the patient and other care providers for future use. More mundane processes, such as reminders for annual immunizations and screening procedures, will also be generated for the convenience of the physician and the patient. Last, claims for services will be processed automatically through the computerized systems, including electronic transmission of data to payers for billing and reimbursement.

THE REALITY

Today's information management systems meet specifically defined data management and interpretation requirements. Systems may include physician office management systems, clinical information systems, community health systems, hospital information systems, and decision support systems for all types of providers (Burke, 1994). Problems in present information management systems are given in Table 11–2.

Integrating information management systems and exploiting information appropriately are the key ways in which provider management groups can address the problems in information management and, thereby, improve the quality and efficiency of patient care. Although safeguards must be built in to assure patient privacy, networking makes available more complete and comprehensive patient information. This approach, emphasizing integrated systems, affects all aspects of health care delivery. The physician has greater opportunity for improving diagnoses and assessing alternative treatment possibilities. The researcher has greater access

TABLE 11–2 Problems in Today's Information Management Systems

Proprietary systems dominate the environment
Systems are labor-intensive
Information flow is fragmented
Administrative costs are high

to data to support decisions about health care delivery and financing for academic purposes, regulations, and evaluations. At the same time, costs decline because duplicative and inefficient functions are eliminated.

ACHIEVING THE VISION

The computer-based patient record is the central component of a strong health information infrastructure. The CPR includes clinical, administrative, and payment information that is specific to the patient. Computerized patient records are linked together through high-speed communications highways. Voice, image, and text data can all be transmitted, provided that appropriate data formats and definitions are used. Additional support for enhanced patient care and outcome management is available by accessing reference data bases and other computerized systems. The latter use decision logic and practice guidelines specifically designed to assist physicians in their evaluative and decision-making processes.

Preparing for future applications means positioning the organization to implement new and better solutions rapidly and cost effectively. Many future applications may incorporate lessons learned during Internet development. The following steps are recommended to guide the organization's growth:

1. Assess current needs and capabilities.
2. Define strategies and objectives for an intra- and inter-enterprise-wide information system.
3. Establish guidelines and standards for hardware and software platforms, communications, and user interfaces.

Many advances have already been made toward the CPR. Longitudinal data bases are being created to represent a broader perspective on health care delivery, and widespread, appropriate access to these longitudinal files is accepted as a given principle. The exchange of clinical and financial data is an example. Networks clearly provide the needed access to individual and aggregated data for providers, payers, administrators, policy makers, and others.

Many items should have a high priority when purchasing new systems for organizations. The following items are the technological building blocks of a CPR system:

- Data base management systems
- Graphical user interfaces
- Work stations
- Data acquisition and retrieval
- Voice recognition/text processing
- Image processing and storage
- Cooperative processing

BENEFITS TO THE PHYSICIAN

Most physicians today are already working with personal computer work stations to manage information in their practices. Connections between individual office practice systems and affiliated hospital systems benefit the physician, the hospital, and the patient. The shift to computerized systems has necessitated *point-and-click* types of interactions, allowing physicians to enter data and otherwise use their systems to greater benefit than labor-intensive typing permits. Other positive results of the linkages between physicians and hospitals include streamlining hospital preadmissions, facilitating access to ancillary test results, and expediting changes in physicians' orders, among other beneficial outcomes. Physicians are also using system linkages in order to collaborate with other colleagues and providers on patient clinical management and academic research.

The CPR is a highly appropriate tool for physicians, who require comprehensive information to deliver care successfully. Using patient data stored in the CPR, along with information supplied through external systems, such as the National Library of Medicine, enables the physician to deliver the highest standard of care.

CROSS-PROVIDER BENEFITS

Information systems have tremendous advantages for integrating and communicating data between departments and providers. How this integration is achieved has clinical and administrative implications.

Clinical Systems

Applications in clinical systems must supply patient data to the CPR and other appropriate providers (Drazen, 1995). The most common examples of clinical applications are order entry and results reporting.

Order entry applications enable providers to enter orders for drugs, laboratory tests, and procedures directly into the system for communication to and action by other departments. Process improvement, cost reductions, support for clinical decisions, and greater efficiency and productivity are some of the key benefits derived from order entry. For example, order entry solves problems of lost orders, illegible handwriting, delays in test result reporting, excessive paperwork for order processing, and inconsistent or lost start/stop orders.

Results-reporting applications retrieve results from other areas, such as laboratory, radiology, and off-site facilities, and deliver them to the care provider's location. Optimally, results are custom-designed to meet the needs of the individual physician as well as to reflect different types of patient diagnostic scenarios.

Medical Decision Support Systems

Applications in the medical decision support area provide diagnostic investigation tools, expert system resources for clinicians, and clinical guidelines. An early example of this application is drug interaction software. Many types of diagnostic tools are now available, and their use varies by practice. Many physicians have links that enable them to send out information for analysis as well as to receive data for independent application to clinical decisions.

TRANSITIONS IN INFORMATION TECHNOLOGY

Within the next few decades, the CPR will be an accepted and universal principle in all health care systems. In addition to planning carefully for the development and implementation of the required standard for the CPR, other tasks must be addressed in this transition.

- User friendliness, ease of accessibility, and patient confidentiality must be strictly monitored
- Proactive discussions must take place on an ongoing basis with health care providers, payers, and patients to assure comfort and confidence with the direction information management is taking
- Systems and processes must be analyzed in preparation for reengineering the operational environment to optimize the use of the CPR
- Associated quality and cost incentives must be developed to encourage use of the CPR
- Technology must be used appropriately to support cost-effective and affordable improvements in the work flow
- Revised legal concepts must be pursued that allow widespread use of the CPR

As individual information system needs are isolated and addressed, one of the key concerns of information management professionals is to identify cross-provider benefits. In addition, enterprise-wide objectives must be clearly defined. They include such objectives as:

- Offering streamlined data capture and storage in a well organized data repository
- Reducing redundant data
- Offering more extensive patient data to appropriate, authorized users
- Delivering data efficiently for day-to-day business tasks
- Standardizing communications and other linkages within the health care community
- Localizing processing while maintaining cost-effectiveness and effective data security
- Developing user-friendly reporting and analytical tools

TYPICAL APPLICATIONS

Today's health care providers are very involved in acquiring or developing applications in administrative and decision support areas and integrating them into the overall business strategy. Some of these applications are reviewed below.

Administrative Systems

Applications in the administrative area are used to operate daily business functions in the organization including scheduling, registration, claims processing, accounting systems, and eligibility and enrollment applications. A wide variety of these applications is available commercially. The challenge is to assure that the applications selected meet the standards set for enterprise-wide use and that they are designed with the CPR in mind.

Decision Support Systems

Applications in the decision support area reinforce the planning functions of the provider. Typical analyses include high-level strategic reviews, contract evaluation, and policy development, as well as simpler analyses, such as cost per patient for specific providers. Access to multiple data bases is necessary to perform this kind of analysis of business planning and strategy.

System Implementation

The organization must define and develop implementation strategies that minimize disruption to professional, quality service. New systems must be instituted quickly and effectively, and comprehensive training must be a top priority. Other critical tasks for system implementation include:

- Customization identification—specific needs for this practice
- Specification development—define exact technical requirements
- Conversion planning and specification—how new system will take over processes
- Interface identification and development—who will assume responsibility for each aspect

- Application testing—quality assurance
- Policy and procedure development—development of written protocols for implementation
- Go-live plan—turning on the system
- Post-live plan—on-going monitoring and management of the system

SUMMARY

Today's health care providers must share integrated patient information within their own environments as well as across all service facilities. Capturing, analyzing, and storing patient information in longitudinal data bases are critical to assuring the optimal use of this information in enhancing the quality of care and maintaining cost effectiveness. Group practices with either managed-care or private-pay patient populations must automate to stay competitive. Following the guidelines outlined in this chapter will enable those practices to manage both costs and care effectively. The new paradigm in technology includes provider communication systems, strong data management functions, interface-enabling tools, and local, enterprise, and community networks. Although the role of information technology is a challenging one, the comprehensive, long-range planning and implementation efforts that the health care industry now demands will be rewarded by better care for patients.

REFERENCES

Ball, M.J. & Collen, M.F. (Eds.). (1992). *Aspects of the computer-based record.* NY: Springer-Verlag Publishers.

Burke, M.K. (1994). *Strategy and architecture of health care information systems.* NY: Springer-Verlag Publishers.

Drazen, E.L. (1995). *Patient care information system.* NY: Springer-Verlag Publishers.

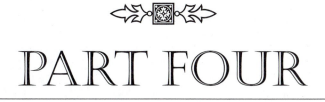

PART FOUR

HUMAN RESOURCES MANAGEMENT

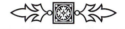

CHAPTER

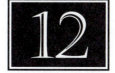

The Physician

Austin Ross

CHAPTER TOPICS

Physician Recruitment and Retention
Intraprofessional Relationships
Quality Assurance
The Impaired Physician
Family and Spouse Relationships
The Challenge of Managing the Physician

LEARNING OBJECTIVES

Upon completing this chapter, the reader should be able to:

- Explain how key factors affect physician recruitment and retention
- Identify important aspects of physician intraprofessional relationships
- Explain the importance of conducting physician evaluations
- Describe several aspects of the physician culture

The physician is the key provider and leader in the group practice setting. Although the roles of administrators, midlevel practitioners, and support staff are important, the role of the physician is the critical element determining the success or failure of the practice. In spite of the growth in the number and variety of midlevel practitioners and other paraprofessional specialists, it is still the physician who is responsible for the overall orchestration of patient care.

This chapter explores the physician's role as a human resource in the practice setting. It addresses such issues as recruitment and retention, physician termination patterns, intraprofessional relationships, performance evaluation, physician leadership development, the impaired physician, and family and spouse relationships. Parenthetically, much of this chapter applies equally to providers in other professions, such as nursing and dentistry.

PHYSICIAN RECRUITMENT AND RETENTION

Because of the importance of the physicians' role, the leadership of the medical group must assure that recruitment and retention practices are adequately designed to attract the best physicians. In the past, there has typically been a shortage of physicians in many specialty areas, particularly primary care, and the geographical distribution of physicians has been uneven. Although more attractive practice settings experienced a surplus of physicians, more isolated or economically deprived settings experienced a physician shortage. From now on, however, there will be a significant surplus of physicians (American Medical Association Council on Long Range Planning, 1989). This surplus is due to several factors, including the development of integrated health care delivery systems that focus on managed care and more efficient use of resources, the unabated output of medical school programs, and marketplace pressures from cost-conscious purchasers of care. This physician surplus will have a profound impact on the recruitment and retention of physicians. Many groups will be able to be very selective in choosing physicians. For their part, physicians will prefer practice groups and hospital-based groups for their job security and their ability to market services and provide physicians with ready-made practices.

Even in an environment of physician surplus, some practices may have difficulty recruiting physicians. In general, the more isolated the practice setting is, the more difficult the recruitment. Physicians appreciate the problem of keeping current with new medical developments in isolated settings because of lack of access to continuing education and limited opportunities for interchange of ideas with other practitioners. The group practice offers an obvious means of addressing this problem. Groups of two or more physicians in rural areas allow physicians to have back up and time away from the practice setting for continuing medical education and relieve the pressure on physicians to always be available.

Not only rural areas have problems recruiting physicians. Inner-city areas serving medically indigent populations always have had difficulty recruiting physicians. One of the more promising models for addressing this problem involves outreach programs for developing primary care-oriented group practices. The latter are sponsored by community hospitals, their medical staffs, group practices, and integrated health care delivery systems. The effective grouping of services associated with group practices and the linking of individual family practice groups with larger practice organizations are phenomena that will occur with increasing frequency. These linkages will be either geographically or financially based. Geographic linkages will involve sponsorship by hospitals or groups of satellite ambulatory care practices. Financial linkages will involve per capita financing (as with health maintenance organizations, or HMOs) or the packaging of medical services to attract insurance or employer purchasers of services.

For purposes of recruiting, the organizational structure of practices will make less difference in the future than it has in the past. In the decades of the 1930s and 1940s, there was considerable resistance to group practice on the part of traditional medical organizations. The rapid increase in the number of group practices and physicians in recent decades, coupled with a new awareness by hospitals of the need to diversify, has led to an explosion of new practice arrangements.

Especially in large or complex practice arrangements, the role of the administrator in the recruiting and retention process is very important. In some practices, the administrator plays a key role in recruitment and orientation. In others, the administrator functions in a more supportive role and the physicians take the lead. Such arrangements need to be worked out in advance between physicians and administrators. It is a fundamental responsibility of the administrative team to work with group physicians in the development and monitoring of the recruitment, orientation, and retention processes.

Recruitment Decisions and Strategies

In group practices, the request to add a physician usually comes from a particular clinical section. The interview and approval processes then typically involve the group's management or executive committee. In smaller groups all the physicians may be involved in the interviewing and approval processes. In larger groups, a subcommittee of the board or managing committee may review and endorse final candidates.

The decision to recruit is important because of the significant cost of recruitment. Management must answer a number of questions before initiating the recruitment process. For example, are the physicians within the specialty practicing at capacity, and how is capacity determined? Can the perceived need for another physician be met by adding physician assistants or other personnel instead of a full-time physician? Do patients have a difficult time obtaining appointments? Do market studies point toward the longer term need to increase physician capacity? Does the practice have the financial resources to compensate the new physician adequately during the period required for the physician to build a practice? Are adequate space and equipment available to support a new physician, or will there be a need to expand? How will the addition of a physician affect the net income of the practice, and for how long?

If the decision is made to add a physician, the next step involves determination of recruitment responsibility. Before the interview visit, one person should be des-

ignated to negotiate compensation and fringe benefits with the candidate at the appropriate point in the recruitment process. Compensation and fringe benefits should also be determined before the visit, and the individual responsible for negotiations should be provided with a range of compensation to allow adequate negotiating room.

In a group practice, determination of the compensation level is usually made by an executive committee or board of directors and is based on consideration of factors relating to internal and external equity. Internal equity means that the new staff member is compensated in a manner that avoids dissension within the group. The initial compensation must provide room for growth and reflect the fact that some specialties are in more demand than others. External equity relates to the relative marketplace value of the specialty. Access to compensation figures and methods of compensation can be obtained through surveys conducted by the Medical Group Management Association, the American Medical Association, or the American Group Practice Association, among others. Some practices commission third-party consultants to conduct annual compensation surveys for them.

Fringe benefits typically include health insurance, moving expenses, life insurance, disability insurance, and time off for vacations and meetings. They also include such benefits as payment of society dues, journal subscriptions, and other services.

It is important that both the applicant and the applicant's spouse be brought to the practice for the interview to assure that the position is a good fit for both of them. The candidate's visit to the practice can be enhanced by carefully structuring the itinerary, providing assistance in travel and housing, and arranging interviews with the appropriate physicians, administrators, and other personnel in the practice. The candidate should meet as many individuals in the group as possible to get a broad picture instead of just a glimpse of the practice. Packets of information concerning policies, practices, and the community should be sent to the candidate in advance of the interview visit.

One fundamental rule in recruitment is always to provide an honest picture of the community and practice environment. Failure to be honest can lead to future problems.

Physician Retention

Retention of the physician begins with recruitment. Commitment made during the recruitment process should be noted in files, and review dates for compensation should be carefully honored. An orientation program should be conducted during the early stages of the physician's affiliation with the practice. In smaller practices orientation may be handled informally, but responsibility for the orientation should be delegated to those best qualified for that task. In informal orientations, care must be taken to avoid the potential drawback of information lacking consistency. Orientation sessions should include the history of the group; financial and statistical profiles; professional practice patterns; and procedural details, including charging practices, proper handling of medical records, risk-management control practices, and a multitude of other topics useful to the newcomer. Administrators or their delegates should maintain close contact with the new physician to assist in the orientation and integration of the newcomer into the practice.

Also important for retention is the early and regular use of performance evaluations. Formal evaluations frequently are conducted at six months and again at twelve months. Evaluations help the new physician know whether his or her professional work quality and quantity are considered satisfactory by peers. The responsibility for conducting the evaluation should be clearly delegated to selected leaders. The role of the clinic administrator is to monitor the process and participate actively in helping provide performance feedback.

When evaluating performance, it is also important to monitor how the physician's family is adjusting to the community. Although a physician may enjoy the practice setting immensely, if the physician's family has not settled into the community, problems may occur that might lead the physician to resign from the group. A well-designed socialization process helps to assure that the spouse and children also are adapting to the new setting.

The expense of replacing a physician who leaves the group is high, not only in the loss of income while a replacement is located, but also in the loss of any patients who follow the departing physician to a new practice. Although restrictive contracts can discourage a terminating physician from establishing a new practice within the immediate geographical area, such contract are not always effective or enforceable. It makes more sense to establish a solid recruitment, orientation, and retention program than to be careless in selecting the physician or to increase the chance of turnover by failing to provide adequate orientation and early evaluation.

If the match between the practice and the physician is not a good one, the decision to terminate should be made in a timely fashion. Groups usually establish a clear point in time when the probationary period terminates, with one or two years being typical. However, long before the probationary period is up, a decision should be made as to whether the physician is performing adequately.

Physician Termination

A survey some years ago of 2,100 physicians in 134 organized group practices revealed some interesting patterns concerning why physicians leave group practice (Ross, 1969). In this survey, 3.6 percent of the physicians left their practice in the year of the study. Physicians entering group practice appeared to be more likely to stay in the practice. Group practice thus seems to be a stable practice environment.

A leading reason for physician termination is personal problems, including family-related problems. A number of physicians in the survey left the practice because it was not satisfactory from their spouse's viewpoint.

Other significant causes of physician turnover relate to practice arrangements, including disagreements over compensation, hours, coverage on weekends, assigned duties, and length of time off. Sometimes these disagreements occur because clinic representatives, physicians, and administrators are reluctant to adequately outline policies and practices that affect the physician's practice life. Another significant cause of physician termination is interpersonal conflict between physicians in the group. Groups should closely study causes of termination in preparing for the recruitment of replacements.

Causes of termination are not always clear, and terminations are often handled awkwardly. Once the physician elects to resign or is terminated, quick closure is best. Policies regarding handling of the terminated physician's patient calls and patient- or practice-related mail should be established well in advance and understood by all parties. Every effort should be made to make the parting amicable. To do otherwise may unfairly impact patients. Group leadership should be careful how the termination is accomplished, because failure to handle the termination in a fully equitable fashion may create other problems within the group and lead to subsequent terminations by others.

INTRAPROFESSIONAL RELATIONSHIPS

Intraprofessional relationships in a practice are often affected by the economics of medicine. Disparity in income among specialties may create friction within groups. Surgeons, for example, are usually paid more than internists.

The tension this creates may be heightened by differences in practice overhead. The surgeon, for example, typically spends more time in the operating suite of the hospital than in the practice setting. The internist, on the other hand, spends the majority of time in the practice office. Thus, in the group practice setting, the internist may have a higher overhead expense than the surgeon. However, the internist may also generate additional practice fees through the use of diagnostic services such as laboratory and X ray. Some argue that giving credit to physicians for services generated through laboratory and X ray tends to heighten the internal economic competition. Others argue that it eases tension.

In the specialties of pathology and radiology, a portion of the work is performed by technologists, technicians, or other paraprofessionals under the specialist's supervision. Although the interpretive and supervisory services of the radiologist and pathologist are vital, direct productivity measured in monetary terms may be difficult to assess, since the work of the support staff adds to the productivity as measured in dollars.

Similarly, anesthesiologists may employ nurse anesthetists and supervise several operating rooms simultaneously. As a hospital-based service, the economics of anesthesiology differ from the economics of the outpatient setting. The anesthesiologist who provides anesthesia for cases requiring short periods of operating time may generate higher total income because of the greater volume of cases than the anesthesiologist who provides anesthesia for longer cases. Thus, in anesthesia groups it may be best to pool income to avoid conflicts based on differences in gross dollar productivity.

These examples provide a glimpse of the subtle ways that economics can contribute to the delicate balance among specialists in a practice. The practice that succeeds in maintaining a balance is characterized by a fusion of staff personalities and group concurrence on practice and compensation goals. An example of such concurrence is the development of a center of excellence, where cardiologists and cardiac surgeons work together to provide a highly specialized service that depends on both groups to produce the appropriate result. Coordination between orthopedic specialists and specialists in physical medicine to develop a strong rehabilitation program, or between allergy specialists and otolaryngologists to solve allergy problems, are other examples of the merging of activities within a group practice.

Another important factor in intraprofessional relationships is the age of the physicians in the practice. It is important to attract young physicians to the practice to provide new knowledge and techniques. This can help older physicians maintain proficiency. Younger physicians, on the other hand, can learn about practice and style from the more senior physicians. Groups that arbitrarily limit their size and do not attract young physicians also may have no one to buy into practice assets when older physicians retire. The recent trend toward the employment of physicians by hospitals and by integrated health care delivery systems minimizes this asset transfer problem.

Social interdependency of the physicians is another factor to be considered when making hiring decisions. Friction can occur if there is a lack of social respect between members, and this problem may carry over from the office setting to the new physician's home. The life of a physician's family is demanding and difficult, and practices should recognize the need to offer support systems through social interchange within the practice.

As a practice increases in size, social interrelationships tend to be transferred from the group as a whole to professional sections or subsections of the group. Members of the group must like each other in addition to respecting one another's professional ability. Lack of compatibility inevitably results in the premature departure of the incompatible physician. Wise leaders promote social interchange, such as section dinners with spouses, because these events enhance both professional and personal communication, and this is reflected in patient care practices.

Some physicians are so driven and dedicated to their patients that their own family relationships suffer. Prac-

tices should encourage physicians early in their careers to be aware of the dangers of this pressure and help them achieve a lifestyle that provides adequate quality time for family projects and activities. Also as a result of practice pressure, many physicians find it difficult to become involved in community activities. This is unfortunate for both the physician and the community. The physician's community leadership potential is substantial, and the rewards of community involvement for both the physician and the community are significant. It is important for groups to encourage such involvement.

QUALITY ASSURANCE

Methods of evaluating physician performance may be formal or informal. Informal systems are based on patient complaints; patient attitudes; professional work patterns; and physician involvement in professional ac-

---

CASE STUDY 12–1

THE RUMOR

Dr. Smith is the medical director of a 15-physician multispecialty practice located in a rural community in central Iowa. The practice serves the population within a 100-mile radius. Staff include certified family practitioners, internists, pediatricians, obstetricians, and general surgeons. Patient activity levels have consistently been strong, and the group has added three physicians in the past year. The group seems happy.

At a meeting of the state medical association, Dr. Smith is approached by a faculty colleague from the state university who asks if there is trouble in his practice. Dr. Smith is surprised at the question and then learns that three members of his group attended a special session, sponsored by the state medical association two weeks earlier, to instruct physicians on how to establish independent solo practices. On his return home, Dr. Smith quickly conferences with John Hardy, the clinic administrator. John seems as surprised by the news as Dr. Smith, but then he recalls hearing rumors of dissension due to income, and they seemed to involve one of the practice's general surgeons.

Case Discussion Questions

1. What practice processes might have forewarned Dr. Smith of problems in the practice?
2. How should Dr. Smith and John Hardy approach the problem?
3. Why might dissatisfaction be more likely to be attributed to a general surgeon than an internist?
4. What factors other than compensation might have a bearing on this case?

tivities, such as continuing medical education, publication of professional papers, or clinical research. This information is supplemented by observations from administrators, supervisors, and others involved in the practice setting. Formal evaluation systems are based on data-integrated quality assurance programs and involve formal peer review processes.

Practice Review

Increasingly, clinics are adopting quality assurance programs based on a total review of the physician practice. These programs are conducted by an organized review committee. Typically, a committee reviews criteria concerning acceptable performance in the handling of both specific cases and randomly selected cases. This requires input from medical records. The committee usually requires input as well from nursing and administrative representatives.

Quality assurance programs vary substantially according to the type of practice, size of group, and interest of the physicians involved in the pursuit of practice improvement. A clinic that is closely associated with a hospital that uses the same medical records is likely to have a more formal quality assurance program than does a freestanding clinic.

Although in the ambulatory practice setting accreditation is voluntary, clinics may elect to be accredited because the accreditation process helps the group establish internal audit standards. Of particular merit in this regard is the pioneering quality assurance program focusing on data comparisons initiated by Dr. Paul B. Batalden and his research staff (Batalden and O'Connor, 1980).

Defining Quality

Most quality assurance programs are based on examining outcomes, structure, or process of care. In the outcome approach, quality is based on determination of whether treatment resulted in improved health status for the patient. In the larger picture, the outcome approach focuses on determining whether the patient received the best value. Value, in turn, is based on the appropriateness of the intervention, the quality of the outcomes and services achieved, and the utilization of resources (defined in terms of charges and/or costs) (Ross and Fenster, 1995).

In the structure approach, a set of standards is established that is then used as a measuring tool. In the broadest sense, professional certification, where a physician qualifies as a specialist by taking written and oral examinations, serves as a standard. In practice, a board-certified general surgeon is allowed to perform more complicated procedures than is a nonboard-certified surgeon. However, recalling information for a certification test may not be the same as recalling information for treating a patient (Batalden and O'Connor, 1980), and this may be a limitation of this approach. The strategy also relies on medical data recorded in the charts, patient complaints, evaluation of care processes, observations of colleagues, and the use of external criteria for comparative purposes. The information gathered may be of questionable consistency, at times difficult to obtain, and rely on professional judgment.

Implementation

Most quality assurance programs rely on a combination of approaches. The goal of any program is to guide physician development. To achieve this end, a quality assurance program should be visible but not threatening, understandable, and based on measurable data. To be successful, programs should focus on the educational aspects of the process rather than on punitive or censuring aspects.

As noted earlier, whereas larger groups tend to develop more formal evaluation programs over time, smaller groups tend to rely more on informal programs of evaluation. To be reliable, however, any program must include adequate feedback from those served—the patients. Thus, most programs use some form of patient survey. Patients may be reluctant to complain because of concern about how this might affect future relationships with the physician. When patients feel strongly enough to complain in writing or by telephone, however, these complaints should be carefully noted and investigated. Administration can play a key role in reporting complaints exactly as they are expressed by patients. Administrators must avoid leaping to conclusions about physicians' practice patterns, however, because patients may occasionally make unsubstantiated claims. The role of the medical and administrative structures is to identify the facts about patient reports and make judgments based on careful analysis. A system should be established to provide feedback to both the patients and the professionals involved. Such a system should not be used punitively but to educate and inform. To succeed, the system must be supported by the medical staff. Such a system can also aid risk management by revealing poor physician-patient relationships that might eventually cause patients to pursue litigation.

Another way of assuring quality is appropriate physician compensation. Good performance by physicians should, ideally, translate into higher compensation. Group members must concur on which factors are important in evaluations of performance. Some clinics establish a point system to rank physicians according to professional competence, patient rapport, employee relationships, involvement in continuing medical education, or other factors that reflect quality of performance.

In summary, quality assurance programs vary in their complexity and comprehensiveness, but the primary aim of most programs is to achieve changes in physician behavior. Correction of problems usually is handled most effectively when they are addressed discretely by practice leaders. Organizations also must be able to act quickly when problems of a serious nature are identified. One advantage of the group practice environment is that the professional who is a poor performer is usually identified early, because his or her practice is scrutinized more carefully by peers than is the practice of a solo practitioner, who functions in relative isolation. The responsibility of the administrator in quality assurance and physician relations involves the practice as a whole. The administrator should recognize that courage will be required to bring physician practice problems out into the open.

Each group should adopt a program of quality assurance that best fits the medical practice and style of the group. Quality assurance programs that work best are usually those that have been developed by the professionals who are being evaluated. Physician leadership in developing such a system is therefore essential.

THE IMPAIRED PHYSICIAN

Physicians can become impaired, and it is management's role to address such problems. The most important responsibility is to protect the patient from harm. Deciding whether a physician has become impaired is very difficult, and a team approach to making such decisions is important. Physician peers must be involved, which can be difficult because of professional and personal relationships (Berman and Townsend, 1980). Some local medical societies maintain 24-hour answering services that can be called by relatives or other concerned individuals to report problems associated with potentially impaired physicians. Such services allow for anonymous reporting and impartial review by professionals competent to investigate such situations.

Several physicians from a local medical society committee may visit the impaired physician and offer assistance in a confidential atmosphere. Such visits have been instrumental in pointing out to the physician the need to take corrective action. A visit by professional colleagues who are not closely related in a professional way to the impaired physician demonstrates the severity of the problem and its visibility and emphasizes the potential hazards to the patient and the professional career of the physician if appropriate action is not taken.

The decision to address a suspected problem can require both care and courage. The degree of impairment is often difficult to determine, and an erroneous accusation can be made. This can have a tremendous impact on a physician's professional and personal life. However, the fundamental responsibility of the group and its representatives is to the patient. It is the patient's well-being that must be protected, and the medical director, administrator, and impaired physician's colleagues must keep in mind that risk-taking may be necessary to assure that the patient's welfare is protected. Responsibility to the physician is secondary. Professional counseling,

CASE STUDY 12-2

TEMPEST IN A TEAPOT

Dr. Christine Goodman is head of the obstetrics and gynecology section in a university-based practice. She is very dedicated to her patients and is known to be one of the finest obstetricians and gynecologists in the region. The only problem is that Dr. Goodman seems to be totally intolerant of even minor mistakes by employees. For example, when Dr. Goodman recently called Sally Stevens, the practice administrator, on the telephone, Dr. Goodman exploded, saying that she "had had it," that the medical record system was "all fouled up," and that she was coming down to see Sally right away. Dr. Goodman arrived in Sally's office seconds later, slammed the office door, and immediately launched into a five-minute tirade about the poor administration, inattention to detail, and lack of follow-through on the part of office assistants, receptionists, and record clerks. She completed the tirade by saying that unless something changed soon and the system improved, she was going to recommend that Sally Stevens be fired. As Ms. Stevens attempted to find out more details regarding the specific problem that had triggered Dr. Goodman's response, Dr. Goodman interrupted and said, "Your attitude is lousy. You don't belong here." She then marched out of the office, slamming the door behind her.

Case Discussion Questions

1. What should Sally Stevens do to resolve the acute problem with Dr. Goodman?
2. How should problems of physicians verbally abusing employees be solved in general?
3. Why might the absence of a medical record have created such a reaction on Dr. Goodman's part?
4. What might be done to prevent similar situations from occurring in the future?

leaves of absence, or other approaches may be used to help the physician deal with the problem. All depend for success on the attitude of the patient, in this case, the impaired physician. Once an appropriate approach has been identified, action has been taken, and the impaired physician has accepted responsibility for resolving the problem, it still remains the responsibility of the organization and its representatives to monitor the course of recovery to assure that solutions are permanent.

In sum, there are few problems more delicate or difficult to solve in group practice than those of impaired physicians whose practice patterns have begun to degenerate. However, failure to face up to such problems usually results in even more devastating outcomes for the impaired physician, his or her family, the patient, and the practice.

FAMILY AND SPOUSE RELATIONSHIPS

The individual physician's family and spouse relationships may be complex, but some generalizations can be made. Generally, premedical students have a different lifestyle than many other college students. Premedical college students tend to become totally and quickly immersed in their studies. In medical school, this immersion in studies tends to become even more

CASE STUDY 12–3

THE IMPAIRED PHYSICIAN

George Carpenter has been practicing in his specialty field of urology for 25 years. He is known as an excellent and compassionate physician and is respected and generally liked by colleagues, patients, and employees. Dr. Carpenter arrives early in the morning and carries on a very busy surgical practice. He is known for his willingness to cover weekends and holidays for other urologists in the 100-physician group practice to which he belongs.

Unfortunately, Dr. Carpenter has experienced a series of family problems, including the death of his son six months ago. Dr. Carpenter took a month's leave of absence following his son's death, and it was soon after his return that problems began. For example, an intensive care nurse reported to the nursing director (who conveyed the information to the clinic administrator) that Dr. Carpenter broke down and started to cry while visiting a critically ill patient in the intensive care unit. On another occasion, several months ago at a cocktail party, another clinic physician noticed that Mrs. Carpenter kept very close to her husband all night long and was very carefully monitoring his alcohol consumption. Although Dr. Carpenter had been known previously as virtually a teetotaler, it was obvious that he was drinking heavily. When the time came for the Carpenters to leave, Mrs. Carpenter drove.

A week ago, Dr. Carpenter suddenly appeared at the chief of surgery's home. He was shaky and confused and indicated to Dr. Crisp, the chief of surgery, that he felt he was losing his mind. He was having a very difficult time making decisions and was not sure he could "take much more." Dr. Crisp was quite concerned and convinced Dr. Carpenter that professional psychiatric help should be sought quickly. Dr. Crisp advised Dr. Carpenter to cancel his elective surgery cases for the following morning, and Dr. Carpenter agreed.

Dr. Crisp arrived at 8:00 A.M. the next day. Just before leaving for surgery, he called the operating room to ask whether Dr. Carpenter's cases had been canceled. The operating room supervisor responded that she had been about to call Dr. Crisp because Dr. Carpenter had shown up at 7:00 to prepare for his first case and seemed to be acting peculiar.

Case Discussion Questions

1. What should Dr. Crisp do now?
2. What steps should a practice take to prepare for the possibility of an impaired physician?
3. What is the responsibility of clinic administrators or other members of management when they suspect a physician is impaired?

marked, and social activities are often curtailed. The medical student is likely to be under financial pressure, and if marriage occurs during medical school, a working spouse usually must carry a heavier-than-normal responsibility to earn a sufficient level of income to supplement stipends or loans. Childbearing is likely to be deferred, especially if both spouses are concentrating on achieving career goals.

The pressures mount when the new physician begins practice. First there is a need to repay loans incurred during medical school and residency. Family expectations mount as the costs of establishing a new practice mount. The expectations of achieving a higher standard of living similar to more established medical partners can add to the problem. The drive of the physician member to cope with a demanding profession that requires long hours and the emotional drain that comes with confronting the problems of others at all hours of the day and night can limit his or her ability to respond adequately to the needs of spouse or children.

The physician's marriage can prosper, but only when these pressures are accepted. Both spouses must also work hard to preserve and nourish the marriage. Quite frequently, the physician's spouse becomes isolated from the physician's professional life. The spouse may also lack supporting relationships in the community if people fear he or she has access to confidential information about patient problems. This may be more a problem in small communities than it is in urban areas.

The role and status of the physician and physician's spouse, their relatively high income, and the special nature of the patient-physician relationship tend to place stress on physicians' family and spouse relationships. Recognition of this fact by administrators and others working with physicians may be helpful in providing support to physicians and their families in a timely fashion.

THE CHALLENGE OF MANAGING THE PHYSICIAN

The physician's role in group practice and ambulatory care clearly is a dominant one. Physician involvement in decision making and leadership of the practice are crucial to the success of the practice. Management's role is to participate with the physician in seeing that the organization is structured to help physicians engage in these roles. For example, management educational opportunities should be provided to interested physicians. The challenge to the administrator is to identify physicians who have the interest and potential for development and to then assist them in crafting programs that enhance their management competencies. Close collaboration between the physician leaders and the administrator in building these involved teams of professionals provides the key to success for the organization and those served.

REFERENCES

American Medical Association Council on Long Range Planning. (1989). *The environment of medicine.* Chicago: Author.

Batalden, P.B. & O'Connor, J.P. (1980). *Quality assurance in ambulatory care.* Germantown, MD: Aspen Publications.

Berman, J.I. & Townsend, C.E. (1980, October). The history of the development of the Physician Rehabilitation Committee. *Maryland State Medical Journal, 29*(10), 40–43.

Ross, A. (1969, July). A report on physician terminations in group practice. *Medical Group Management, 16*(5), 15–21.

Ross, A. & Fenster, L.F. (1995). The dilemma of managing value. *Frontiers of Health Services Management, 12*(2), 7–12.

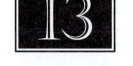

CHAPTER

13

The Administrator and the Physician Executive

Austin Ross

LEARNING OBJECTIVES

Upon completing this chapter, the reader should be able to:

- Describe the roles and responsibilities of the group practice administrator and physician executive
- Identify several unique organization conditions found in the group practice setting
- Explain leadership issues in group practice
- Describe the basics of performance review
- List the advantages and disadvantages of serving a management role in group practice

This chapter focuses on the group practice administrator and the physician executive. There are unique conditions found in the group practice setting that affect how administrators and physician executives function. The relationship between the two must be carefully crafted. The chapter identifies some of the key aspects of that relationship.

ORIENTATION OF GROUP PRACTICE

Group practice is based on the principle of shared resources. It is considered more efficient for physicians to practice medicine together, sharing staff, facilities, and equipment and providing each other with professional backup, than it is to practice as individuals in solo practice. However, to function in a group setting requires a degree of sacrifice by the physician. Instead of being the sole proprietor of his or her own practice, the physician must share decision-making responsibilities with others. In smaller groups, all physicians tend to participate in decision making. However, as the group grows in number of staff, decision making usually is delegated to an elected executive or managing committee. Physician executives in smaller-sized groups, and even in many large groups, continue to function in a dual capacity, practicing medicine but assuming administrative responsibilities as well. As the group continues to grow, more organizational and management formality is required. Full-time administrators are retained to direct certain business and administrative activities for the group. The administrator is employed by the group as an executive, to plan, identify, and solve problems and to implement new programs. The administrator serves as a business specialist for the group.

Describing the roles and functions of those who manage group practices is difficult, because group practices vary so substantially in organizational structure. In the typical private for-profit group, the owner (the physician) is also the producer of the primary service product—patient services. In the not-for-profit or corporate-owned groups, the physician executive and the administrator may find that they must answer to a board, which includes public and community members. In either type of group practice, leaders find themselves in unique organizational situations. Group practice is unique in that the physician board members are charged with determining policy and are subject themselves to that policy. This creates an interesting exercise for those in management. They are involved in implementing "what is best for the organization" to the "owners" who are affected by those very decisions. Because physicians tend to value personal practice independence and autonomy highly, this sometimes creates internal conflict and turmoil in the organization.

The system or hospital-based group practice may function with a different orientation. The mission of system or hospital-based group practices is closely tied to broader corporate goals, and the physicians may be salaried employees. Interrelationships between physicians and the management and governing boards of the system or hospital can create additional tensions if there is conflict between the autonomy of the physicians in practice and the broader organizational needs. These conflicts must be resolved in order to assure highly integrated and coordinated service.

The development of group practice proprietary chains that provide emergency room or short-stay surgery services, with a staff of salaried physicians, places yet another demand on administrators and physician executives: the need to coordinate geographically separate smaller units. Health maintenance organizations (HMOs) require that extra attention be paid to the consumption of health service resources, because failure to monitor resource use can financially disrupt plans that survive on per capita payments.

ORGANIZATIONAL CONDITIONS

There are several organizational conditions specific to group or clinic management. Reviewing these helps clarify the management role. In general, they relate to the potential conflict between individual physician autonomy and the needs of the organization.

Practice leadership must be responsive to those who own or control the practice. In the case of the private for-profit clinic, this is the physicians; in the case of the non-profit hospital-owned satellite clinic, this is hospital management. Responsibility in the group differs from the responsibility of the corporate business executive, who is not personally involved in directly serving the customer. Executive officers in the clinic have the challenging task of allocating personnel, equipment, and other resources to support the individual (physician) who not only consumes these services but also judges the executive officer's ability to facilitate access to the services.

Another organizational condition specific to the group or clinic relates to split supervisory responsibility. This is common in the group practice but less frequent in the corporate business world. For example, an office assistant assigned to work with the physician may be accountable to more than one supervisor (the physician and a manager of a department). Such dual reporting can lead to conflicts between the wishes of the physician and the policies of the organization.

Specialization is another condition specific to groups or clinics. In the corporate setting, the chief executive officer is usually responsible for the overall direction of the organization. In the clinic, however, the administrator operates as a specialist in business and management, whereas the physician executive has accountability for the medical practice. Other tasks are shared between them. The administrator may encounter conflicts between the prerogative of the physician and the good of the clinic. The hierarchical structure of the group may also create tension. The administrator often must resolve issues by persuasion, based on personal credibility and good will, rather than by authority, based on organizational structure.

Another condition relates to the allocation of available resources. Should resources be allocated for new technology and growth or should they be used to enhance the compensation of the staff? The balancing act by management is continual. All businesses face similar balancing acts, but they are accentuated in the medical group practice setting. Budgeting decisions for both operating capital and equipment are not always made on a rational, business-oriented basis.

Meeting Changing Needs

Health care reform is well under way. Regardless of the final details of any federal legislation, market forces are at work to reduce health care costs and to increase access. Group practice leaders, both medical and lay, need to prepare the way for change in the organization. It is important, for example, that when an event such as an economic downturn is predicted, the organization is prepared for it before it occurs. This requires that leadership refine environmental surveillance techniques in order to improve forecast accuracy. Internal and external economic trends should be monitored closely. Board members should receive full disclosure of information, with carefully prepared interpretations of the implications of trend lines.

Physicians also should be encouraged to become more involved in management. This will make it easier to address needed changes in practice or operation. Some physicians enjoy dealing with management issues, while others prefer to remain aloof. Leaders should seek out those physicians who have a genuine interest in participating in management. This may require a blurring of the line between business management and medical practice issues to help create a management team approach rather than a compartmentalization of tasks. It is through such joint management efforts that cost-effective, high-quality, and value-focused services can be provided.

THE ROLE OF THE PHYSICIAN EXECUTIVE

Managing the group practice requires a management team that collaborates well. The physician executive and the administrator must know their specific tasks and their shared duties. These are listed in Figure 13–1 (Mitka, 1994).

The role of the physician executive is changing rapidly with respect to the conduct of affairs in hospitals, group practices, and integrated health care delivery systems. The demand for physician executives is increasing greatly. There are four main developments leading to the increasing need for physician executives, including (Merry, 1993):

1. The rise of complex health care delivery institutions
2. A fundamental restructuring of health care financing, including a change from cost-plus to value-based purchasing

3. A progressive move from inpatient to ambulatory care, with the concomitant need to develop vertically integrated systems
4. The introduction of a series of leadership and management practices, known collectively as total quality management, which focus upon maximizing value in any production-of-service environment

Physicians concerned about the future are inclined to take active roles in management in order to have an impact on their future directions. Physicians are taking a greater interest in the structuring of decision making within organizations, and those with a bent for man-

The physician manager's tasks:
• Maintaining quality in the group practice
• Assuring adequate work effort and efficiency of the physicians
• Assuring retention of physician staff
• Developing an adequate physician compensation plan
• Determining physician recruitment needs and recruiting competent staff
• Resolving physician personnel issues
• Dealing with exceptional and problematic physicians
• Managing the group's external relationships
• Developing future leaders and managers

The administrator's tasks:
• Maintaining quality in the business office functions and procedures of the organization
• Managing the business office functions
• Managing nonphysician personnel
• Developing and implementing an adequate compensation plan for nonphysician staff
• Developing appropriate financial plans
• Negotiating contracts
• Being aware of and keeping the practice in compliance with government regulations
• Developing an appropriate fringe benefit package for physician and nonphysician staff

Shared tasks:
• Assuring customer satisfaction
• Directing strategic planning
• Maintaining marketing systems
• Assuring information systems development
• Developing proper procedures
• Assuring adequate communication within the organization
• Developing a fee schedule
• Determining the allocation of resources to practice development, fringe benefits, and current income for practice members

FIGURE 13–1 Division of Management Duties in Group Practice

agement are concerned with improving their management skills. Group practice increasingly is viewed as a safer haven; one-third of the nation's physicians are now in group practice as compared to less than one fifth in the late 1960s (De Lafuenta, 1994). Over 40 percent of physicians completing residencies now join group practices, multihospital systems, or HMOs as salaried physicians instead of entering physician partnerships or solo practices (Cejka, 1993).

The effectiveness of the physician executive rests on the executive's professional credibility; he or she must be viewed by peers as a competent doctor. Personal integrity is also important in a physician executive; the person has to be trusted by colleagues. Physician executives also must have effective communication skills and the ability to think in terms of systems and processes (Mitka, 1994).

Physician executives in group practices typically provide patient care in addition to their management activities. This dual role is driven by the need for the physician executive to maintain credibility as a physician in order to enhance his or her acceptance by other physicians. This credibility is important and serves as a basis for the acceptance by group physicians of the physician executive's leadership. Because the physician executive is subject to appointment and evaluation by a group's governing board, it is also important for the physician executive to maintain clinical proficiency. This provides a fall-back position when leadership is rotated or changed.

Currently there are a number of options for physicians interested in developing management skills. A first step is to become involved in professional association activities that focus on management issues. Physician leaders might become involved in activities of such associations as the American Group Practice Association, the Medical Group Management Association, the American College of Physician Executives, or the American College of Healthcare Executives.

The enlightened group practice administrator should promote physician involvement in these organizations. Doing so stimulates physician awareness of the need for formal training in management. Formal management training can be accomplished in a variety of ways. Professional associations and universities offer a

---

CASE STUDY 13–1

SABOTAGE

In a very successful 120-physician group practice, all patient appointments for return visits are handled by the office assistant in each physician's office. The office assistant also is responsible for coordinating patient visits with other consultants in the group and for all laboratory, radiology, and special test requisitions. Six months ago a computerized system was installed to provide centralized scheduling. The office assistant no longer has to make telephone calls to coordinate the schedule because the schedule of the physician needed or the test ordered can be called up on the computer screen.

Members of the department of medicine fought the installation of computerized scheduling because they felt it was an invasion of their scheduling prerogatives. They did not want someone else to determine how they spent their time in the office. To sabotage the new system, a handful of physicians decided to reserve many appointment times on their computers. As a result, the credibility and effectiveness of the system is suffering.

Case Discussion Question

1. Assume you are the administrator of this practice. What steps would you take to resolve this problem?

---

diversity of certificate courses. Internal management training programs are provided by larger organizations to give in-house training to their physician leaders. Universities also conduct both extended degree programs, which permit the physician to continue practicing while attaining a graduate degree, and full-time in-residence master degree programs in health administration departments or business schools.

THE ROLE OF THE NONPHYSICIAN ADMINISTRATOR

The nonphysician executive in group practice can be characterized in a number of ways. For example, titles vary widely. In smaller group practices the executive may carry the title of clinic manager. As the size of the group increases, the title may change to administrator or executive director. The tenure of lay executives in group practices also varies widely, and in these days of rapid change due practice mergers and other consolida-

tion ventures, tenure figures are generally unreliable as indicators of stability. Compensation also varies by size of group, and the ranges are wide. Benefits for lay executives generally parallel those of physicians in the group.

Lay executives come from varying educational and vocational backgrounds. Typically in the past, executives of larger groups were male, but this pattern is gradually changing as more female executives gain experience and professional recognition. Most groups of more than about eight physicians have nonphysician leaders with a bachelors degree. In larger groups, nonphysician leaders typically have a masters degree. The most current and valid source of information on tenure, compensation, benefits, and educational profiles of lay executives can be obtained from the Medical Group Management Association, which conducts regular surveys of clinic nonphysician executives.

As a practical matter, groups seeking administrators today seek individuals with degrees in business or health care administration or their equivalent in

CASE STUDY 13–2

ADJUDICATING PATIENT COMPLAINTS

Elsie Schultz, the administrator of a clinic, first learned of a patient complaint when she received a letter from the local newspaper's "troubleshooter," a weekly column that responds to consumer complaints. The troubleshooter wrote to Ms. Schultz, attached copies of letters from Marion Smith, a patient of the clinic, and asked for an immediate response.

The patient, Marion Smith, complained that Dr. Black of the clinic had charged an exorbitant amount for a procedure she had thought was going to be very minor but which turned out to be much more extensive. Ms. Smith also alleged that she went to a physician in another group who quickly diagnosed the problem and treated it with a very minor office procedure.

In attempting to obtain the facts in the case, Ms. Schultz discovered that Dr. Black and the patient had been feuding over the bill for six months but that the business office had not been aware of the problem. A review of the medical record suggested that the patient had a legitimate complaint, and the record was forwarded to the chairman of the quality-of-care committee, who agreed that the case may not have been handled well. Ms. Schultz also discovered that the case had been reviewed, at the request of the patient, by the local medical society grievance committee, which concluded that Dr. Black had not acted inappropriately and that there had obviously been miscommunication in the case.

Ms. Schultz reviewed the situation with Dr. Black, knowing that a response to the troubleshooter was required. Dr. Black had repeatedly refused to talk to the patient, but he called the patient and told her there was a difference of opinion on the facts of the case and that Ms. Schultz, the clinic administrator, would "solve the problem." Upon hearing this from Dr. Black, the patient promptly wrote a letter to Ms. Schultz requesting not only that the bill be cancelled but also that a payment of $5,000 by made for the pain and inconvenience associated with the poor treatment.

Case Discussion Question

1. What steps should be taken by Ms. Schultz to resolve the problem and respond to the troubleshooter?

experience. Obviously, administrative orientation in the field of health care is highly desirable.

Administrator Responsibilities

The administrator must relate well to the medical staff and be capable of representing the clinic publicly through involvement in community activities. The administrator acts with a considerable degree of independence, subject to policies set by an executive committee or governing body. In the broadest sense, the administrator's job is to support the framework within which the physician works. Overseeing financial affairs is a major responsibility. The administrator is responsible for controlling the receipt and disbursement of funds and must be capable of forecasting profitability, capital expenditure needs, cash flow, and tax implications. The assets of the group also must be protected from risk through insurance and security.

Management of patient accounts is a basic responsibility. The identification and accumulation of charges and credits, preparation and mailing of statements, and other financial activities all fall within the administrator's area of responsibility. The selection of equipment for business functions, including data processing systems, is a further responsibility. The administrator also recommends fee schedule changes and monitors the charging of fees to assure policy consistency. Understanding the implications and importance of managed care contracting is very important.

Another responsibility of the administrator is to supervise nonphysician personnel. Satisfactory recruitment, interviewing, orientation, salary administration, job enrichment, record-keeping, and application of laws affecting personnel are all responsibilities of the administrator. The administrator also must assure equitable treatment for all personnel. In addition, the administrator is responsible for the system integrity of medical records, the timely procurement of supplies and equipment, and building and facility maintenance.

Any successful group participates in the activities of the community in which it is located. Along with medical leaders, the administrator shares responsibility for civic affairs. The image of the clinic should always be of concern to the administrator. He or she must be conscious of the overall appearance of the clinic and be aware of the manner in which patients are served by lay and professional staff. Form letters, instruction sheets, and other forms of written communication with patients should be carefully reviewed and edited as necessary. The administrator should also be expected to be a person of stature within the community. Stature is earned over time through a continual demonstration of ability, perseverance and emotional stability during times of confrontation, and especially adherence to personal standards of integrity and honesty.

Although not carrying direct medical responsibility for the functioning of physicians within the group, the administrator is involved in matters that indirectly affect the quality of medicine practiced. For example, the administrator helps recruit and orient new physician staff members. Employment relationships between medical staff members are often developed with assistance of the clinic administrator, and the administrator

has responsibility for compiling information regarding medical staff policies. Beyond this relationship there is a high degree of personal contact between the physician and the administrator. The administrator possesses information essential to the physician in conducting both professional and personal business affairs, such as current bank interest rates for buying a new home, how the practice economy looks for the year ahead, and any tax law changes. However the administrator should be cautious about giving advice on subjects he or she is uncertain of because the wrong advice can rebound badly.

As a business specialist, the administrator fulfills a role as a conservator of the practice interest. The administrator is responsible for curbing the tendency to overexpand or buy too much equipment or facilities. The administrator is also responsible for assuring there is adequate medical liability insurance or insurance to cover other potential and catastrophic incidents, ranging from embezzlement to natural disasters. It is also often the administrator who plays a quiet counseling role to the young physician who finds that he or she is financially overextended.

One of the administrator's critical responsibilities is to manage human resources in support of the clinic's mission. The recruiting of members of the team to support the physician is an essential function. Group practice is inherently a combination of dozens of miniteams: teams consisting of physicians and office assistants, record personnel, business office staff, or laboratory or radiology technologists. There is an average of four to five employees for every physician in the group. It is the development of teamwork that oils the machinery and supports the objectives of quality patient services. Knowledge of the personal characteristics of the physicians, together with sensitivity in attracting and motivating paraprofessional staff members, are key ingredients to success. Likewise, the ability to work out differences of opinion and to know when to implement change is critical to the administrative process.

Managerial Characteristics of Administrators

Regardless of group size, the same five managerial characteristics are needed by administrators. These are technical competence, resource management, good communication, leadership, and innovation. The administrator must have a thorough knowledge of good business practices and accounting. The administrator does not have to be an accountant but should be capable of supervising accounting personnel. The administrator must be able to anticipate problems, apply analytical techniques to identify solutions to problems, know when and how to make decisions, and be capable of marketing a decision to the group's principals. Most importantly, the administrator must be capable of implementing change.

The administrator also must have the ability to communicate verbally and in writing. The administrator must be mature, emotionally stable, and get along well with others. He or she must be tuned in to nonverbal communications and be sensitive to the complex relationships among team members. Highly developed writing skills are desirable for communicating matters of importance to busy physicians and others because frequently it is not practical to convene all parties in one place at a time. Actions taken by executive committees, advisory committees, or other groups must be written and transmitted quickly and accurately.

In the group practice setting, authority is earned rather than inherited, and the administrator must be a pacesetter and effective leader. Leadership involves putting in long working hours, often matching the physician's long day. Leadership is an elusive quality. Recognition as a leader in a group practice setting comes slowly and it may require a period of apprenticeship.

Finally, the administrator must be an innovator if the group is to meet new challenges successfully. Not only must the administrator be able to recognize the need for change, but he or she also must be able to persuade others of the need for change.

Administrator Compensation

Administrators are compensated in a variety of ways. Key methods include straight salary, percentage of the net revenue of the group, and a combination of the two. Compensation by straight salary is established on entry and reviewed periodically. Salary ranges are used as guides. From the administrator's viewpoint, the primary advantage of a straight salary is that it provides a guaranteed income.

A compensation formula calculated as a percentage of net revenue provides the administrator with an incentive for assuring profits. Participating in the risk of the organization also identifies the administrator more closely with the physicians, which is viewed by most administrators as advantageous. However, in hospital-based group practices, HMOs, and practices where physicians are salaried, it is unusual to find an administrator who is compensated as a percentage of net revenue.

In the third system, which is probably the most common, the administrator receives a base income plus a percentage of the net revenue. This combination approach provides incentive as well as protection and stability of income.

Administrator Performance Review

The governing board of the practice should establish an organized process for review of the administrator's performance. Absence of a regular performance review schedule can be hazardous to good job performance. It is important for the group practice administrator to obtain this type of performance feedback, just as it is essential for physicians and other employees. Such a review normally should include a comparison of the position description against performance, a process and schedule for reviewing performance, and the use of surveys to determine marketplace levels of compensation, including fringe benefits.

Preparing an adequate job description for the chief administrative officer is a difficult assignment because of the variety of tasks that may be involved. Nevertheless, a position description is essential to clarify relationships between the administrator on the one hand and governing boards and subordinates on the other. The description also serves as a baseline against which the performance of the individual can be measured.

Because physician executives in group practice settings may not be familiar with the importance of performance review, it is often the administrator who must initiate the process. A structure must be established to provide the administrator with an opportunity to meet regularly with the executive committee or selected members of the governing body to receive feedback on performance.

A growing practice in the group practice field is the use of contracts between the administrator and the group. Contracts have the virtue of providing protection for the administrator charged with making changes in the management of the group, changes that may not be well received by all involved. Whether use of a contract between a group and an administrator is applicable might hinge on whether the group maintains contracts with physicians in the group.

In group practice, fringe benefit schedules for administrators should closely parallel fringe benefit schedules for physicians. Benefits might include term life insurance, health care benefits such as major medical, disability income plans, and accident or dismemberment policies. Additional benefits might include vacation time, sick leave, time to attend professional meetings, and retirement plans. Benefits such as dues for professional organizations and professional journal subscriptions are also common, depending on the setting, size of group, and role of administrator. Because the fringe benefit list can be extensive, a clear-cut understanding of benefits must be in place between the group and the chief administrator. Sometimes benefits are paid entirely by the group; in other cases, benefits are paid partially by the group and partially by the individual. These arrangements must be spelled out clearly in writing.

OTHER ASPECTS OF THE ADMINISTRATOR ROLE

The administrator role differs in hospital and group practice settings. Being a good administrator, especially in the group practice setting, requires certain personality traits. Although being a group practice administrator has several advantages, it can also be stressful. Each of these points is addressed in this section.

Contrasts Between Hospital and Group Practice Management

There is a subtle difference between hospital and group practice management in how management re-

lates to its governing board. In a hospital, the chief executive officer is responsible to the governing board for all actions taking place within the hospital. In a group practice, or clinic, the administrator has more limited responsibilities because the physician principals function as both board members and employers. The administrator of the clinic serves as a facilitator and colleague of the physicians in accomplishing the goals of the practice, but, unlike the executive officer of the hospital, does not usually carry overall responsibility for the functioning of the organization.

The nature of relationships with colleagues and subordinates depends on the management style of the administrator. In general, however, the administrator of a clinic tends to have a closer relationship with subordinates than the administrator of a hospital of similar size or scale. The clinic administrator usually must rely more on persuasive powers to accomplish results and must function in a more democratic and less structured fashion. In contrast, the administrator of a hospital, which is a more highly structured organization, relies more on formal relationships with all parties, including medical staff, colleagues, and subordinates.

The clinic administrator is directly accountable to individual physicians within the group and is evaluated by each as to performance. The authority of many different physicians can make the administrator's position challenging. The hospital administrator may be slightly better protected from conflict with physicians because he or she reports to a board of directors (often outsiders) who are not as well versed in internal operating problems. If the hospital administrator alienates a physician, there may be some protection from the board. The clinic administrator is protected, too, but in a different way. Clinic managers administer policies set by the clinic board, so physicians who are antagonistic to a new policy or procedure must hold their physician colleagues, rather than the clinic administrator, accountable.

An additional advantage for clinic administrators is that they typically share more information with each other than do hospital administrators, whose organizations seem to be more competitive with one another. Clinic administrators may share considerable information with each other in order to assure that their group physicians are well informed.

Management Style

Basically, the administrator functions as an allocator of resources. He or she serves as a coordinator, an innovator, and a steward. Stewardship involves developing and implementing policies and procedures.

The administrator's leadership is accomplished through the consent of others. Although authority may be based on structure, in practice the administrator tends to handle conflict or controversy by seeking equitable compromises. To be a successful leader of this type, the administrator must have a base of good will and respect. The ability to persuade, based on a reservoir of good will and respect, is probably the keystone to success in the management of group practices.

Administrators in the group practice setting must also have a high level of interpersonal sensitivity. To bring about change requires achieving the physicians' endorsement and support through logic and persuasion rather than through title or position. Fortunately, most physicians recognize the administrative complexities of the group practice setting, and special bonds often develop between administrators and physicians. The physician is in an excellent position to monitor the end result of the administrator's performance, and once the physician staff is comfortable with the administrator (and vice versa), a strong relationship may develop that allows the administrator to move easily into decision making.

An administrator who is personally ambitious and wants top organizational billing may not be suited for group practice. A physician elected as chairman of the board (or executive or managing committee) quite properly is the individual at the top of the ladder. The administrator's function is as a management specialist, bringing to the group a dimension essential to organizational success. The healthiest relationship between administrator and group is found in those groups where the administrator is recognized as an administrative expert, just as the chief of surgery is recognized as a surgical specialist.

Advantages and Disadvantages of the Administrator Role in Group Practice

One advantage of functioning as a group practice administrator is the satisfaction that comes from using management expertise to assist physicians in accomplishing patient service-related goals. The administrator is an important member of the team, and close identity with the physician tends to produce a healthy level of compensation. The physician respects the administrator's expertise, and once the administrator proves his or her capability, the administrator's judgment and counsel are sought by physicians, producing a satisfying relationship for both parties. The challenge for practice administration lies in the need to communicate persuasively with many individuals.

There are also several disadvantages associated with the group practice administrator role. The group practice administrator's performance is subject to constant evaluation. Sometimes this evaluation is not fair or rational, because each physician tends to judge the administrator's competency based on personal observations. The practice administrator must always carefully assess the impact of his or her decisions on a number of physicians, keeping in mind it is neither possible nor necessary to please everyone all of the time.

Another disadvantage in the administrator role is the stressful, pressured nature of the position. The practice administrator is subject to frequent interruptions and must respond quickly to a wide variety of requests. Good time management is an essential skill for the administrator role.

Stress and Survival

The pressures of the administrator role can cause burnout. The position often requires long hours, leaving too little time for recreation and vacation. The administrator who tries to keep a hand in everything becomes bogged down with details and unable to complete projects on time. In trying to please everyone, the administrator may find it increasingly difficult to make decisions. He or she may tend to lose emotional control, have few close friends because there is no time to cultivate friendships, and find it difficult to communicate with spouse and children. The administrator may be tired much of the time and not really look forward to the future. He or she may feel uneasy, uncertain, and even panicky on occasion.

Stress can be negative, especially if it is caused by fear, anger, insecurity, poor health, financial pressure, or similar stressors. Stress can also be positive, especially if it is caused by such desirable stressors as love and marriage, rearing children, sailing a race, or climbing a mountain. Just about all of the good things in life result in some degree of stress. The Rembrandts and Picassos of this life certainly faced many forms of stress. Beethoven's hearing problem certainly must have been stressful. Some stress is even necessary for normal existence. It would be catastrophic to be totally insulated from any external stimulus.

Individuals respond to stress in different ways. Although this may be due in part to genetic differences in constitution, it may also be due to different attitudes toward stress. To be successful, an administrator must have a commitment and willingness to understand and accept stress as an inherent characteristic of the position—and of life in general. The individual who has really learned to accept and cope with stress usually stands out in a crowd of average performers.

Tools for Survival

How does the administrator survive in these difficult times and cope with job stress? There are several strategies worth considering. One is to maintain a sense of routine. It is also important to set decision-making priorities. When the administrator finds it difficult to make decisions, it is a signal to sit down and reflect on overload. Sometimes clearing the desk of routine matters provides a sense of accomplishment and clears the deck for tackling tough issues.

Another strategy is to resist the temptation to fill every minute with activity and create time just to think. Administrators also need to identify and find time to pursue enjoyable activities. Unfortunately, because of the predominant Protestant work ethic, many people feel guilty if they are not busy all of the time. Being busy all the time can itself be stressful. In terms of managing time, the administrator must learn to tap his or her own personal

rhythm, to sense when the creative juices are flowing. Not every day can be equally productive, and some of the most productive days follow the least productive ones.

Another strategy is striving to foster physical and mental health. The individual who is physically active tends to be more alert mentally and to have more energy to cope with pressure.

Knowing When to Quit

A problem some administrators must face is the question of whether or not to quit. In some cases, the decision is made by others, but this is rather unusual. It is more likely that the administrator is able to pinpoint landmarks along the career path against which to assess his or her own accomplishments and then make a valid decision. The administrator also must consider whether the position is worth the sacrifices it requires.

Little has been written about how to decide when it is time to quit and move on. There are several questions administrators should answer in making this decision. For example, is work an agreeable challenge or an unpleasant chore? If the answer is the latter, it may be time to move on. Has work become so routine that the quality of work is at risk? If the answer is yes, it may be time to quit before the decision to quit is taken from the administrator's hands.

Have poor decisions or correct but unpopular decisions resulted in a loss of good will? If so, it may be time to resign and move on. Although good will can be rebuilt, if enthusiasm and vitality are low, it may not be worth the effort. Finally, does the position compromise ethical principles? If it does, it is time to reflect about the future. A professional manager should not stay in a position in which principles are being compromised.

ORGANIZATIONAL SUCCESS

The successful executive team in group practice thrives on trust among the principals, adherence to the same vision, and vigilant attention to group values. A group practice has a complex organizational structure, and managing a group practice presents many opportunities for failure. Thus, those who elect to become involved in managing and leading group practices must have a strong sense of dedication and the determination to succeed.

REFERENCES

Cejka, S.A. (1993, August). Physician trends. *Health Care Strategic Management, 11.*

De Lafuenta, D. (1994, February 28). Market forces dictate group growth. *Modern Healthcare, 44.*

Merry, M.D. (1993). Physician leadership for the 21st century. *Quality Management in Health Care, 1*(3), 33.

Mitka, M. (1994, May 16). What you need to lead. *American Medical News, 27* (19), 23–26.

CHAPTER

14

Managing the Employee

Austin Ross

LEARNING OBJECTIVES

Upon completing this chapter, the reader should be able to:

- Describe basic human resource management practices
- Explain the importance of employee empowerment
- Identify some of the management/employee subtleties unique to the group practice setting

In a labor-intensive industry, the effective manage-ment of human resources assumes considerable im-portance. Management of human resources in such an organizational framework encompasses many func-tions, the extent of which depends on the size and scale of the organization. However, there are a number of human resource functions common to all organiza-tions, including:

- Recruiting, selecting, and training employees
- Maintaining records to meet legal requirements of employment
- Developing procedures and policies relative to work performance and performance evaluation
- Establishing equitable compensation and fringe ben-efit processes
- Monitoring and administering employee health and safety standards
- Formalizing grievance procedures to resolve employee-employer conflicts
- Collective bargaining activities when unions are in-volved

Although clinic executives or their delegated repre-sentatives are directly responsible for personnel program implementation, including productivity en-hancement, cost containment, and human resource al-location, the management of human resources is a strategic function performed by managers at all levels in an organization. Smaller organizations and units with-out their own personnel specialists still require servicing of all personnel functions. Larger organizations often have full-time directors of human resources. The direc-tors usually report to the chief executive officer or chief operating officer, which reflects the importance of this function, especially in a labor-intensive industry. In this chapter, human resources management is considered both as a distinct function and as an integrated function, essential in the support of an organization's mission.

HUMAN RESOURCE ISSUES IN THE HEALTH CARE SETTING

The health care setting possesses several unique char-acteristics that bear on the management of human re-sources. These include supervision, specialization, edu-cational differences, diversity, and duality of roles.

Supervision

There is often ambiguity in supervisor-employee re-lationships in medical practices. This is because each employee is supervised by several people. The office as-sistant, for example, may be accountable to both the physician and the office manager. Close coordination between the physician and the manager minimizes con-fusion for the office assistant. It is important that physi-cians support personnel practices and policies and make decisions that are consistent with fairness for all em-ployees. Absence of cohesion and coordination between representatives of management, including physicians, may create opportunities for the individual employee to manipulate the system, such as when an office assistant asks for special privileges.

Specialization

The care of patients requires the employment of people with many different specialty skills. The regis-tered nurse or the laboratory technician has little in common in terms of their specialty knowledge base. This lack of a common knowledge base creates poten-tial conflicts, because the boundaries of service to the patient are not always clear. Where, for example, do the office assistant's work assignments begin to im-pinge on the professional prerogatives of the registered nurse? Thus, specialization can create problems, be-cause each group of employees tends to become cen-tered on a different set of operating concerns. Furthermore, highly specialized employees who termi-nate due to burn out or some other reason are not eas-ily replaced. Specialization also contributes to a lack of internal mobility and advancement between positions in ambulatory care, and this leads to higher turnover. The employee who wishes to advance has few rungs in the ladder of advancement in a specialty. In order to achieve professional goals in life, the employee may be forced to leave for a position in another, perhaps larger, organization.

Educational Differences

As with specialization, the variance in educational levels within a practice can create special personnel challenges. The backbone of any organization rests with the first line of supervisors, but difficulties are created by variations in educational backgrounds. Some first-line managers may have high school educations while others have masters' degrees. Although supervisory training programs can focus on generic human resource issues, it can be difficult for the executive to structure continuing education programs to meet the particular needs of each specialty.

Diversity

In this context, diversity refers to two dimensions—gender and race/ethnicity. With the exception of physicians, the vast majority of those employed in the health care industry are women, and the percentage of women physicians is increasing rapidly. Although more women are moving into management ranks, chief administrators of larger groups are typically males. The glass ceiling is showing some cracks, but the predominance of males in positions of power means that human resource managers must be vigilant to gender discrimination. Such discrimination can creep into the hiring, promotion, and daily life of the practice. For example, when a physician keeps referring to his office assistant as "my girl," he should be corrected, no matter how well-intentioned he may be. Racial/ethnic issues also require proactive responses by human resource personnel. Problems must be identified early and resolved quickly. The health care setting is too fragile to allow diversity issues to fester.

Duality of Roles

In group practice, lead medical personnel often double as managers of their departments. The more highly specialized the field, the more likely the departmental supervisor's role will be filled by a person who is trained first in the specialty and second, if at all, as a manager. Frequently, the technician or professional supervisor learns to manage on the job. Often it is assumed that if the individual is technically qualified, he or she will be able to manage. Although this may be true, it is not necessarily so. It is a challenge to executives to identify the management competencies of the technologist and professional supervisor. The department manager is usually paid more than the technician, so there is a perverse incentive to move the brightest technicians into management. This may not meet the career needs of the individual, who may be more challenged within the specialty. One of the human resource deficiencies in the health care field is lack of parallel compensation systems in specialties and management to avoid this siphoning off of the best clinicians into administration.

THE JOB

The individual job is the starting point in managing the employee. Each employee's job must be completely described, specified, and analyzed and its role in the organization clarified.

Job Description

The job description is a statement providing an overview of the job and its relationship to the organization. For example, the description of a medical records filing clerk position would include a title, summary statement of the job, list of specific duties, and delineation of the limits of authority and responsibility. The format of the description should be standardized for all positions.

Job Specification

The job specification carries the description one step further and outlines required qualifications for the job. Generally, the job specifications include:

- Education and technical qualifications
- Experience levels required
- Responsibility limits, including authority to make decisions and organizational accountability
- Physical effort, including dexterity, special skills, and degree of effort required
- Mental effort, including level of initiative required
- Number of employees directly managed
- Chain of command, including an outline of relationships with other departments

Job Analysis

Job analysis takes the description and specification another step and provides a factoring or ranking system that assigns values to each of the specification categories. The total value over all categories provides a weight that is useful in comparing jobs on the basis of responsibility and performance. Job analysis can also provide a system of measurement to assist in establishing performance standards for productivity. Such analysis can be conducted by existing staff or outside consultants. Properly conducted, job analysis studies produce very useful management tools (Bell, 1989). However, with less than a full commitment to them, undertaking the studies can be disruptive. The studies are detailed and need to be approached with a full commitment by supervisors and an understanding of them by employees.

Role Clarification

Role clarification is an ongoing assessment of employee relationships within working sections or between departments. The relationship of the office assistant to the front desk receptionist and of the receptionist to the record-filing clerk are examples of relationships requiring role clarification. Role clarification delineates these relationships through written policies and verbal understandings.

THE EMPLOYMENT PROCESS

The employment process involves recruitment, employment applications, reference checks, hiring, advancement and promotion, and separation. Each of these aspects of employment is addressed next.

Employment Applications

Employment application forms completed by job applicants serve as the initial record of employees. Application forms should include questions on personal data, experience, education, previous employment, and references. It is important to remember that laws determine the type of questions that employers may and may not ask on application forms (Gellerman, 1989). Questions relating to race, color, religion, national origin, age, disabilities, or marital status are usually illegal.

Recruitment

Employee recruitment can take the form of advertising in the local newspaper or in professional journals. Search firms can also be retained. Local college and vocational training programs can also be very useful sources of recruits.

Reference Checks

Reference checking is an important part of the employment process. Telephone reference checks are far more reliable than written references, but it is important to make adequate notes of telephone reference checks. Questions should be asked about the applicant's performance strengths and weaknesses and reason for leaving the employment of the reference. It is useful to ask if the reference would rehire the applicant. It is important that the applicant provide written permission for reference checking. Federal credit laws place restrictions on the scope of questions that can be raised, and the executive should review these limitations with an attorney to assure conformance with the law.

Hiring

Hiring constitutes employer commitment, and the commitment should spell out clearly the new employee's compensation, benefits, and methods and timing of performance evaluation (Zemke, 1989). The commitments made at hiring should be in writing and carefully filed. Most organizations have a probationary period during which the employee can be terminated for noncompatibility or inadequate performance. It is usually easier to terminate an employee then than after the conclusion of probation.

Adequate orientation of the new employee is a critical aspect of hiring. In smaller organizations, orientation is often based on a buddy system, with the new employee assigned to a senior employee for orientation and training. Supervisors should oversee orientation to assure that good work habits are established. In larger organizations, the personnel department, in collaboration with administrators, provides formal sessions at which policies and procedures are reviewed in detail. Such sessions also cover the history, mission, and organization of

CASE STUDY 14-1

DISCRIMINATION

Jean Smart is the personnel director of a 42-physician health maintenance organization (HMO) located in upstate New York. The director of nursing services, who has been employed by the HMO for five years, is resigning to spend more time with her family. Knowing that replacing the director of nursing in a group practice is a difficult task, Ms. Smart has initiated an extensive recruitment process. The clinic administrator, Fritz Baker, has authorized advertising in national professional journals and retaining a prominent executive search firm in New York City. He has also requested that the search be accelerated because of staff unrest in the absence of nursing leadership, with the departure of the previous director who was popular with the other employees.

The candidates have been few and far between, and Jean Smart now appreciates how great the differences in job requirements are for nursing directors in ambulatory care settings as compared with those in hospitals. However, a candidate with excellent credentials has been found, and she is currently interviewing. The candidate is bright, has excellent references, and seems comfortable with the physicians and supervisors who are interviewing her. The candidate is more experienced than some, and she has experience as a nursing unit director in a very large ambulatory care unit in a major Midwestern hospital.

When Fritz Baker asks the current assistant directors of nursing for their opinion of the candidate, they seem reluctant to comment. After gentle prodding by Mr. Baker, they state that they think the candidate is a lesbian. Mr. Baker reports this comment to Jean Smart, the personnel director, who agrees with the nurses' conclusion, but knows that the law does not allow for discrimination on the basis of sexual preference.

Case Discussion Questions

1. Does this HMO have a problem, and, if so, what is it?
2. What if any action should Mr. Baker take with the two assistant nursing directors? Justify your approach.
3. Is this a matter that should be brought to the attention of the group's executive committee? Why or why not?

---

the group; its relationship to hospitals or other health units; and other appropriate information.

Advancement and Lateral Transfer

Adequate record keeping and a clear understanding of employee work performance are important for advancement and promotion decisions, particularly when comparisons are made between existing employees and applicants from outside the organization. Employees who exhibit initiative and demonstrate growth potential should be monitored and provided with opportunities for advancement.

Procedures for transfer from one position to another within the organization should be developed carefully. Lateral transfer can sometimes solve problems of incompatibility between employees within a particular section. Also, an employee may request a lateral transfer because the change in work is perceived as a promotion. For example, a change from the record department to reception might be perceived in this way. Such transfers can work to everyone's advantage. However, if transfers encourage the best employees of a department to leave for another position within the practice, the message this sends to remaining employees can be misinterpreted. Job enrichment is important, but reasons for transfers should be clearly understood. Care should also be taken not to transfer an employee who is a proven poor performer. Chances are high that the poor performance will be repeated in the new department.

Separation

Administrators, directors of human resources, personnel directors, and supervisors must have the courage to take action when separation is required. Whenever an employee is placed on probation, it is essential that a decision be made at the end of the probationary period whether to terminate the employee, extend the probation, or remove the employee from probation. The separation process for an employee who is past the probationary stage must be handled even more carefully. Personnel records should clearly document conferences held with employees who are not performing up to expectations. Such documentation should refer specifically to the employee's probationary status and deficiencies. The employee should also acknowledge in writing that the problem was discussed. Documentation of a problem with no proof that it was discussed with the employee has little or no value.

Reasons that employees voluntarily separate from the organization should be determined with exit interviews conducted by the supervisor and personnel director. Employees may be reluctant to state their real reasons for leaving (perhaps for fear of jeopardizing job references), so probing questions may be needed. Follow-up of employees after voluntary separation with mail questionnaires may be useful, because employees may be more willing at a later date to share the real reasons they left the practice.

Turnover rates should be monitored regularly as an early warning signal of supervisory and personnel problems. It must be kept in mind, however, that turnover rates also reflect the economy. A recession, for example, tends to reduce the rate of turnover. The turnover rate is computed by dividing the number of employees terminating by the total number of employees and then multiplying by 100.

COMPENSATION AND BENEFITS

The level of compensation and the duties associated with the position are closely related. The qualifications of the employee are also important. Ideally the compensation levels and the qualifications have a close relationship. Placing an overly qualified applicant in a position that is viewed by the employee as unreasonably low contributes to unnecessary turnover. Clarification of duties and responsibilities assigned to a particular position in the organization is therefore important.

Compensation

Factors affecting compensation include the rate of compensation in the marketplace, the financial goals of the institution, the relationship between supervisors and employees in the practice, and assessments of employee capabilities. In terms of the marketplace, the level of compensation should be similar to that offered by other organizations for similar jobs. Salary surveys are often undertaken on a cooperative basis between institutions and serve to delineate equitable compensation ranges. The salary ranges for a particular position also should relate to internal job structures. Ideally, jobs carrying the same level of responsibility should receive equivalent compensation. Even under the most rational compensation system, however, exceptions may be necessary in order to attract or hold employees who are particularly skilled or to recruit replacements if these are difficult to find.

The financial goals of the institution also influence compensation levels. The short-range financial advantage gained by compensating employees minimally usually creates long-range and continuing personnel problems. This is because turnover may be accelerated if a group tries to compensate its employees below the rates of the competition.

Compensation relationships between supervisors and employee staff must also be considered in compensation decisions. At times, supervisors working on a straight monthly salary are at a salary disadvantage. Hourly workers in the same department may receive higher pay if they are working overtime hours at premium rates. Such factors should be considered in revising salary ranges.

More capable employees may be paid better in recognition of the quality of their work. Evaluation systems that are used to set pay ranges must be understood by employees. Otherwise, differences in pay may be interpreted as favoritism or special privilege, and this may lead to dissension among employees. Although systems oriented toward merit or incentive pay for special performance are highly desirable, they are difficult to implement and maintain in group practice. For example, in evaluating an office assistant who is responsible to a specific physician, the evaluation may be heavily weighted by the physician's personal opinion of the employee. The evaluation may include such statements as "best office assistant I ever had" or "worth more than anyone else on the floor."

An inability to evaluate employees accurately and objectively in comparison with other employees can lead to compensation based on favoritism. Because of the difficulty in establishing merit systems that are fair, larger organizations increasingly use step-and-range pay systems. Step-and-range pay systems compensate employees on the basis of tenure. A range of pay is established for each position, and then pay increases are given regularly until a maximum rate of pay is reached. The ranges are also adjusted to compensate for inflation and other marketplace factors. Within the range, pay differences among employees reflect differences in tenure, not performance. When such a system is used, employees must be monitored particularly closely in the first 90 days of employment so that weaker employees can be weeded out before they move into tenured positions.

The administration of any compensation system requires attention to a number of procedural factors. An important one is confidentiality. From the organizational viewpoint, keeping salaries confidential is important to avoid internal friction. However, adoption of a step-and-range pay system, as well as the process of recruitment, requires salary ranges to be made public. Although a given individual's salary is confidential,

considerable information about salary may still be exchanged by employees. Thus, it is important that the salary system avoid any practice that might be construed as leading to favoritism or special privilege.

In maintaining equity, reevaluating existing positions, and establishing pay for new positions, a credible salary administration program needs a compensation committee. The committee should be composed of both senior and middle managers. It must be a consistent group of individuals who have the organizational scope and commitment to maintain the system fairly.

Benefits

Managers and employees sometimes focus too much on direct compensation and fail to recognize the importance of fringe benefits. Benefits may vary according to employee position, tenure in the job, and other factors. Benefits may include retirement, life and accident insurance, disability insurance, medical and dental health insurance, vacation time, worker compensation, tuition reimbursement, sick leave, subsidized child care, and other benefits.

The type of benefits most attractive to employees may depend in part on the age of employees. Younger employees may be more interested in dental coverage and wages, for example, than they are in retirement benefits. Older employees, on the other hand, may be more interested in retirement benefits than in life insurance. Structuring of benefits also must take the marketplace into account, and benefit and compenstion surveys should be carefully performed and analyzed.

Compensation Volatility

Organizations should decide how they wish to position themselves in the employment field, that is, whether their compensation and benefit levels will be at the median level, in the upper third, and so on. This will depend on organizational goals and objectives. Employers usually try to maintain competitive compensation and benefit packages. It is important to remember that enrichment of a single benefit increases the total employee cost. Thus, the decision must be made whether to put additional compensation into direct pay or benefits or both.

CASE STUDY 14–2

EMPLOYEE EQUITY AND FAIRNESS

Dr. Jim Swarthmore, a board-certified internist, has always dreamed of having a family practice clinic that is so sensitive to the needs of patients that it is a genuine family center. Dr. Swarthmore believes that the key to success in such a center is to attract the most highly qualified individuals and pay them better than other employees in town. Only employees who believe that personal patient service must be of the highest quality should be selected, in Dr. Swarthmore's view.

The group that Dr. Swarthmore has developed has grown to 10 physicians. Dr. Swarthmore is still the lead physician and serves as both medical director and administrator of the practice. Salary increases are determined annually, and the economy is stable. Although the 35 employees generally have been accepted as important members of the team and seem happy, a rumor recently has reached Dr. Swarthmore that the compensation system has been criticized for favoritism.

Dr. Swarthmore consults with the head office manager, John Ragen, who also serves as the credit manager, and discovers that the rumor is true. Mr. Ragen gives the example of the registered nurse working for Dr. Swarthmore; she received a 14-percent increase in salary last year when most other employees received a 3-percent increase. Dr. Swarthmore responds that the nurse has worked with him since the inception of the group, and that the increase reflects her importance to the practice.

Case Discussion Questions

1. How should an administrator respond to physician-owners' salary increase requests for employees' whose performance does not justify the increase?
2. What type of a rational evaluation system could be established that would minimize this type of conflicts and be acceptable to employees?
3. Assume that Dr. Swarthmore's nurse is indeed worth the extra pay. Should this be explained to supervisors and employees, and, if so, how?

Caution should be taken to avoid too rapid a change in benefit or compensation systems, because this can throw a balanced internal equity structure into disarray. For example, if a particular section of the group is having a difficult time recruiting, there may be a tendency to concede to the section's request for higher compensation. Should this take place, other employees may believe that their compensation and benefits are substandard. If an organization develops job parity in compensation that is based on detailed studies of job specifications, exceptions to the established system can be made but only after careful scrutiny. As in other salary administration matters, if equity relationships are not monitored, the system may lose credibility and support.

PROBLEM IDENTIFICATION AND EMPLOYEE COUNSELING

Problem Identification

Problems can be identified by a variety of mechanisms that are broadly classified as either operational or environmental. An example of a mechanism for operational identification of a problem is an employee complaint to a supervisor or other member of management about a specific problem. An example of an environmental mechanism is review of employee turnover rates and exit interviews. Other mechanisms for identifying problems include monitoring absenteeism rates, which assumes that unhappy employees tend to take more time off from work, and reviewing regular operating reports, in which supervisors and managers are asked to list problems.

Personal contact with employees can also reveal problems with job satisfaction. The enthusiasm of employees can be measured in many ways if managers are attuned to this aspect of job performance. In some organizations, employers use employee attitude surveys. To be most effective, these should be administered by an outside party. Such surveys can produce excellent information about employee perceptions of the effectiveness of supervisory structures and the level of job satisfaction. A commitment to change based on findings of the survey is essential to the success of this process.

These and other indicators provide managers with a sense of the state of employee morale. It should be cautioned that lack of specific problems on a day-to-day basis should not be taken by itself as an indicator of high morale. It is possible for managers to be so distant from the operation that they are not attuned to employees' feelings. The lack of recorded problems, such as failure of the supervisor to monitor employee absenteeism, may in fact be an indicator of a serious problem.

Counseling

Job-related counseling helps build a productive, smoothly working team. Essentially, there are two different counseling approaches, directive and nondirective counseling. Directive counseling is a fact-finding process relating to a specific problem. The supervisor weighs the facts, advises the employee, and attempts to motivate the employee to adhere to the advice given. Nondirective counseling focuses on the person being counseled rather than on the problem to be resolved by the counselor. A broader view is taken. Typically, a counseling approach is selected that matches the prob-

lem being addressed. However, a good counselor tends to favor approaches that build rapport and contribute to the employee's understanding of the larger picture. The counselor must sort out the facts of the problem from the projected attitudes of the employee. It is important to distinguish between factual information and information that is biased by the employee's viewpoint.

There are several requirements for effective counseling. The most important are to set the stage carefully, create rapport, and permit the employee to engage in meaningful dialogue with the counselor. It is also important to determine in advance, whenever possible, where and how closure should take place. This requires that the counselor carefully think through useful strategies to meet the employee's needs.

EMPLOYEE EVALUATION

Any evaluation process involves three basic components: understanding by both employer and employee of the employee's assignments that are subject to evaluation; processes and procedures for conducting the evaluation; and feedback to the employee about the outcome of the evaluation. Obviously, the evaluation process depends on adequate job descriptions and agreement among all parties regarding the objectives to be evaluated. The absence of feedback on performance can seriously jeopardize the evaluation process. Ideally the evaluation should be in writing and signed by the supervisor and employee, because what is heard in an evaluation conference by the employee may be selective.

Discipline

Disciplining an employee is a complicated process that includes recognition of the problem and careful assessment as to whether the policy or practice has been violated. When it has been determined that disciplinary action is in order, disciplinary policies must be followed carefully to maintain morale and equity of personnel relationships. The first step in disciplinary action is often a warning. Careful documentation of any verbal or written warning is essential. The timing and degree of further

---

CASE STUDY 14–3

ATTITUDE PROBLEMS AT HAPPY VILLA

Anthony Organized, the chief administrator of Happy Villa Group Practice, a 50-physician partnership located in downtown San Francisco, just completed reading an article in *Medical Group Management.* The article suggested that undertaking employee attitude surveys can aid immeasurably in the early identification of morale problems. This sounded like a tremendous idea to Mr. Organized, so he spent all day Saturday designing a survey questionnaire to measure the attitudes of the 221 employees of the practice.

On Monday, Mr. Organized called a special meeting of his 14 administrative colleagues and key department heads to explain the survey. He indicated that monitoring employee morale was extremely important so the survey should move forward quickly. Mr. Organized called the project "Blue Binder." He felt that providing the project with a name would help create identification with the survey process. Mr. Organized also indicated that he wanted to have the questionnaire form printed and distributed by the following Monday, with the survey results to be compiled and ready for discussion at a meeting in two weeks. Because Mr. Organized was busy with so many other activities and believes in delegation, he then went on to other business.

At the end of two weeks, attitude survey forms had been issued to all employees and the responses compiled. The scheduled meeting has convened, and Mr. Organized questioned his second in command, Susan Helpful, about the results. She informed him that only 17 percent of the questionnaires had been returned. Of those returned, 63 percent indicated a very favorable response to management supervisory processes. They also indicated a high level of morale. The remaining 37 percent of those returned indicated that there were problems. Mr. Organized assumed there would be a 100-percent response on something as important as a measurement of employee attitudes, so he was surprised by the low response rate.

Case Discussion Questions

1. How could Mr. Organized have better handled the implementation of the survey?
2. Were the results of the survey helpful and, if so, how?
3. Given the poor rate of return, what if anything should Mr. Organized do about completing the assessment process?

---

intervention by management in disciplinary matters depends on the magnitude of the problem. Management also must assure that a deviation from norms is in fact taking place. Sometimes many employees are violating the same rule for which only one employee is being disciplined. Once disciplinary action has been initiated it is very important to set a timetable for resolution of the problem. For example, if the employee is put on proba-

tion, a definite length of time for the probationary period must be specified.

UNIONIZATION

If management can maintain good communications with employees and be responsive to employee concerns and issues, it may be unnecessary for unions to evolve

CASE STUDY 14–4

CLOGGING THROUGH THE CLINIC

In a prominent specialty-tertiary group practice in Texas, the receptionists are uniformed, the physicians wear ties, and at least five percent of the patients arrive in limousines. One of the most successful physicians in the clinic is Dr. Heartache, a prominent cardiothoracic surgeon who contributes heavily to the gross productivity of the group practice. Dr. Heartache employs a very bright office assistant named Jane Smiley, who performs all of her professional duties with great care and enthusiasm.

The only problem is that Ms. Smiley refuses to conform to the nursing department manager's dress code. Her skirt is four inches too short, and due to a foot arch problem, she wears wooden clogs instead of shoes. Carol Fit, the nursing director, believes that her inability to enforce the dress code with this employee is seriously detracting from her ability to manage the nursing department. On two separate occasions, Ms. Fit has met with Dr. Heartache about the problem. Dr. Heartache refuses to step in because he values Ms. Smiley's nursing skills over enforcement of the dress code.

Case Discussion Questions

1. What steps should Ms. Fit take to try to resolve this problem?
2. What might have been done earlier to avoid the problem?
3. If Dr. Heartache refuses to budge, how far should Ms. Fit go to correct the situation?

to resolve employee problems. However, the occasional memorandum from the front office will not do the job. It is a responsibility of supervisors and managers to work with physicians and other professional personnel to clearly communicate and resolve employee problems.

Major employee problems that lead to union representation include:

- Inadequate pay levels
- Unsatisfactory working conditions
- Absence of well-defined grievance procedures to resolve problems
- Lack of clarity, in general, in personnel practices and policies
- Failure to communicate the mission and objectives of the institution to employees

If labor does make an effort to organize employees, a practice has two key responsibilities to its employees: to see that representation is not forced upon them, and to assure that employees have a free choice in which union represents them.

Usually there is advance notice of a union-organizing program. For example, organizing leaflets may be passed out to employees, or there may be rumors of off-site meetings. Administrators who anticipate union-organizing activity should get legal advice about how to respond. For example, if an administrator accepts or reviews employee-signed cards, indicating representation rights from a union organizer, this may legally constitute acquiescence of union prerogatives. Good legal advice can help prevent such problems from occurring. Preparing in advance for union intervention can also contribute to a healthy, free-flowing, and productive relationship between management and employees.

EMPLOYEE TRAINING

The complex process of adequately orienting a new employee so that the employee becomes a valuable, well informed member of the staff is just the beginning of employee training. Recruiting experienced health professionals makes this initial training easier, but it is still necessary to provide the new employee with an adequate sense of the organization's culture. Once the employee is well oriented and productive, the practice must provide continuing education opportunities so the employee can remain current in the conduct of professional and practice activities.

Educational opportunities are nearly limitless. Professional societies, colleges, vocational schools, workplace consultants specializing in continuing education, and suppliers all provide access to on-the-job training and job enrichment. There are several general principles that can help narrow the alternatives in designing an educational program:

- Provide integrated training toward specific objectives based on employee weaknesses and strengths and training objectives of the organization
- Include money in the training budgets to cover the significant costs in employee time of training programs
- Establish policies for selecting employees to attend training
- Require that employees who attend meetings at practice expense share what they learn with others on the staff

LEGAL ISSUES ASSOCIATED WITH EMPLOYMENT

Regulations affecting employment practices are extensive and beyond the scope of this book. The reader is directed to the Medical Group Management Association (MGMA) for excellent resource advice. MGMA's *Personnel Postscript,* for example, provides an outstanding overview of the many key pieces of legislation at both federal and state levels. An inventory of key laws at the federal level includes the following six (Price and Stickler, 1994):

1. The Fair Labor Standards Act (FLSA)
2. The National Labor Relations Act (NLRA)
3. The Occupational Safety and Health Act (OSHA)
4. The Family and Medical Leave Act (FMLA)
5. The Americans with Disabilities Act (ADA)
6. The Age Discrimination in Employment Act (ADEA)

The reader is also directed to the article by Vecchioli and Gassman (1993) as an excellent resource on labor and employment issues. It provides solid advice on avoiding liability.

THE CHALLENGE OF MANAGING PEOPLE

In a service industry the work force component assumes great importance. This is particularly true in the health field. The process of managing employees is complicated by the environment in which the patient and health care provider interact. In the small-sized organization, the administrator must assume a wide variety of tasks essential to the process of bringing aboard new employees and managing the environment in which they practice. Human resource management is so complex that, with any growth, specialization occurs and human resource specialists must be employed. While it is hoped that some simplification in the multitude of applicable laws and regulations will take place, it is the wise executive who consults with the practice's attorneys for help in sorting out the maze.

REFERENCES

Bell, A.H. (1989). *The complete manager's guide to interviewing: How to hire the best.* Homewood, IL: Richard D. Irwin, Inc.

Gellerman, S.W. (1989, Summer). The art of management selection. *Recruitment Today, 40.*

Price, C. & Stickler, B. (1994, Spring). Personnel policies and procedures update. *Personnel Postscript, 9*(2), 1–12.

Vecchioli, J. & Gassman, A. (1993, Winter). Structuring group medical practices: Labor and employment issues. *The Medical Staff Counselor, 7*(1), 19–31.

Zemke, R. (1989, August). Employee orientation: A process, not a program. *Training, 33.*

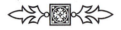

CHAPTER

15

Managing the Patient: Patient Relations

Austin Ross

CHAPTER TOPICS

The Patient
Dealing with Patient Complaints
Avoiding Medical Malpractice
The Importance of Patient Relations

LEARNING OBJECTIVES

Upon completing this chapter, the reader should be able to:

- Describe patient likes and dislikes
- Identify the dynamics of physician-patient relationships
- List the elements of a patient relations-monitoring program
- Explain the administrator's role in monitoring patient relations

As a health care administrator, it is important to keep in mind that the patient arrives at the physician's office with some level of anxiety, regardless of how well it may be concealed. How the patient handles this anxiety depends on the patient's level of confidence in the health care provider and the care provided. From the first phone call to the last bill, whether the patient is aware of it or not, he or she is monitoring how things are going. Unpleasant contacts at the reception desk, a curt radiology technician, or an unexplained long wait in the examining room can contribute to a loss of faith in the system and create obstacles for the physician who deals with the patient directly. To some patients, considerable courage is required to visit the physician and be subjected to the authority structure of traditional medicine. To others, a visit to a physician provides a release, an opportunity to review real or imagined symptoms and get attention that may be lacking at home. Understanding the diverse needs of patients is important. Ways to maintain good patient relations are the subject of this chapter.

THE PATIENT

In caring for the patient, the physician often must address both the patient's needs and the needs of the patient's family. It is difficult to predict how patients and family members will react to medical advice. Patients may respond differently from one visit to another depending on the situation, severity of illness, and other factors. The role of the physician in managing complex interactions with patients and their family members can be trying and exhausting. Those in support of the physician should keep in mind how difficult this task is.

Group practice personnel need to focus on identifying and resolving patient concerns and complaints. The anticipation of patient concerns and the development of operating processes that help bring the patient into contact with the physician, without registration, parking, billing, or other problems, contribute to the willingness of the patient to accept medical advice from the physician. This is because the patient judges contact with all the staff, not just contact with the physician, when forming an opinion about the group practice.

When patients feel they are not getting anywhere with a physician, they often respond positively to a manager or patient advocate who is a good listener. This does not mean that patient advocates should agree with everything the patient says concerning problems. Nonetheless, they must convey a valid and humane interest in the patient's perspective, even when, on occasion, patients express considerable anxiety or anger about alleged disservices.

The primary oversight for resolution of patient complaints normally rests with the physician, because it is the physician who supervises the patient's care. In a group practice, this responsibility may be shared by a number of professionals, as the primary care responsibility is shifted from one member of the team to another. Optimally, the relationship should be solid enough for the patient to feel that concerns can be registered with the primary care giver. However, patients may elect not to complain to their physician for fear that doing so might jeopardize their relationship with the physician. Hence, it is important for systems to be in place to address these concerns in a way that helps protect the essential physician-patient relationship.

Patients may be quite accepting of functional system problems, such as delays in appointments, billing errors, or similar problems, providing there is a perception that the problems are being addressed by the physician or staff. Management must recognize that a timely response can make a great deal of difference in patient satisfaction, but so can physician attitudes. Some physicians are always behind schedule, yet they never receive complaints from patients because the physicians are so skilled at focusing attention on the patient that the patient overlooks the lengths of the wait. Other physicians run precisely on schedule yet receive complaints because they are perceived as aloof, cold, or distant. Clearly there is an art to medicine, and "bedside manners" apply to the ambulatory setting as well as they do to other settings for patient care (Shorter, 1995).

Often, a patient complaint is merely a symptom of a broader problem (Watrous et al., 1994). A complaint

---

CASE STUDY 15–1

A CASE OF PATIENT SENSITIVITY

Joe Jinx, a clinic administrator, received a telephone call at 9:15 A.M. from the irate husband of a patient. Mr. Knox, the caller, expressed great displeasure with the fact that his wife, Henrietta, who had come to the clinic for a scheduled first-time diagnostic workup, was sitting in the outer lobby cooling her heels because she didn't have her check book and was unprepared to make the $250 deposit being requested by a credit clerk.

Mr. Knox attested that he is wealthy and for this reason does not carry health insurance. He and his wife also do not believe in carrying credit cards. Mr. Knox was highly critical of the clinic's policy that assumes that he and his wife are credit risks because they do not have health insurance. Joe Jinx responded that he was unaware of the requirement for an advance deposit if the patient is uninsured. Meanwhile, Henrietta was still sitting in the lobby.

Case Discussion Questions

1. What should Mr. Jinx do right now?
2. How could this problem have been prevented?
3. What questions should Mr. Jinx ask to familiarize himself with credit and collection policies of the group?

---

about a bill for professional services, for example, may reflect dissatisfaction with services rendered by the physician or with the clinic as a whole. Or it may simply reflect the fact that professional findings were poorly communicated. Determining the real cause of a complaint can be helpful in identifying system problems that may affect a number of patients. It should be remembered that relatively few patients ever complain, even when they are dissatisfied with the care received. Many just "vote with their feet" instead and do not return. Relatives of patients often act as patient advocates. Although some patients and professionals may resent this, it is a healthy process. Contact with family members helps provide a more complete picture of the patient's situation. The physician's primary responsibility is to the patient, however, so the involvement of others in care decisions depends on the wishes of the patient.

Most organizations recognize that their employees can be their best or their worst public relations agents, because they represent the organization both at home and in the community. Administrators should develop in each employee a sensitivity to patient opinions and awareness of the effect of their actions on public relations.

DEALING WITH PATIENT COMPLAINTS

Figure 15–1 lists the top eight complaints made by patients. In dealing with patient complaints, the administrator first must recognize that all patients cannot be satisfied all of the time. Patients with complaints must be listened to and dealt with using common sense. Even angry patients should not be confronted until the facts are known.

Dealing with patient complaints requires an understanding of the personalities and objectives of both the provider and the patient. The administrator is not usually authorized to settle problems without checking with the appropriate medical professional for review and advice, and administrative skill is needed to

Top Eight Patient Complaints

1. Too little time was spent with the physician
2. The physician wasn't listening
3. The staff has an uncaring attitude
4. Waiting time in the lobby or examining room was too long
5. The physician took telephone calls during the examination
6. Physical findings and test results were not explained adequately
7. Billing and insurance procedures were confusing
8. Specialists were slow in sending reports to primary care physicians

FIGURE 15–1

translate patient complaints into terms that are acceptable to the physician. The best approach is to gather the facts carefully, determine the magnitude of the problem, and focus on assuring that the patient is dealt with fairly. Physicians typically respond well to such an approach. However, some physicians may resent staff members who bring complaints to their attention. Others may respond to complaints by withdrawing from providing the patient with further service. The goal should be for practitioners to respond thoughtfully, carefully, and sensitively to each patient concern.

Practices should implement an effective patient-oriented complaint system. The system should be designed not just to defuse single complaints as they arise, but to monitor patient satisfaction over time to reveal significant problems. To be effective, the system must be endorsed and supported by the medical leadership and staff. The importance of supporting an effective, impartial fact-finding system in resolving patient complaints should not be minimized (Dolinsky, 1995). Such a system includes the following five attributes:

1. Identification of problem areas through surveys, focus groups, or other techniques
2. Recording and analyzing of data from patient complaints in order to identify trends
3. Reporting of complaint summaries to leadership and staff
4. Implementation of actions to reverse negative trends
5. Regular revisiting of actions taken to assure that improvement is taking place

The objective of such a monitoring system is not to find the "bad apples" on the staff but to involve the staff in developing processes to improve patient care and satisfaction. Monitoring systems can also demonstrate to patients that the staff and organization care about and are accountable to them. The most compelling objective of a well-functioning complaint-monitoring system is to improve the overall quality of care and enhance patient goodwill.

The Written Survey Instrument

In the written patient survey, patients are asked to fill out a questionnaire regarding their experiences with the practice. The patient should be contacted by a letter explaining the purpose of the questionnaire, and the questionnaire itself should be designed for easy response. Also, a prestamped return envelope should be enclosed. The staff must be oriented and involved if the results of the survey are to be of value. If 30 to 40 percent of the questionnaires are returned, the survey instrument can be considered successful. Requiring patients to sign the survey form may be intimidating. Approximately 15 to 20 percent of the returns are likely to be signed if the signature is optional. Any patient who does identify himself or herself by signing the survey instrument should receive a personal response.

The written questionnaire can aid in the overall evaluation process by increasing staff awareness of the types of problems patients have. It can also help to put complaints in perspective, because the process may yield compliments as well as complaints.

Physician Peer Review Process

If a physician review process is established in which physician department heads receive copies of factual reports on the performance of physicians in their departments, the success rate for resolution of problems increases significantly. With such a process, physicians respond to patients, information about the solution of problems is much more readily conveyed to administration, and department heads seldom have to intercede. The positive use of peer review in resolving patient complaints in this fashion cannot be underestimated.

CASE STUDY 15–2

PATIENT COMPLAINT BASKET TEST

The administrator of a clinic has received the following series of patient complaints:

1. The parents of a patient alleged that the physician rudely rushed off their daughter's symptoms; shortly thereafter, the daughter was diagnosed elsewhere with a malignant brain tumor
2. A patient complained that the physician refused to provide a letter to her employer stating she needed more time off from work, and she threatened to sue if the letter was not forthcoming
3. A patient complained that his bill was too high, that the physician had misinformed him about one of his test results, and that this caused a delay in treatment
4. A patient was angered when her biopsy was put off because of the physician's vacation plans, delaying a diagnosis of metastasized breast cancer by four weeks
5. A patient complained that confidentiality was breached by an employee who discussed his case outside the clinic in a social setting; the patient demanded that the employee be fired
6. A patient requested a refund because the clinic lost X-ray films depicting progress of his pituitary tumor
7. A patient accused a physician of improper sexual conduct
8. A patient relayed a series of minor complaints against the physician and the clinic, requesting that the remaining bill of $38.00 be written off

Case Discussion Questions

1. Classify the complaints by severity on a scale from one to three, where one is the most severe.
2. Select one of the severe complaints and recommend a solution.

There is tremendous opportunity for innovation in developing sensitive patient-physician response systems in order to resolve conflict and enhance the diagnostic and treatment processes.

Complaint Resolution Process

In summary, the administrator should apply the following six steps in implementing a complaint-resolution system:

1. Delegate responsibility for collecting factual information about patient complaints
2. Obtain medical leadership endorsement of the process
3. Meticulously follow procedures and policies established for resolving complaints
4. Recognize the role of administration in collecting facts and focusing attention on the problem rather than on judging the facts of the case
5. Use physician peer review processes as much as possible
6. Report the nature, type, and resolution of the complaint to the physician leadership and staff

AVOIDING MEDICAL MALPRACTICE

There are a number of factors that can trigger specific claims of medical liability or malpractice. One major factor is alleged careless practice of medicine. Carelessness can relate to any member of the medical team. It is not only the physician who can trigger an incident, but supporting personnel as well. Disputes about care between physicians, or between physicians and other members of the professional team such as nurses, can be detrimental in the case of malpractice claims. Physicians or others who make entries in the medical record that criticize other professionals provide the litigating patient's attorney with a field day.

Although the best defense against the possibility of malpractice claims is obviously the practice of good medicine, this is not always an effective defense against a litigation-minded patient. Often equally important is a high-quality relationship between the physician and the patient. Some of the best qualified professionals in a technical sense can be subject to considerable malpractice liability exposure if they approach the patient or the patient's relatives with professional arrogance.

THE IMPORTANCE OF PATIENT RELATIONS

In summary, administrators should pay close attention to patient concerns. Administrators are in a unique position to help improve health care services by providing essential feedback to the staff. In an era characterized by self-awareness, health promotion, and more openness in communication between the physician and patient, it behooves the administrator to establish systems that are structured to encourage patient questioning of processes and procedures.

Physicians also should encourage patients to "bother the doctor." Patients should be encouraged to think about the visit before they arrive and to be prepared to discuss symptoms and concerns. This openness of contact between the patient and the physician can only result in improved communication. From the moment the patient enters the system until the process is completed, it is essential that supporting systems are attuned to patient needs and expectations. The role of the administrator and of the administrative processes is to provide support to the physician in accommodating the diversity of patient expectations and needs.

REFERENCES

Anderson, E. (1995, February). How to deal. *Physicians Management, 35*(2), 38–40.

Dolinsky, A.L. (1995, May). Complaint intensity and health care services. *Journal of Health Care Marketing, 15*(2), 42–47.

Shorter, E. (1995). *Beside manners: The troubled history of doctors and patients.* New York: Simon and Schuster.

Watrous, J., Pettis, J., & Hobson, A. (1994, November/December). A systems approach to gathering and analyzing patient and family complaints and suggestions. *Journal for Health Care Quality, 16*(6), 14–16.

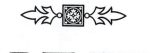

PART FIVE

PLANNING FOR AND MARKETING THE GROUP PRACTICE

CHAPTER

16

Strategic Planning

Stephen J. Williams and Austin Ross

LEARNING OBJECTIVES

Upon completing this chapter, the reader should be able to:

- Describe the historical context of planning and regulation of health services
- Identify a general formulation for institutional strategic planning
- Explain the steps and principles of strategic planning
- Describe the political and procedural aspects of strategic planning

The essence of long-term survival for any organization is strategic planning. The health care environment has changed so radically—and undoubtedly will continue to do so in the future—that every practice administrator must attach high priority to planning.

This chapter focuses on the strategic planning function: what it requires and how it is done. To provide a complete picture, the chapter includes historical perspectives on community planning and health services regulation. It also discusses the design of organizational missions and strategies for organizational growth and development. The chapter emphasizes the philosophical and practical importance of planning to the successful operation of ambulatory care organizations and to the personal success of administrators. Administrators who fail in this arena will not succeed in their jobs for long.

The information in this chapter is integrally related to facilities and financial planning and to the marketing of services, topics that are discussed in detail in separate chapters. In fact, virtually every chapter in this book is related to strategic planning.

A FRAMEWORK FOR STRATEGIC PLANNING

Planning can be externally imposed through regulation, or it can be an internal strategic process conducted by management (Williams & Torrens, 1993). Furthermore, planning can be viewed from both community, or societal, and institutional perspectives.

Mandatory planning is a manifestation of national, state, and local policies designed to manipulate the health care marketplace and modify the health care delivery system in individual communities. Many, but certainly not all, of these mandatory planning efforts have fallen by the wayside in recent years. It is still important for the administrator to understand and adapt to these external planning pressures.

They require compliance with governmentally imposed rules concerning the way in which organizations may function. Societal perspectives are met through zoning ordinances, building codes, and other similar requirements.

Internal strategic planning, on the other hand, is primarily a voluntary activity, although it may have mandated components. It involves establishing organizational priorities and determining ways to meet them. The aim is to maximize the organization's success, but community needs may also be considered in determining the organizational priorities. The priorities must be translated into objectives, and specific strategies must be developed for meeting these objectives.

HEALTH SERVICES REGULATION IN THE UNITED STATES

In the United States, the modern era of government intervention began in the 1960s, primarily as a result of a perception by government that the health care system had failed to meet the needs of certain population groups. Governmental intervention in the health care system has assumed a number of forms. One is the direct provision of services through such agencies as the Indian Health Service and the Veterans Administration. Government also supplies money to both providers and clients. Examples of the former include federally funded community health centers and other organizations. There are also programs that receive grants from federal, state, or local governments in return for providing defined sets of services to eligible populations. Examples of providing funds directly to clients include federal, state, and local entitlement programs for health care, primarily Medicare and Medicaid. Again, the purpose of these programs is to alleviate market imperfections, at least from a social perspective.

Other governmental interventions have taken the form of attempts to influence perceived structural imperfections in the provider system itself. These interventions have addressed such major problem areas as too few or too many hospital beds, skyrocketing health care costs, and poor quality of care. The interventions have involved mandated planning and regulation, primarily instituted by the federal government in cooperation with the states. Four major avenues for intervention have included subsidies, entry controls, rate or price regulation, and quality controls.

Subsidies

Subsidy interventions have primarily been designed for one of two purposes: to facilitate the development of provider organizations so that they can offer more services; or to provide financial subsidies to clients so they can use more services. These awards increase the supply of providers and, hence, of health care services. Subsidy awards to institutions include grants to hospitals to develop additional physical resources, primarily through the Hill-Burton Act. They also include funds from local governments to develop health care resources through such mechanisms as hospital districts that are vested with taxing authority. In addition, many institutional providers have been granted tax exemptions, thus substantially increasing the subsidy they receive from federal and state governments.

Subsidy awards to individuals take two forms. The first form includes such major programs as Medicare, which was designed primarily to provide health insurance for individuals aged 65 and above. The second form includes Medicaid, which has assumed program responsibility for medically indigent individuals in a federal-state partnership, as well as other programs that exist for needs ranging from end-stage renal disease to assistance for pregnant women. In addition, employers can deduct the costs of providing health insurance benefits to their employees, who usually receive this benefit on a tax-free basis.

Market Entry Controls

Market entry controls consist of personnel licensure and institutional licensure for hospitals and long-term care facilities. Although licensure interventions are designed to assure a minimum level of quality of care, they also limit entry of additional providers into the medical care marketplace. The other major area for entry restrictions is capital expenditure controls, the most prominent of which have been certificate-of-need programs. Capital expenditure controls limit the freedom of institutional providers to expand or modify their physical facilities and, hence, the services they offer.

Rate Regulation

Rather than intervening directly in providing services, rate regulation is aimed at controlling the charges incurred for the care provided. For physicians, the most common rate controls are fee schedules. For institutions, rate setting by hospital cost commissions and reimbursement regulations under Medicare, Medicaid, and private insurance programs serve to define and limit the types of services that are covered, to set fees and define allowable costs, and to otherwise delineate the obligations of the insurer.

Quality Controls

Institutional quality controls include certification of care, such as that required under government entitlement programs, and a wide range of quality-promoting programs, such as that of the Joint Commission on the Accreditation of Health Care Organizations, certification of medical residency training programs, and building code and fire safety rules and regulations. Other regulatory mechanisms range from regulations on prescription drugs to labor rules on the employment of individuals. Specific regulations vary, depending on local jurisdictions.

Summary and Implications

Clearly, then, there is a long and important history of governmental intervention in health care. The market driven environment still contains many important elements of governmental involvement, and further changes are likely in the future. Recognizing how government intervention affects the provision of ambulatory care services is obviously important, but what is even more important is the development of long-term and short-term planning that recognizes the broader environment within which services are provided. Equally important, as discussed in other chapters, is the recognition that this environment changes and that planning must be a dynamic function. The manager of an ambulatory care practice must be actively involved in identifying and interpreting changes in this environment.

HEALTH SERVICES PLANNING IN THE UNITED STATES

Health planning originated as a voluntary, cooperative effort by hospitals. Early health planning efforts can be traced to the 1930s and 1940s, when voluntary hospital councils were started in some cities to coordinate selected hospitals' services and provide some measure of cooperation among facilities. Voluntary planning represented a significant commitment to the philosophical concepts of cooperation and rational allocation of resources. Health-planning legislation, at both the federal and state levels, had origins in well-intentioned approaches to distribute limited resources in recognition of social needs.

Congress passed the Hospital Survey and Construction Act of 1946, also referred to as the Hill-Burton Act, to promote the construction of hospitals in areas of identified community need. To facilitate the identification of need for hospitals, the act also mandated and provided federal funding for certain health-planning activities. Congress passed a number of other health-planning initiatives after the Hill-Burton legislation.

The first large-scale federal initiative to develop substantive health-planning agencies throughout the country was the Community Health Planning (CHP) legislation, which was passed in 1967. This legislation established state and local agencies with responsibility for conducting health planning. The state agencies, often referred to as CHP(a) agencies, were responsible for overseeing planning throughout the state. The local agencies, or CHP(b), were responsible for overseeing planning in local communities. Client involvement was important in the design of the CHP legislation and the subsequent development of the CHP agencies. Both state and local agencies were charged with developing health services plans, assessing the need for new resources, and playing other advisory roles in facilitating health planning. Unfortunately, these agencies did not have any mandated regulatory function and therefore had little substantive impact on the health care system, other than to encourage the development of some health-planning methodologies.

A number of other initiatives were passed over the years to encourage planning and facilitate the relationship between planning and regulation, but none was as visible, comprehensive, or significant as Public Law 93–641, the National Health Planning and Resources Development Act of 1974. Under this legislation, the statewide planning function was delegated to an agency similar to the CHP(a) agency, whereas the local function was delegated to Health Systems Agencies (HSAs), which were somewhat similar to the CHP(b) agencies. A complex network of federal, state, and local advisory bodies and coordinating councils was also established to provide client perspectives and oversee the entire effort. There is mixed evidence on the success of these agencies, but they did increase health care providers' awareness of the importance of conducting institutional strategic planning and of relating institutional growth and development to community needs.

INSTITUTIONAL STRATEGIC PLANNING

Institutional strategic planning is the development of an organization's strategies for coping with the future, including the definition of goals and missions and delineation of specific pathways for achieving organizational objectives. Strategic planning requires thinking about and anticipating the future course of events in the environment within which the organization functions. It also involves assuring that the organization is prepared to advance to meet the challenges of the future.

Through strategic planning and related activities, the administrator can position an organization so that it can compete in the health care marketplace and provide needed services in appropriate facilities with the right types of personnel. Strategic planning assures that the practical political processes of the organization's functioning do not raise barriers to successful performance (Henderson & Williams, 1994). Strategic planning provides an opportunity to develop a consensus of opinion among members of the practice concerning the direction in which the practice should move in the future. Such a consensus helps assure that the administrator is not faced with political opposition at every decision point. Figure 16–1 presents an overview of strategic planning in the ambulatory care setting.

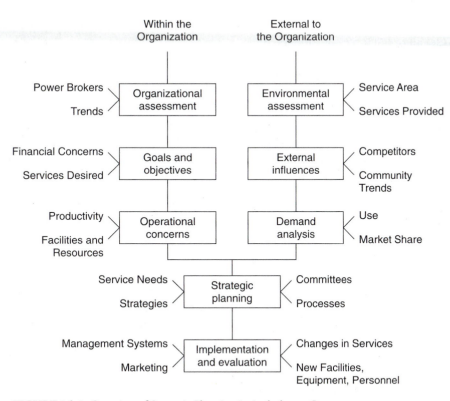

FIGURE 16–1 Overview of Strategic Planning in Ambulatory Care

Strategic planning depends on the development of processes and specific strategies for coping with the organization's environment. The organization's environment includes the external environment, which is the service or delivery arena within which the organization functions, and the internal environment, which is the organization itself, including its own politics. It should be noted that, in many competitive environments, strategic planning may lead to downsizing. The approaches necessary to pare operations and maintain market share while also promoting employee morale are different from the approaches used to expand the organization.

The Administrator's Role in Strategic Planning

The administrator's overall role in strategic planning is one of coordinator, initiator, and implementer (Bracker, 1980). Indeed, most ambulatory care prac-

tices rely on the administrator to perform the bulk of strategic planning functions.

Specific responsibilities of the administrator in strategic planning include monitoring the external environment, assessing the internal environment and current services and facilities, and providing leadership in the conduct of all strategic-planning activities. The involvement of other individuals and committees is essential in order to achieve a consensus of opinion about the organization's strategic alternatives, and all employees should be involved in implementing specific strategies. Although it is critical for the administrator to provide leadership for planning activities, involvement by other administrators and the medical staff is also essential.

First Step in Strategic Planning

The first step in strategic planning for an ambulatory care organization is to assess the external environment within which the organization functions. The external environment includes all of the forces outside the organization that affect the organization's functioning. These forces include regulatory agencies, competitors, insurers, clients, and any other people, entities, or organizations that impinge directly or indirectly on the functioning of the practice. Because strategic planning is an ongoing process, this information should be reassessed periodically. If information on the environment is kept current, it is relatively easy to run through a checklist of all environmental factors that are relevant to particular decisions. For example, a new service may be proposed, but the environmental assessment checklist may indicate that there are regulatory or competitive constraints suggesting it would be a mistake for the practice to offer the service. Such an analytical approach helps assure that administrators do not overlook any significant factors before making recommendations.

As part of the environmental assessment function, the administrator must carefully analyze all other providers who compete for patients, including providers of specific services such as laboratory services. In communities where health care is changing rapidly, it is important that the administrator also anticipate new providers and services that may be entering the marketplace. Competing providers obviously are a major source of external influence on any practice, and very detailed analysis is required to assure that the organization is aware of what the competition is doing. For example, a competing provider that is planning to offer a new service could represent a serious challenge if the administrator's own facility provides the same service. Alternatively, such a factor could be significant in deciding whether to add a service that is now being adequately provided by the competitor. As the health care industry has become much more competitive, these considerations have become increasingly important.

Monitoring Sociodemographic Change in the Community

Changes in the community may affect the operation of the ambulatory care practice, even though the changes are not in health care per se. The most significant of these are sociodemographic changes. These changes must also be monitored by environmental assessment.

Sociodemographic characteristics of the organization's service area include such important factors as age, sex, race, income, education, employment, and marital status. Information on most of these variables is available from census data. The data should be arrayed so that they are readily understood and can be easily related to the practice's decision-making processes. The data also should be listed separately for the total service-area population and for the patients now using the ambulatory care facility. This allows the administrator to compare characteristics of the community the practice intends to serve with characteristics of the population currently being served. Such a comparison can be used to determine which segments of the service-area population could be reached with a more aggressive marketing approach.

In addition to the census, sociodemographic information can be obtained from a number of sources. If the service area can be fairly well defined, information on the characteristics of the population may be obtainable from local banks, telephone companies, and other commercial organizations, as well as from the demographic departments of local government agencies. National census data also can be disaggregated to the local level, but this approach requires a lot of work and may be inexact. Another drawback in relying on census data is that they are collected relatively infrequently and become outdated quickly, especially in communities with rapid population change. Therefore, wherever possible, other sources of data should be used.

Sophisticated adjustments of population data may be needed to account for underrepresentation of population groups such as minorities. Demographers use data from a variety of sources, including school enrollments, automobile registrations, and voter registrations, among others, as well as sophisticated mathematical techniques in order to adjust census and other statistical data to improve the accuracy of the information. Such methods are also important for estimating population characteristics between censuses and for projecting population trends.

Information on the dynamics of population, including data on fertility, morbidity, mortality, and migration,

---

CASE STUDY 16–1

STARTING TO IMPLEMENT STRATEGIC PLANNING

A group practice administrator with many years of experience is used to a seat-of-the-pants approach to running the practice. In the past, with a rapidly growing health care marketplace and relatively few competitors, she was able to succeed admirably with this approach. After attending a continuing education session on the future of health care sponsored by the Medical Group Management Association, however, the administrator realizes that her management style has to change to face future realities. In the past, hard work and an ad hoc approach were adequate for dealing with events as they happened; in the future, it will be necessary to anticipate events.

The practice and its board and physicians have followed the administrator's seat-of-the-pants lead and taken things pretty much as they have occurred. They too are aware that health care is changing, but they are less aware than the administrator of what these changes are and how fast they are occurring. The administrator now recognizes that if the practice is to be successful in the future, it will have to be much more aggressive in many ways and especially in conducting top-notch strategic planning. The administrator also recognizes that many of the physicians in the practice, especially the older ones, are set in their ways and will not jump on the bandwagon for planning, marketing, and similar activities, even though there is really no alternative.

Case Discussion Questions

1. How should the administrator go about getting everyone in the practice interested in and involved with planning?
2. How can the administrator build for the future with people whose thinking is based on a past that no longer exists?

---

is also important for projecting population trends. In addition, data on mortality and morbidity reflect causes of illness and death in the community. An ambulatory care practice should offer services to meet the specific health care needs of the community as determined from these data. It should be noted, however, that problems with the quality and format of these data somewhat limit their applicability. Morbidity data are especially difficult to obtain and use for practical planning. For morbidity data, the administrator may have to rely on surveys conducted by the federal government.

Data on migration are extremely limited. Migration patterns are reflected by school enrollments, job or employment patterns, and some other secondary sources, such as automobile registrations. Some migration information also may be available from local sources. In communities with high rates of in- or out-migration, this information is essential for long-term planning, even when the data are not as accurate as might be desired.

Other Relevant Information

Other relevant information may be available from special surveys. It includes illness levels or health status and the relationship between these and the need for health services. Attitudinal information, measures of the population's propensity to use services in response to specific symptoms, and other relatively complex and sophisticated measures of social, cultural, and psychological characteristics of the population may also be available from special surveys. Although such information is important, it may be difficult to translate into a form that is useful for planning.

The health care industry is not immune to the economic ups and downs of national and local economies. Anticipated demand for some services, for example, may be very dependent on the economic vitality of the community. Information of particular relevance in this regard is the trend in employment, including number of people employed, major employers, and employer sponsorship of health care benefits. Expansion or retraction of housing, education, industry, and other economic activities in the community also relates directly to ambulatory care practice.

It is also important to recognize that third-party reimbursers, including government and private insurers, represent a form of regulation, in that they dictate the types and levels of reimbursement as well as the mechanisms for receiving payment for services provided. This is especially important for managed-care plans, where the practice's approaches to care may have to conform to contractual specifications. Thus, it is important to identify those insurers to which the ambulatory care organization relates. Important data in this area include identity of the insurers, the fraction of the population in the community that they insure, the fraction of the ambulatory care facility's patient load that is covered by each insurer, the scope and level of benefits covered under each policy, and limitations in payments or processing.

Changes in medical technology can be dramatic and severely impact ambulatory care practice. An example is the rapid growth of ambulatory surgery. This is due to the shifting of procedures out of the hospital and to technological innovations, particularly the use of fiberoptic surgical techniques.

Changes in national, state, and local health care policies can substantially impact the funding, and hence delivery, of health care services. Examples include changes in national entitlement program such as Medicare and Medicaid and changes in local programs to provide medical services and financial support to the medically indigent population of the community. Changes in national, state, and local economic conditions can also se-

verely impact health care services through changes in insurance coverage, employment levels, economic growth, and other considerations. The impact of cyclic changes in the automotive industry is a good example.

Illness and injuries are other areas requiring constant monitoring. New disease patterns and threats are introduced into the environment and require responses by health care organizations. An example in recent years is the epidemic of AIDS.

Finally, changes in the essential structure of the society and of local communities can severely impact health care services utilization. These include changes in family structure, the dissolution of families, increasing numbers of births to single mothers, and changes in smoking and other lifestyle behaviors, among other relevant factors.

Organizational Assessment

Identifying trends in the community through the external environment assessment process must be complemented by a similar effort directed toward understanding the ambulatory care organization itself. This process is termed organizational assessment, and, like external environmental assessment, it should be an ongoing activity led by the administrator. Organizational assessment is a very important function that can help assure that the administrator understands the strengths and weaknesses of his or her own organization. Organizational assessment also requires a careful analysis of the existing and projected future financial trends of the practice.

Organizational assessment is directed toward the internal structure and function of the provider organization and has a number of major components. The first is identifying the services currently provided. These include both clinical and support services and any other products. It is useful to measure the degree of use of each service or product, to rank the relative prominence of each service, and to assess the potential for expansion, particularly when these data are related to information on the number and productivity of physicians and other employees. A larger organization or a more comprehensive provider, such as a hospital, should include in the list of services provided those that could potentially impinge on or interrelate with ambulatory care services.

Another major function of organizational assessment is to determine the effectiveness and appropriateness of the ambulatory care organization's internal structure and management. To facilitate this analysis, each administrator should review the organizational chart to clarify management, medical staff, and governing body relationships. The governing body members should be listed and the key players identified, including their substantive interests and political strengths, and the characteristics of the medical staff should be detailed, including each physician's age, patient volume, and specialty. After outlining the organizational structure, the administrator should analyze it, especially with regard to informal organization and individual power brokers. For administration, the analysis should include an examination of each manager's strengths and weaknesses, relative performance, and areas of expertise and knowledge.

Service Area Definitions

The application of quantitative methods to strategic planning and particularly to the analysis of potential demand for services requires that the ambulatory care practice's service area be defined. The service area is the geographic region from which patients currently are, or potentially could be, attracted. The service area is usually defined at a point in time because it can change over time as the practice changes its scope and quantity of services. Defining the service area is an important function that the administrator should perform in conjunction with medical staff and other key individuals, with the objective of targeting marketing efforts and service delivery strategies toward specific population groups.

Identifying a geographic service area may not be easy. The administrator first needs to define the geographic area from which patients are currently drawn. One method for doing this is to obtain, from medical or administrative records, the addresses of all current patients (those who have used the practice during the past one or two years). This should be compiled by geographic subregion and number of patients per region. The use of zip codes can be particularly helpful for this purpose, although it is important to recognize that zip code geographic boundaries frequently do not coincide with those of census regions. This can complicate the use of demographic data in interpreting patient-origin information. The compilation of patient-origin data by city or country may be feasible, depending on the practice's location, but frequently these political divisions are too large to provide enough detailed information to define the service area usefully. In some instances, such as large metropolitan areas with high population density (for example, Manhattan), a practice may want to restrict the service area to a few city blocks.

It is frequently useful to physically plot on a map the locations from which patients are coming. Color codes can be used to show the relative percentage of the practice's patient population coming from each geographic area. Alternatively, patient-origin information can be combined with census data to demonstrate changes in the market-penetration rate. Whichever approach is used, information should be displayed so that the geographic location of patients attracted to the practice is clearly evident.

Service areas can be defined in a variety of ways other than the geographic location of patients. Frequently, demographic rather than geographic definitions are used, particularly by managed-care plans. For specialty services as well, certain patient demographic characteristics may be important in defining the service area population. Other characteristics of the target community that may influence service area definitions include patterns of employment, housing, insurance coverage, and transportation. Transportation patterns, for example, including highways and public transportation, can define existing and potential utilization patterns. Similarly, in defining its service area, an urban hospital providing ambulatory care to local workers during the day would need to differentiate this population from the same area's residential population, which might use the facility on evenings or weekends. As another example, the development of new housing close to a facility could substantially affect its service area definition.

CASE STUDY 16–2

THE POWERS THAT BE

Organizational assessment is of particular interest to the administrator of a medical practice. He took a lot of organizational theory courses in graduate school and has always been fascinated by the policies of management. As an administrator, he has looked informally at the policies and power plays around him. The interactions between people have been especially interesting to watch, and he has noticed that the physicians seem to have their own internal policies in addition to their often unique interactions with others in the practice. As part of the organizational assessment he is initiating, the administrator decides to look at the politics of the practice more formally. He wants to examine who has power, how that power is used, and the consequences to the organization of the formal and informal structures in the practice.

Case Discussion Questions

1. How should the administrator proceed? Whom should he involve, and what techniques should he use?
2. What are the problems and pitfalls he might experience?
3. What are the risks and benefits of this type of analysis?

In changing its mix of services or expanding its operations, the practice aims to increase its potential market share. This may require identifying new target service areas, using a more community-based analytical approach. Maps and other visual displays that identify existing service areas can be used to identify new target areas that may be amenable to marketing. Deciding where to draw the lines however, requires data on such factors as housing, employment, transportation, migration patterns, and the other types of information discussed in this chapter. The subjective judgment of the administrator and other key individuals may also be useful in refining the boundaries of new target service areas.

By using a map or a computer simulation of community characteristics, the administrator can readily define the geographic areas that are accessible within specific travel times or distances. Obviously, in such an analysis, it is important to consider whether the facility is located in an urban or a rural area, to recognize the geographic and physical barriers that may affect travel patterns, and to consider carefully the practical aspects

of patient movement, such as rush hour traffic. This type of analysis can be valuable to understanding both the sources of current patients and the potential for expansion of services in a more market-competitive environment, which is a key aspect of strategic planning.

Market Demand and Use of Health Services

Use of health services is not identical to demand for health care. Demand is usually defined as including all potential use that the patient desires, whether it actually occurs or not. In other words, demand includes use that never occurs, because people lack access to care for financial or other reasons. Use is usually defined as the actual number of visits, days of care, or other similar measures that a population experiences. Need for health care is defined as the underlying level of health care use that should be utilized to meet all health care needs, although various barriers, or the patient's or physician's lack of recognition of need, may mean that need exceeds use.

Market Demand

The importance of understanding the nature and extent of demand for services in a practice cannot be overstated. Estimates of market demand should be conducted for time periods that are appropriate to the strategic planning processes of the practice. Many practices make short-run plans for one-year periods and long-run plans for up to five years. It is probably not practical to plan beyond five years except for capital expansions.

Demand for ambulatory care services is a function of the number of people in the target or covered population, stratified by their characteristics, and multiplied by expected utilization rates per person. The demographic characteristics used in demand forecasting are usually limited to those available from census information, including age, sex, and certain socioeconomic factors such as income. Place of residence may be used as well if it is available for appropriate geographic subunits.

The selection of variables used to stratify the population should be based on those that are known to be associated with differences in the use of health care, such as age and sex. In addition, only those variables for which local, or at least national, utilization data are available can be used to make projections. Thus, attitudinal information, such as the percentage of the population that thinks medical care can improve their health, is not a practical variable to use in demand analysis, because these data are not available except through special, expensive surveys.

Use of Health Services

The usual starting point for computing use of health services is to identify the age and sex characteristics of the population that is currently being serviced or, in the case of a new or expanding practice, the population that is being served. Estimates of use are based on surveys of population using special questionnaires or interview techniques, or on observations of actual use. For each population characteristic, the estimated numbers of visits are computed based on the number of visits expected for people with those characteristics.

Next, it is necessary to determine the percentage of all office visits or other use that the practice can expect to obtain as its market share or enrolled population for a managed-care plan.

Where possible, projections for the use of health services should be service specific. This increased level of detail is helpful in designing strategies for offering new or expanded services. However, more detailed computations are likely to be limited by the availability of data, and the cost of collecting the needed data may exceed the value of planning.

Increased productivity should enter into use projections because this can have a significant effect on the ability of a practice to increase its capacity without expanding staff. Physician productivity is usually measured by the number of patients seen per unit of time. It varies depending on physician specialty, the complexity of cases cared for, and the support services available. There are numerous other considerations that could be built into the forecasting methodology presented here. There are no hard-and-fast guidelines for how far an administrator should go in the sophistication of the planning effort. When justified, the use of consultants to assist in the planning effort may be worthwhile.

Planning Implementation

Implementation includes preparing strategic plans and distributing them to appropriate people in the organization. Figure 16–2 shows the content of a sample group practice strategic plan. The plan is a blueprint for all managers and providers in the organization to follow, and it is a means of achieving consensus and political support for the group's agreed-upon directions for the future. Implementation requires developing a strong degree of support for the strategic plan through ongoing meetings and briefings of individuals important in the internal formal and informal organizations of the practice. In addition, the plan should provide for periodic assessment of the extent to which the practice is meeting its goals and objectives. Modification of each group's specific environment, including both external and internal components, is essential to the process.

Implementation may also involve developing other, highly relevant planning documents, such as financial plans and budgets (discussed in earlier chapters) and a

CASE STUDY 16-3

METHODOLOGY FOR PLANNING

Although John Doe has always considered himself to be a good manager, he knows that he is weak in applying quantitative methods to management. In the past, his statistical abilities were never really used in the practice, and he shied away from using the computer and sophisticated approaches to management functions. However, he is beginning to recognize that these approaches and methods are valuable and that the administrator of the future will need to apply them.

As a result, John Doe recently completed two continuing education courses for ambulatory care managers, one on the use of statistics and other quantitative techniques, the other on the use of computers in physician practices. He was surprised at how easy many of the techniques were to apply, especially when using packaged programs. He bought a personal computer for his office and has begun to try out some programs he bought, including an electronic spreadsheet. He has been thinking about using the computer for strategic planning, but he is not sure how applicable it might be. In general, he wonders how much he and the practice should move into the application of quantitative techniques in management, especially in the strategic planning process.

Case Discussion Questions

1. How would you assess the extent to which quantitative methods are applicable to strategic planning, and which techniques do you think are likely to be most useful?
2. How would you introduce these methods to the medical staff and especially to the more skeptical members of the staff who do not appreciate the value of computers?
3. What specific steps in strategic planning are amenable to computers and quantitative methods?

---

marketing plan (discussed in the next chapter). Specific written documentation of the group's implementation of its agreed-upon missions and goals helps everyone work toward common objectives and eliminates confusion about where the practice is headed and how it is going to get there.

Planning in the context of the competitive environment that is now predominant in health care requires special consideration. Joint ventures and other activities involving multiple organizations must be carefully designed and monitored on an ongoing basis. The financial commitment and rewards of participation must make sense for each organization within the joint venture. The synergies of alliances and joint ventures must

eventually yield overall significant benefit to all the participating organizations.

Strategic planning also must tie into the marketing activities of the ambulatory care organization. Marketing and its associated activities must be formulated in a marketing plan that logically falls out from the overall strategic plan. The relationship between marketing and strategic planning is discussed in greater detail in Chapter 17.

In sum, the most sophisticated planning processes and written plans are useless unless they are implemented effectively. Implementation is a technical, political, and human leadership activity. The administrator must provide an ongoing commitment to planning on behalf of the

Table of Contents

i. **Overview**
   Statement of purpose
   Executive summary
I. Mission and distinguishing characteristics
   Mission
   Distinguishing characteristics
   Values statement
   Strategic planning challenges
II. Environmental assessment
   Health care industry trends: next 10 years
   Summary of previous responses to industry trends
   Competitor analysis: strengths and weaknesses, market share profile.
III. Internal assessment and data analysis
   Financial plan goals and constraints
   Data profile for past 10 years, including volume and activity, patient origins, visits per discharge analysis, etc.
   Service line analysis
   Portfolio analysis, including background of analysis and identification of next 5 years' service priorities
IV. Strategic goals: next 5 years
   Strategic goals
   Strategic annual operational, budgeting, and marketing objectives
V. Key issues and obstacles
   Questions to be discussed to define strategies and implementation plans (these identify obstacles and concerns that may prevent strategy implementation)
VI. Examples of possible, specific strategies and actions
   Regional issues, including policies and potential impacts on organization structure and facilities
   Satellite development plans, including their future role in facilities' needs and policies
   Projected facilities' requirements impacting master plan activity and properties
   New programs and services, including an ongoing process for evaluating proposed new programs and existing programs and prioritizing them for resource allocation
   Others

FIGURE 16–2 Illustrative Strategic Plan

organization, must recognize that planning is a dynamic and continual process, and should involve in this process everyone who has a stake in the group.

THE CHALLENGE OF STRATEGIC PLANNING

Strategic planning has evolved from a combination of internal and external practice perspectives and a variety of governmentally encouraged community-planning perspectives to an institutional focus within a competitive market-driven environment. Managed care has greatly increased the importance of strategic planning. However, the fundamental principles of strategic planning remain intact, dependent upon the assessment of the external environment and the internal current and potential future response on the part of the organization. The implementation of planning efforts will continue to help all groups to cope with an increasingly difficult and complex market (Shortell, Morrison, & Friedman, 1990).

REFERENCES

Bracker, J. (1980). The historic development of the strategic management concept. *Academy of Management Review, 5*(2), 219–24.

Henderson, C., & Williams, S. (1994). *Medical group practice assessment manual.* (3rd ed.). Denver, CO: Medical Group Management Association.

Shortell, S.M., Morrison, E.M., & Friedman, B. (1990). *Strategic choices for America's hospitals: Managing change in turbulent times.* San Francisco: Jossey-Bass.

Williams, S.J., & Torrens, P.R. (1993). Influencing, regulating, and monitoring the health care system. In *Introduction to health services* (4th ed.). Albany, NY: Delmar Publishers.

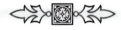

CHAPTER
17

Marketing in a Changing Environment

Meryl D. Luallin and Kevin W. Sullivan

CHAPTER TOPICS

The Nature of Marketing
Internal Marketing Strategies
External Marketing Strategies
Developing the Marketing Plan
The Importance of Marketing

LEARNING OBJECTIVES

Upon completing this chapter, the reader should be able to:

- Explain the nature of marketing in ambulatory care
- Design internal marketing strategies, plans, and programs for a practice
- Design external marketing strategies, plans, and programs for a practice
- Evaluate the effectiveness of marketing strategies
- Develop a marketing plan

One of the greatest management challenges in any industry is to guide the progress of an enterprise through changing times. The health care environment continues to evolve, both in terms of the market forces affecting practice profitability and the skills required of practice managers. Simultaneously, the pace of change is accelerating and the future has become less predictable. In coming years, as physicians and managers seek more effective strategies for achieving the goals of their practices, management meetings will devote a significant portion of time to analyzing these changes and developing strategies to cope with them.

This chapter focuses on marketing the medical practice. It discusses the essential elements of a marketing program and explains why this function is different from other practice management systems. The chapter also explains what marketing is, how it contributes to revenue, and why it is needed in an industry that formerly was exempt from competitive pressures. A review of basic internal and external marketing programs focuses on the purpose and application of specific techniques. Case studies show how specific techniques produced results for solo physicians and medical groups in various competitive situations. Finally, the chapter shows how formal marketing plans are integrated with strategic business plans discussed in the preceding chapter.

THE NATURE OF MARKETING

In a competitive marketplace, patients are subjected to dozens of attempts daily to get their attention and their business. In such an environment, physicians need to be known by their target publics, preferred by those who come to the practice, and recommended by satisfied patients, payers, and referral sources. Accomplishing this is largely the role of marketing.

Marketers are concerned with all decisions made and actions taken to generate and retain patient volume. They operate at the highest management level because their contributions are measured on the revenue line of the profit-loss statement. With so broad a charter, it is not surprising that marketers find themselves working with their peers in other clinic functions, including operations, personnel, data processing, employee training, and others.

It is important to recognize that marketing is neither all art nor all science but contains elements of both. Marketing problems do not lend themselves to textbook solutions, primarily because, for any given situation, marketers cannot make accurate predictions regarding two major variables—the actions of payers and the moves of competitors. Therefore, what works in one set of circumstances may not produce the desired results in another. A newspaper series that builds public awareness of a multispecialty group in Peoria, for example, may not produce similar results for a multispecialty group in Memphis. Similarly, a fast-track scheduling system may satisfy patients who desire quick in-and-out service but antagonize those who want more time for asking questions about their illnesses or injuries.

In short, marketing requires flexibility. Lacking hard-and-fast rules, marketers must develop strategies using the best available information. Marketers also must monitor progress closely so they can modify their programs according to the results generated.

The Ethics of Marketing

In the minds of many people, questions persist about the ethics of marketing. In one public opinion survey conducted by the authors' firm, nearly one in five respondents felt that "doctors shouldn't need to market themselves if their medical skills are any good."

Although some people are unaware of physicians' needs to communicate with their target audiences, marketers *must* consider both the ethics and the tastefulness of their programs and materials. Medicine still occupies a level of prestige in the minds of American consumers, and ethical communications are essential to pursuing business opportunities in a crowded and competitive marketplace.

Basic Marketing Objectives

Some marketing programs are designed to retain current patients, others seek to introduce current

---

CASE STUDY 17–1

THE MANAGEMENT-MARKETING COMMITTEE

HealthCare Partners, based in Los Angeles, has established a formal management-marketing committee to monitor progress and recommend programs for generating and retaining patients. Department heads from human resources, clinic services, marketing, and information systems are among the members of the committee, which also includes physicians, supervisors, and frontline employees.

Each month, the committee reviews patient satisfaction reports, employee suggestions, physician input, and other relevant data, and the members discuss alternative solutions for addressing the problems identified. Recommendations are presented to administrators or the board of directors and, upon approval, are carried out by the committee.

One positive result of this marketing structure is that managers are brought together in an atmosphere in which joint problem solving is more important than protecting one's own turf or worrying about who gets credit for marketing successes. The result is a dynamic, ongoing process that keeps the focus on marketing issues.

---

patients to new services, and still others are intended to reach out into the service area and attract new patients to the practice. In all three cases, marketing for the medical practice has two basic objectives: to protect the current revenue base and to generate new patient volume. Protecting the current revenue base means maintaining patient loyalty. Patients today are more mobile and more willing to seek other providers if their expectations are not being met than were patients in the past, so this is an increasing challenge. Protecting the loyalty of existing patients should take precedence over generating new patient visits for new or traditional services, and expansion of the patient base should never be attempted unless the current revenue base is secure. The pages of business publications are littered with the corpses of organizations that turned their attention to new markets without making sure of their hold on existing customer bases.

Target Audiences

Target audiences of the marketing program include all of the groups and individuals that currently or po-

tentially affect the revenue and profitability of the business. These include:

- Patients, who represent the practice's current revenue base and a principal source of referrals
- The general public, particularly those people who do not have personal physicians and someday may need the practice's services
- Referring physicians, who send the practice all, part, or none of their patients needing specialized services
- Special demographic groups, which are targeted for existing and future services (for example, executives, private-pay patients, seniors, and HMO members)
- Local press contacts, who need to know what is special and newsworthy about the group
- Area employers, who pay for the health benefit programs of current and prospective patients
- Health plans, whose members and policyholders are desirable potential patients
- Local governments and regulatory bodies, whose decisions can affect the business
- The practice's own physicians, who need to understand their multiple roles in owning, directing, and participating in a group practice

- Staff members, whose performance determines patient satisfaction, department productivity, and many other measurements of marketing success
- Other providers with whom the practice does business (for example, hospitals, testing laboratories, pharmacies, and therapy centers)

Two Types of Marketing

To reach these target audiences, marketing activities are organized into two basic channels: internal and external programs. Internal programs deal with systems, policies, procedures, and performance inside the practice. External programs reach out into the marketplace to promote the practices to existing and potential patients.

Internal Marketing

Internal marketing is vital to the success of the practice, because its primary concern is patient-payer satisfaction, which leads to return visits and word-of-mouth referrals. For this reason, internal marketing occupies a premier position in the total marketing program. Internal marketing programs assure that patients' expectations regarding medical quality, accessibility, convenience, and service are fulfilled.

Internal marketing, in turn, encompasses two critical dimensions. First, practice systems must provide a smooth, hassle-free experience for the patient. Second, the performance of physicians and staff members must be responsive to the patient's desire for personal concern as well as effective medical care.

External Marketing

External marketing occurs outside the practice. Its purpose is to reinforce the loyalty of existing patients and to capture the attention of new patients by communicating the benefits of the practices. Advertising, newspaper stories, community presentations, and direct mail campaigns are examples of external marketing programs. Once the marketer is assured that the internal product measures up to patient expectations, external programs are developed to convey the message.

Marketing Resources

With continuing pressures on pricing and reimbursement, practice growth and profitability depend heavily on the skill of marketers to maintain patient loyalty and attract new business. There are many resources available for marketers to achieve these ends, as indicated in Table 17–1.

INTERNAL MARKETING STRATEGIES

At one time, when patient volume was dependable and pricing was retrospective, physicians' incomes were assured regardless of how they chose to structure their practices and deliver their services. The marketplace has changed, however, and physicians in solo and group practice have entered a world in which there are rarely enough patients to go around; hospitals and other physicians are competing aggressively for a disproportionate slice of the pie; and/or legislators, regulators, and managed-care plans are lowering the reimbursement of physician-delivered services. The result is a user-driven, competitive arena in which marketing is essential for maintaining or increasing physician income.

This section discusses five key internal marketing strategies. Separately, each performs an important function in helping to achieve the marketing objectives noted earlier. Together, they form a matrix of complementary programs that assure the responsiveness of the practice to patients, payers, and referral sources.

TABLE 17–1 Marketing Resources

Internal Resources:	*External Resources:*
Physicians and staff	Advertising (all media)
Operating systems	Press coverage
Pricing/credit strategies	Direct mail
Practice policies	Brochures and pamphlets
Collection procedures	Billboards
Physical amenities	Community events
Tracking systems	Newsletters
Job descriptions	Yellow-page listings
Performance evaluations	"Welcome Wagon" packages
	Neighborhood weeklies

Strategy 1: Assessing Patient-Responsive Systems

The operating systems and patient-handling protocols of the practice can enhance patient satisfaction. Comfortable, well-lighted reception areas can make patients feel welcome. Timely communication systems can encourage referring physicians, employers, managed-care plans, and others to send more patients to the practice. Discounts for cash payment at time of service can appeal to cost-minded consumers as well as simplify collection procedures and lower the number of receivable days.

Working every day in the same surroundings, physicians and managers can lose a sense of how physical surroundings and practice policies affect their patients. Figure 17–1 gives a sample checklist that can be used at appropriate intervals to analyze the performance of the practice in responding to patient preferences. As an administrator walks around the clinic, he or she will see other items that should be included in the checklist.

What is important is for inspections to be conducted at least twice each year and for negative items to be addressed quickly. Some managers even enlist an outsider to identify weaknesses that might antagonize patients.

Strategy 2: Selecting High-Potential Employees

Many staff members come in contact with patients, payers, and referrers, and their performance affects the reputation of the practice. Telephone operators, receptionists, nurses, physician assistants, lab and X-ray technicians, business office people—all these professionals can make important publics feel good, or not so good, about dealing with the practice.

The first step in assuring that staff members contribute positively to the marketing effort is to select the right people from among the many job candidates who enter the interview process. Too often, the emphasis is on technical proficiency, proper credentials, or experience in

Item

What To Do About It

Accessibility
1. Are patients satisfied with lead times for appointments?
2. Are all patients treated as valued clients when they call?
3. Are patients seen quickly once they reach the reception area?
4. Do patients complain about waiting in the exam room?
5. Are office hours convenient for working patients?
6. Is the office telephone answered quickly?
7. Are calls returned quickly and predictably?
8. Is the after-hours answering service courteous and responsive?
9. Is adequate, close-in parking provided for patients?
10. Are all exterior and interior signs attractive and legible?
11. Does the entryway accommodate elderly and handicapped patients?
12. Are the lobby and reception area clean?
13. Is the waiting area comfortable?

Patient Flow
14. Is there open access to the receptionist?
15. Are patients greeted quickly on arrival?
16. Are waiting patients kept informed of their status?
17. Are front office personnel professional, helpful, and friendly?
18. Are reception-area magazines current and appropriate?
19. Is there a bulletin board for patient information?
20. Does the "no smoking" sign say "please"?
21. Can patient confidentiality be maintained?
22. Are the furniture and carpeting clean?

FIGURE 17–1 Practice Performance Analysis

23. Are the plants and wall art presentable? _____
24. Can thirsty patients obtain water, coffee, or juice? _____
25. Are patients escorted to the exam rooms? _____
26. Do patients wait a long time in the exam rooms? _____
27. Does the staff bid a pleasant "good-bye" to departing patients? _____

Patient Communication
28. Do patients understand instructions? _____
29. Do nurses explain procedures before starting? _____
30. Are there educational materials for patients? _____
31. Does the staff handle patient problems with compassion? _____
32. Are test results reported as soon as possible? _____
33. Do patients understand all billing/credit procedures? _____
34. Is there a reliable way to obtain patient feedback? _____
35. Is there a protocol for responding to patient complaints? _____

Staff Management
36. Is staff acountable for meeting performance standards? _____
37. Is good performance recognized? _____
38. Do patients overhear private conversations among staff members? _____
39. Does the staff recognize that patient satisfaction is important? _____

FIGURE 17–1 Continued

similar positions. Too seldom do managers check to see whether applicants possess the "people" sensitivity and skills needed in the specialized medical environment. Figure 17–2 shows a worksheet that can be used to elicit statements from prospective employees that relate to these attributes.

By listening carefully to the responses to these statements, the manager can evaluate the candidate not only in terms of job performance, but also in terms of how he or she is likely to react to pressure situations and unforeseen crises, such as overloaded schedules and pa-

tients needing special attention. Notes in the Remarks column on the interviewing worksheet can be used to differentiate among several applicants to assure that the best person is selected for the job.

Strategy 3: Installing Performance Standards

Most medical position descriptions concentrate on the technical, procedural aspects of the job and devote too little attention to the service aspects, which are im-

Item
1. Tell me about your last job.
2. What did you like about it?
3. If you could make one change to improve your current job, what would it be?
4. What kind of things frustrate you on the job, and how do you deal with them?
5. What do you think would be the most important skills you would need to work at a medical clinic like ours?
6. What would you do if you heard a patient say: "This is a terrible place; I'll never come back!"?
7. How would you handle a patient who complained about some aspect of care at our clinic?
8. How would you handle frightened patients and put them at ease?

Remarks
_____
_____
_____
_____
_____
_____
_____
_____

FIGURE 17–2 Interviewing Worksheet

Telephone Procedures

Our patients expect a prompt response to their calls.

1. Answer telephone within three rings when possible and say "(Department), (your name), may I help you?"
2. Speak to callers in a friendly, helpful tone of voice
3. When putting callers on hold, ask "Will you hold, please?"
4. Keep callers apprised of their status by saying at 60-second intervals "I'm sorry, (reason). Can you stay on hold?"
5. When returning to the line, thank the caller for holding

Patient Handling

Our patients expect that they will be greeted and treated with a "how may I help you?" attitude by all our people.

6. Greet patients immediately on arrival and establish eye contact
7. Introduce yourself by name to every new patient
8. Use the patient's name during the visit
9. Walk with the patient to the exam room
10. Keep all patients in the exam room informed of their status at 10-minute intervals
11. Conclude every patient encounter with a "thank you"

Communicating with Patients

Our patients expect to receive quick, courteous, and accurate responses to their questions and concerns.

12. Make sure the information you give to patients is accurate
13. Use layperson's language when speaking to patients
14. Explain procedures to patients before you begin
15. Ask for questions and repeat instructions as often as necessary
16. Look for ways to reassure anxious patients

Responding to Patient Complaints

Our patients expect that we will solve their problems in a responsive and professional manner.

17. Stay calm and don't take complaints personally
18. Listen for the facts and let patients tell the whole story
19. Immediately refer abusive patients to your supervisor
20. Make a statement of regret or empathy but avoid making excuses
21. Tell patients what you plan to do and never make promises you can't keep
22. Follow through on all promises made to patients

Professional Standards

Our patients expect us to present an image of top quality health care and dedication to our profession.

23. Follow the dress code and wear your name badge correctly
24. Be courteous with physicians and staff members and don't complain in front of patients
25. Limit personal telephone calls and chatting
26. Observe department rules for food, drink, etc.
27. In the community, represent the clinic positively and professionally

FIGURE 17–3 Patient-Centered Performance Standards

portant in patient satisfaction. Figure 17–3 shows patient-centered performance standards that can be integrated with current job descriptions. They can also be used as a checklist when managers are preparing formal evaluations of employee performance.

The standards can be customized to each department or job classification in the practice, with special sections for employees in support departments such as medical records, transcription, and maintenance. The standards should be reviewed with each applicant during the initial interview and with the new employee during orientation. Department meetings can be used to discuss department-specific standards. When merit increases are associated directly with performance evaluations, the standards are particularly useful for helping employees see the link between patient satisfaction and their own personal progress.

Strategy 4: Installing a Performance Recognition Program

Busy managers often spend time with problem employees and neglect those whose performance meets or exceeds standards. As a result, top-performing employees may feel under-recognized and unappreciated for their contributions by management and physicians. Although most medical practices have an "Employee of the Month" award to recognize outstanding staff members, this does not reinforce the behavior of every employee who goes out of his or her way for patients, payers, or referral sources.

Thanks for Helping!　　　Date _____

We appreciate your willingness to _____

_____

_____

_____

_____

A copy of this form has been inserted in your personnel file so that your performance evaluation will reflect your extra contribution to our practice.

FIGURE 17–4 Employee Recognition Form

A form such as the one shown in Figure 17–4 can be used by physicians, managers, and unit supervisors to give instant recognition to deserving employees. Such informal recognition lets top performers know that their efforts are valuable and welcome. This is important because behavior that is recognized and rewarded tends to be repeated, whereas contributions that are ignored tend to disappear.

Strategy 5: Maintaining a Patient Relations Program

A patient relations program is a formal effort to help patients differentiate the practice from others. A variety of techniques can be used by solo physicians as well as by single and multispecialty clinics to establish good patient relations, which in turn help maintain patient loyalty and promote return visits and referrals. Some of these techniques are illustrated in Case Study 17–2.

Patients often judge the responsiveness of the practice by how easily they can access and get through the system. This reality can be reflected in the patient relations program by focusing on clinic systems in addition to the performance of physicians and staff members. This is illustrated in Case Study 17–3.

A further example of patient relations involves promotional items, which many physicians use to enhance their relationships with current patients and spread the word about their practices. Gone are the days of lollipops at the reception desk. Today's giveaway items, such as patient education materials, exemplify creative marketing at its best. An example of how one clinic used a promotional item is given in Case Study 17–4.

The foregoing are examples of innovative and tasteful ways to tell patients that the practice welcomes and appreciates their business and their trust. Figure 17–5 provides a systematic listing of proven techniques for maintaining patient loyalty.

EXTERNAL MARKETING STRATEGIES

When Ralph Waldo Emerson said that the person with a better mousetrap would find the world beating a path to his door, he did a disservice to medical marketers. Emerson was suggesting that the superiority of a product or service is sufficient to guarantee success in attracting and retaining customers. He may have been right for his day, but his advice does not apply to physicians competing in volatile marketplaces where criteria

---

CASE STUDY 17–2

SKEMP CLINIC WELCOMES NEW PATIENTS

Skemp Clinic, located in LaCrosse, Wisconsin, shares its marketplace with three huge competitors—one in the same city and two within reasonable driving distance. To bring home its marketing strategy of "caring concern," Skemp Clinic offers a modest discount to patients on their first visit. To help realize its business objective of establishing long-term relationships with patients, Skemp management enlists the cooperation of physicians and staff members in welcoming new patients and making an excellent first impression.

A large, plastic paper clip is affixed to a new patient's chart, which is readily seen by everyone who comes in contact with the patient during the first visit. The extra-friendly smiles tell the patient that Skemp Clinic appreciates the visit and is willing to go out of its way to create a permanent customer.

At the same time, Skemp physicians participate in a formal effort to recognize people who support the program. The recognition can be as formal as receiving the "Employee of the Month" award or simply a "well done" comment in a hallway.

CASE STUDY 17–3

BRENHAM CLINIC EXPRESS

Nestled in the Texas ranch country about halfway between Houston and Austin, Brenham Clinic Association built its new offices on the crest of a hill. In the heat of summer and the cold of winter, many patients had to struggle up from the parking lot and arrive breathless at the reception desk.

Brenham Clinic physicians chose to turn this potential disadvantage into a vehicle for demonstrating their concern for their patients. They bought two comfortable golf carts and hired the part-time services of several retired gentlemen to conduct a valet shuttle ride to whisk patients from their cars to the front entrance and back again when their visit is over. Not only are Brenham Clinic's current patients pleased with the extra effort, but surveys indicate they also tell their friends about the concern of the physicians at the clinic.

CASE STUDY 17–4

DR. RADA DELIVERED ME!

Memphis, Tennessee, has more than its share of obstetricians and gynecologists, all of whom are alert to ways to attract new patients to their practice. The management of the group Ob/Gyn Physicians of Memphis has installed all the usual patient-sensitive protocols designed to assure the comfort and satisfaction of the new parents, from their first visit through postdelivery checkups.

In addition, management of the group decided to take a novel approach that would clearly set their practice apart from competitors. To each newborn, the practice gave a set of infant T-shirts emblazoned with a silkscreened stork cartoon and the legend: "Dr. Rada Delivered Me . . . With T.L.C.!" Feedback from surveys showed that a significant number of new patients saw the T-shirt in a park, church, or supermarket, and decided that their expected heirs deserved the same treatment.

---

for selecting a physician are complex and patient expectations are not easily predicted.

Regarding physician-selection criteria, many studies have demonstrated the power of word-of-mouth referrals for both primary care providers and specialists. In Sullivan/Luallin patient surveys over a nine-year period, more than 60 percent of respondents said that their selection of a physician or clinic was heavily influenced by the recommendation of a family member, coworker, or friend. In other words, more than half of a primary care physician's new business is likely to come from the referrals of satisfied patients. Further, the willingness of referring physicians to send patients to specialist practices is dependent, at least in part, on feedback from patients who have reported positively on their experiences, important in managed care as well.

Patients are willing to give referrals when they perceive that their expectations have been met. People consulting a physician want to get well, but they also expect service not only from the physician but also from all the people who play supporting roles in the delivery of medical care. Patients may not understand the intricacies

Physician Techniques

1. Make sure that appointments begin on time: no more than 20 minutes late and never late on two consecutive occasions
2. After the exam, communicate with patients by sitting down at their eye level and using plenty of eye contact
3. Use patients' last names unless they give you permission to be more familiar
4. Ask patients whether they understand all instructions and your answers to their questions
5. Note something personal in the chart and refer to it at the next visit
6. Introduce yourself, your staff, and your specialty by letter to newly arrived physicians in the community
7. Pay attention to committee work and informal opportunities for networking at the hospital

Physician and Nurse Techniques

8. Use layperson's language whenever possible
9. Return patients' telephone calls as promptly as possible
10. Escort patients whenever possible

Practice Manager Techniques

11. Send welcome letters to new patients
12. Send get-well cards to patients in the hospital
13. Send timely thank-you notes for referrals
14. Track all referral sources to reinforce growth, and take corrective actions with any falloff in referrals
15. Make a personal visit to administrators in referral physician offices (for feedback as well as public relations)
16. Include referring physicians on your mailing list
17. Provide educational materials for referring physicians to use with their patients
18. Install a separate telephone line for referral sources

FIGURE 17–5 Patient Relations Strategies: Techniques for Maintaining Patient Loyalty

of medical technology, but they are acutely aware of the attitudes of the medical professionals who come in contact with them. The criteria they use for selecting, staying with, and recommending a provider are based almost exclusively on these service criteria.

External marketing programs reach out to and influence important target audiences in the community and convey the message that their expectations for both medical quality and service will be met by the practice. Each external marketing strategy has an appropriate cost, based on its ability to help achieve the objectives of the total marketing effort, and a specific job to do. Contrary to the better mousetrap fallacy, it takes energy

and resources to compete with the hundreds of printed and broadcast messages aimed every day at a practice's target audiences.

Some external marketing strategies benefit the entire practice and lead prospective patients to any of the services offered. For example, an advertising campaign might be used to build public awareness of the medical group's size, diversity, length of service to the community, and reputation for high quality. Other strategies promote patient volume for specific service lines. One example might be arranging an interview by a local newspaper editor with the manager of the clinic's newest satellite. All the external marketing strategies, taken together, have a cumulative effect in creating an image of the practice.

Image

Every business has an image, or mental picture that people get when they think about the organization. A medical group can have different images, depending on the perspective of the target audience. For example, a clinic might be seen by the following target audiences as serving the diversity of purposes listed:

- Patients, as a convenient source for one-stop medical shopping for many specialty and ancillary services
- Physician/partners, as a top-quality practice dedicated to providing the very best medical care
- Referring physicians in the same city, as a good place to send patients who temporarily need specialist care
- Employees, as a good place to work
- Managed-care plans, as an organization that practices better-than-average utilization control
- Competitors, as a threat
- The general public, as a possible source of medical care if they ever need a physician's services

Image can be a temporary phenomenon. Public awareness might be heightened for a time by the first ophthalmologist to advertise radial keratotomy, the psychologist who gives a press interview on a recently published book, or the hospital that generates publicity by staging a free Father's Day aerobic testing program.

Five External Marketing Strategies

This section reviews the major premises of external marketing and presents five distinct external marketing strategies. It describes the strategies in terms of their value to medical practices, their typical costs, and basic considerations needed to put them to work. Not all of the strategies must be used in every situation. The appropriate mix of strategies should be chosen that is most likely to produce the desired results, especially in managed care environment.

Strategy 1: Maintaining Community Visibility

One of the least expensive and often most effective external marketing strategies is to have physicians or other professionals speak before local audiences. This strategy often is useful in building awareness of individual services in a specific target audience. An example might be a slide lecture by a cardiologist on new angioplasty techniques. Another example is given in Case Study 17–5.

Case Study 17–5 not only describes a successful community visibility program. It also demonstrates the potential of exploring more than one medium. Through the efforts of South Bend Clinic marketers, each lecture had potential for media coverage and provided an opportunity for clinic physicians to get acquainted with walk-in attendees. Such community presentations are simple to arrange and coordinate. Figure 17–6 shows a basic checklist for contacting a target organization and handling the logistics of a typical presentation.

Strategy 2: Using Press Coverage To Publicize the Group

Years ago, when news stories appeared about physicians and medical practices, they were often seen as

---

CASE STUDY 17–5

CELEBRITY LECTURES PAY OFF

Although it had served approximately half of all area residents at some time in their lives, South Bend Clinic in South Bend, Indiana, found that its public profile was low and that most people were unaware of the full scope of its services.

Clinic management proposed a series of free lectures on such subjects as nutrition, heart disease, and techniques for avoiding fatigue. For each subject, the kickoff presentation featured a well-known health authority, with follow-up lectures conducted by panels of South Bend Clinic physicians. The lecture series was publicized through modest newspaper announcements. In addition, 5,000 pamphlets were distributed to patients in the community.

The lecture series now draws more than 1,000 persons annually—nearly two-thirds of whom are not clinic patients—and 90 percent of the evaluations by attendees are in the "excellent" category. An added bonus is heavy media coverage by major newspapers, interviews on local evening news shows, and invitations to participate in radio call-in shows. Best of all, through the lecture series, the clinic has significantly enhanced its public image. It is now seen as a contemporary, public-minded, major medical provider in the area.

1. Determine what makes the physician/organization interesting to the specific audience
2. List available subjects, with an interest-generating title and brief descriptive paragraph for each
3. List all target organizations (business, civic, social, etc.), with names and telephone numbers
4. Initiate contact by telephone, with a specific offer of a speaker and subject; keep it noncommercial and also offer group physicians as last-minute substitutes
5. Follow-up with a letter confirming the offer
6. Ascertain equipment needs and who will provide equipment; prepare handouts or arrange for free literature
7. Let everyone in the medical group know about the opportunity through a bulletin board announcement, flyer, etc.
8. Prepare a brief article for the organization's newsletter, if applicable; prepare an introduction for the program chairperson
9. Produce reprints of remarks to the local press
10. Use the presentation as a story in the practice newsletter, if applicable, and make reprints available in the reception area
11. Write a thank-you letter to the program chairperson and offer to direct inquiries to the appropriate people

FIGURE 17–6 Ways To Put Physicians on the Podium

ego-serving. Today, however, in response to public demand for health care information, print and electronic media are hungry for good stories about interesting medical developments. Nearly every major daily newspaper, radio station, and network television channel has a health reporter eager to use information about new developments, innovative procedures, techniques for staying healthy, and similar topics.

Press coverage gives marketers the ability to reach large audiences across their entire service area, and it carries the extra impact of a third-party endorsement by the station or publication that presents the story. However, news has an amazingly short life span. It is supplanted by tomorrow's edition. Further, marketers have little control over the length of the story, because editors may cut the copy to fit the space available. Another disadvantage is that stories may sit in the editor's in-basket for long periods of time before publication, or they may never be used.

Despite these disadvantages, press coverage can be a valuable part of the marketing mix, especially for building the image of the practice. A close look at the local television news or the local newspaper's lifestyle section

1. List all print and electronic media in the practice service area, including editors and/or health writers
2. Monitor the media to learn what types of stories the editors want
3. Introduce yourself in person, leave a press kit (information folder or brochure, physician resumes, reprints or articles, etc.), and offer to serve as a source for roundup, or news summary, articles
4. Hold a monthly public relations meeting in the practice to identify newsworthy subjects, such as:
   • a new location (tie to patient advantages)
   • a new technique (if your physician uses it)
   • human interest stories (e.g., pro bono services)
   • new equipment (benefits to patients)
   • general health improvement advice
   • new physicians or staff
   • a new program or service
5. Prepare for and follow up press releases by:
   • Calling ahead to announce that a release is coming
   • Hand-delivering material if possible
   • Calling later to make sure the material was received
6. Plan feature stories by:
   • Working with principals to produce a fact sheet
   • Targeting the publication/station
   • Taking the fact sheet to the editor/writer
   • Asking for an indication of interest
   • Coordinating additional information if needed
   • Checking in periodically with the editor/writer
7. Telephone a "thank you" for feature articles

FIGURE 17–7 Strategies for Press Coverage

is likely to reveal several examples of successful press placements. Figure 17–7 provides a brief checklist for identifying newsworthy subjects and coordinating with local media sources.

Strategy 3: Publishing a Patient Newsletter

The American public has acquired a hearty appetite for information abou.t medical care, and many patients try to extend their time with the physician to ask questions and discuss their health problems. Others expect that the physician will take the initiative in providing information that will help them stay healthy or cope with existing problems.

Patient newsletters have proven to be highly effective external marketing tools—external because they can be used to communicate not only with current patients,

Distribution

1. Establish the publication cycle (quarterly, semiannually, etc.)
2. Decide whether the newsletter will be sent to all patients or just those with selected demographic characteristics
3. Determine nonpatients in the service area who are targets for services (e.g., growing communities, specific demographic segments, etc.)
4. List all area individuals who should also be on the mailing list (e.g., political, business, and media contacts)
5. Obtain a bulk mailing permit from the postal service
6. Order extra copies for distribution via department counters and other clinic locations

Editing

7. Schedule a meeting of physicians and appropriate managers at least eight weeks prior to the desired mailing date
8. Use patient surveys to identify subjects of greatest interest to patients
9. Survey practice physicians and technical people to identify interesting subjects or events they could write up
10. Draft the stories and revise the drafts with appropriate subject experts in the practice
11. Adopt a policy of using layperson's language wherever possible

Design

12. Retain the services of a designer and produce a dummy version of the newsletter (title, masthead, sample page layout, etc.)
13. Decide what photographs and artwork are needed, and arrange for production
14. Arrange the stories so that readers can see a mix of longer and shorter articles
15. Allow some blank space around copy blocks and do not crowd information
16. Use large headlines and legible typefaces

FIGURE 17–8 Producing a Patient Newsletter

but also with patients who have not visited the practice in recent months. Newsletters also tend to have a widespread distribution because satisfied patients pass them along to their family members and friends.

The cost of producing and distributing a newsletter is low compared with advertising. Although some clinics produce high-gloss newsletters with color photography and original illustrations, most practices can achieve good results with two-color printing and black-and-white pictures.

Writing and producing a newsletter requires the involvement of physicians and practice managers, partic-

ularly in the early stages of deciding editorial content. Figure 17–8 shows the steps involved in producing a patient newsletter. A typical production schedule for a patient newsletter is shown below.

Week 1:   Editorial content approved
            All background material to writer
Weeks 2–4: First draft to physician(s) for review
            Photos and illustrations to physician(s) for review
            Revision deadline
            Copy to typesetter
Week 5:   Art boards completed for review
            Approval deadline
            Art boards to printer
Week 7:   Blueline approved
Week 8:   Copies delivered by printer
            Mailing house makes distribution

The range of possible newsletter topics is extensive. Possible topics include:

- Updates on health research (e.g., a new report on smoking and lung cancer, advances in cardiac surgery)
- Newsworthy, current health topics (e.g., AIDS, Alzheimer's disease, retin-A, surgery for snorers)
- Seasonal stories (e.g., spring allergies, back-to-school immunizations, what to do about flu season)
- Biographies of physician(s) and key staff members
- Announcements of new facilities, equipment, or procedures
- Explanations of new services or programs
- Announcements of changes in hours or operating policies
- Positive approaches to managed care
- Question-answer column

Strategy 4: Publishing a Practice Brochure

One of the best ways to convey information about the practice is through a formal brochure. In other industries, this marketing vehicle is called an *identity and capabilities brochure,* because its chief functions are to establish the image of the organization and describe its services. Medical groups have an additional objective

1. Welcome/introduction: begins with a statement that reflects the practice's appreciation for having been selected to provide medical care and includes a commitment to keeping patient trust
2. Mission statement: describes the philosophy of medical practice, including the intention of physician and staff members to provide the highest quality medical care while respecting the dignity of each patient
3. Services: describes services, including all ancillary departments and affiliations with other providers
4. Physicians and key staff: includes one-paragraph biographies of physicians, nonphysician providers, and others
5. Practical policies: describes such information as how to make an appointment, how to obtain a same-day appointment, how to use the hospital emergency room, and how and when telephone calls are returned
6. Payment and credit issues: summarizes how fees are set, the extent to which staff members help complete paperwork and/or file insurance claims, and policies for collection and extending credit
7. How managed care plans are facilitated

FIGURE 17–9 Elements of an Effective Practice Brochure

for this brochure: to educate patients regarding basic operating policies, including how to access the services; payment and credit policies; and procedures, such as how to obtain prescription refills.

To establish a practice's image as a caring and concerned group of highly skilled professionals, the patient brochure should contain the elements listed in Figure 17–9. The practice brochure should be distributed not only to new patients, but also to all key target audiences, including referring physicians, area employers, managed-care plans, and other parties who influence patient volume.

Strategy 5: Advertising for New Patients To Increase Volume

Advertising is the most visible and most expensive part of the marketing budget. But some marketing goals cannot be reached except through this medium. Advertising can build awareness among large demographic groups or in large communities of a practice's service area. It can also help reach newcomers and build market share by attracting patients, referral sources, and payers who currently use other resources.

Advertising is expensive even for a one-time placement. Because consumer buying decisions are usually made on the basis of multiple impressions, most advertising campaigns require consistent placements over periods of time to produce results. The advertising message matches a service with an identified need of the target audience(s). It answers such questions as: What problem will the practice solve? What is special about the way it will solve this problem?

Newspaper advertisment can be an important advertising medium. Newspapers reach every community and demographic segment of the marketplace. People read newspapers for quick access to such information as local news, sports, special interests, television listings, and weekend events. The same copy may be read by several people, and newspaper ads are frequently clipped and saved by interested readers.

This medium should be used to educate people because it can include more details, selling points, or specific advantages of coming to the practice. Response coupons may be included to elicit a reply or publish schedules for free seminars.

Magazines tend to have longer lives than newspapers, sometimes sitting on coffee tables, desks, or kitchen counters a full month or longer before being tossed out. Most service areas contain a variety of magazines and periodicals suitable for medical advertising: upscale publications with a high-fashion or town-and-country readership; hotel guides that help visitors get around the city; and monthly magazines published by political, social, business, or civic organizations.

In many cities, it is possible to make a zone or regional buy of national magazines such as *People, Reader's Digest, Sports Illustrated,* or other high-readership publications. In this format, advertising appears only in copies of the magazines that are distributed to selected zip codes or subscriber categories. The cost of this type of magazine advertising is substantially lower than national or regional rates.

Radio advertising goes everywhere: in cars, offices, and homes; through joggers' headsets; and blaring out

---

CASE STUDY 17–6

ADVERTISING HELPS A NEW SATELLITE

Wausau Medical Center in Wausau, Wisconsin, needed to increase walk-in traffic for a new satellite, which it was opening in a growing community approximately eight miles from its main clinic. Working with a local advertising agency, management assembled a marketing plan that included quarter-page display ads in the area newspaper and a large sign at the construction site announcing the planned opening date.

During the first eight months of operation, volume exceeded initial projections. Feedback from new patients indicated that the announcement ads caught their attention and kept them aware of the new facility.

---

of boom-boxes at the beach. In addition, radio is consistently rated first in terms of drive-time and weekend market coverage, round-the-clock listeners to news updates, and total reach throughout a community.

The number of radio listeners varies by stations, type of programming, time of day, and other factors. Some radio stations are more appealing to various segments of the public than to others. There are rock music stations, easy listening stations, and all news or news/talk stations, and each type attracts a different audience.

Radio ads must be quick and simple, with copy that zeroes in on the target audience and communicates the benefits of the practice to the listener. Messages can be prerecorded at the radio station or in an independent sound studio, or they can be announcer-read live spots.

Television is the most successful mass medium in history, and no medium can surpass television in terms of audience reach. Cable channels, all-news and all-sports stations, shopping channels—all carry a heavyweight impact: sights, sounds, color, and live action in a single package. With all these features, television advertising enables the practice to reach viewers with forceful messages.

Costs for air time vary greatly for television advertising, with advertising on evening prime-time programs and daytime soap operas or quiz shows being much

more expensive than late-night movies. In addition, rates of network affiliates are significantly higher than those of local cable stations. The cost of television advertising is increased further because of the need to repeat an ad many times in order to reach and influence an audience.

Television commercials are very brief; within a few seconds, a commercial spot is replaced by programming or other commercials. Commercials are perfect opportunities for viewers to visit the refrigerator or powder room.

Yellow pages advertising can consume a large portion of the marketing budget. Some clinics are located in regions where they must appear in many local directories to be able to reach all the communities in their service areas.

Telephone directories have lives of a year or more, and they are the most frequently used references for finding numbers and addresses of physicians and medical groups when a consumer decision must be made. Nonetheless, most medical practices overspend on telephone directory advertising, often listing each physician in the individual physician/surgeon section, again under the specialty section, and yet again in a display ad. Figure 17–10 contains guidelines for developing a display ad in the telephone directory.

Billboards have become an extremely popular means of reaching large numbers of people. They are well

1. Get the reader's attention by using:
   - Clear headline and logo
   - Easy-to-read type style
   - Compatible typefaces throughout the ad
   - Plenty of space around the copy
2. Compete effectively with other ads on the page by using:
   - Sufficient size of ad
   - Eye-catching but tasteful illustration
   - Larger type size for telephone number
   - Map showing clinic location
3. Give the reader a reason for contacting the practice by providing:
   - List of services
   - Physicians' names and specialties
   - Special information (e.g., "serving our city for 40 years")
   - Major managed care plans
4. Make sure advertising is in the right directories by checking:
   - Patient origin reports
   - Patient demographics

FIGURE 17–10 Guidelines for Yellow Page Advertising

Planning
1. Determine the message to be conveyed and the desired response
2. State the target audience(s) for the campaign
3. Identify the best media for carrying the message, and establish a budget large enough to obtain the frequency and continuity needed to get the message across

Creative Considerations
4. Determine the most important thing the target audience(s) should remember about the clinic or service
5. Work with an agency to develop the ad layout (including headline, body copy, illustration, etc.)
6. For continuity be sure logo, signature, and telephone number appear in the same place on every advertisement, brochure, and other media, and use the same typeface for all ads
7. Include telephone number in a larger type size

Related Activities
8. Send advance ad slicks to all key decision makers and influences in the service area
9. Evaluate the performance of the ad by tracking responses
10. Keep physicians and staff apprised of results

FIGURE 17–11 How To Create an Effective Print Ad

suited to large organizations and to building public awareness of new facilities. Not surprisingly, billboards in high-traffic locations cost substantially more than those on less frequently traveled streets.

Billboards have little room for wordy or cluttered ads, because people in vehicles moving in traffic usually have only a few seconds to notice and focus on the message. Illustrations should be large and eye-catching, and copy should be restricted to a single statement and the clinic's name.

Producing an effective advertising campaign is a logical and businesslike process that considers the target audiences to be reached, the desired response to be created, and the media that are most likely to reach the target audiences. Figure 17–11 contains a checklist for an effective advertising campaign. It includes developing the advertising message, choosing the appropriate medium, and supervising the production of a print ad.

DEVELOPING THE MARKETING PLAN

The income security of physicians practicing in a provider-driven marketplace has been severely disrupted by rapid changes in the health care industry. To protect existing revenue sources and develop new pa-

tient volume, practice managers are developing formal business plans that focus on realistic strategies for maintaining revenue and increasing profitability.

The marketing plan is a road map that helps a practice achieve its business objectives. Developing the plan takes the time and effort of several people, including physicians, practice managers, and perhaps outside consultants and other resources. However, the results are well worth the effort, because a formal marketing plan provides the structure for analyzing strengths and weaknesses and identifying internal and external strategies for achieving business goals. The marketing plan also ties directly into the strategic planning process discussed in Chapter 16. The marketing plan accomplishes the following specific objectives:

- Helps determine for physicians, managers, and staff the mission of the practice
- Helps administrators and managers set objectives in light of organizational goals
- Provides a road map for practice development that keeps everyone on track toward agreed-upon goals

1. How is the marketplace changing? What new opportunities are opening up for medical providers?
2. What is the market potential for patients in various pay classes (e.g., private-pay, HMOs, PPOs, Medicare)?
3. Which health plans should we contract with?
4. What does the general public think of us? Are people aware of our reputation, services, locations, other features?
5. What do our patients think of us? Where are our operating strengths and weaknesses, and what parts of our systems or performance need improvement?
6. Do our patients go elsewhere for some of their care?
7. Who are our competitors, and what are they doing?
8. Where are our referrals coming from?
9. How sensitive are patients/payers to price as opposed to service?
10. Are our external promotion campaigns producing results?
11. What specialties or new services could we add to serve growing health needs in the coming years?
12. What issues are important to our physicians regarding current directions and strategies?
13. How do our staff members feel about working in our practice?
14. Are our governance processes effective? How easily and quickly can we make decisions and commit to action?

FIGURE 17–12 Questions for Market Planning

- Relates proposed programs and expenditures to specific objectives with measurable criteria
- Gets physician approval because recommendations are based on solid thinking and relevant data
- Emphasizes that marketing is everybody's business
- Helps evaluate practice performance in dollar terms

Figure 17–12 lists specific questions that should be addressed as a practice prepares its marketing plan.

Steps in Developing a Marketing Plan

This section reviews practical steps for developing a marketing plan, including how to obtain the involvement and support of physicians and staff, and how to monitor programs to assure that practice objectives are reached.

Step 1: Interviewing Physicians

A series of private interviews with physicians should be scheduled to determine their goals for the practice and to obtain their views on practice directions, oppor-

tunities, competition, and other issues. Specific topics to be addressed might include:

- Strengths and weaknesses of the practice
- Areas that require attention/improvement
- Attitudes toward managed care
- Working relationships with administration
- Governance and decision-making processes

In these interviews, each physician's level of commitment to the marketing process also should be ascertained. It is best to learn as soon as possible how willing physicians are to change practice habits or allocate dollars for a marketing budget.

Step 2: Studying the Service Area

Market plans require reliable information about the practice's service area. (See Chapter 16 for a more detailed discussion of service areas.) This phase of market planning involves obtaining information to identify opportunities in current and potential service areas and developing specific strategies to take advantage of the opportunities. Four key areas that are relevant in this regard are market analysis, patient origins, new health services, and other providers.

Analyzing demographic trends in the current and projected service areas helps position the practice for the future. A local newspaper or chamber of commerce may be an inexpensive source of data on population trends (for example, by age, gender, and income), new building permits (indicating commercial or residential expansion), and other information that suggest growth opportunities.

Comparing patient origins with demographic estimates and projections for various communities helps identify current and projected strengths and weaknesses in market share. For example, the practice may serve a high percentage of an established neighborhood but only a small percentage of a fast-growing new suburb. Or the practice's share of older patients may be concentrated in a small radius surrounding the facility, with few older patients coming from other areas.

Demographic projections also help identify opportunities for developing new services within the practice.

For example, if the senior population is growing faster than other age groups, the practice might consider developing gerontology services, a skilled nursing facility, or even a hospice to serve elderly patients.

As opportunities become evident from the demographic projections, the competition must be analyzed in terms of physicians and facilities already serving those needs. Managed-care health plans in the area should also be contacted to learn their marketing programs for the coming years. Additionally, meetings should be held with hospital planners to identify services that might be pursued jointly.

Step 3: Surveying Critical Publics

At this step in the planning process, it is valuable to obtain feedback from patients whose evaluations of practice quality and service influence the volume of return visits and referrals. Figure 17–13 shows a sample patient survey questionnaire that can be used for this purpose. Surveys can be mailed to patients or distributed directly through departments of the practice. They can be cross-tabulated to identify differences in opinion among various pay classes, age categories, or other sample strata, and reports can be tailored to department and/or location.

Note that the first two questions on the questionnaire relate to selection criteria—how the patient came to the practice. Question three is for analyzing survey responses by physician, department, location, or other similar criteria. Question four asks the patient to evaluate specific dimensions of the practice. This provides the details needed for interpreting the overall rating in question five. Question six gives the referral potential of the current patient base, and question seven helps identify patient-perceived needs for services.

A second valuable source of information about practice can be obtained by surveying the general public in existing and potential service areas. Figure 17–14 lists questions that might be included in a general public survey, which is normally conducted by a professional research firm that employs trained interviewers and has the facilities to monitor and validate telephone calls.

Q1. When you think of health care providers in your area, whom do you think of first? (unaided awareness)

Q2. Which health care providers have you used in the past 12 months? (utilization)

Q3. Do you have a personal physician? (buying patterns)

Q4. How did you select your physician? (selection criteria)

Q5. How satisfied are you with the services of your current physician? (satisfaction levels)

Q6. How could your physician improve services to you? (satisfaction levels)

Q7. I'm going to mention some medical groups in the area. From what you've heard or read, please rate the services of each group. (differentiation)

Q8. I'd like to probe further regarding your perceptions of (your name). (specific image/knowledge)
    Locations/size/diversity of services
    Orientation toward fee-for-service vs. HMO patients
    Convenient locations/hours
    High-quality medical treatment
    Friendly, competent staff
    Specific services (out patient surgery, urgent care, etc.)

Q9. What kind of health coverage do you have? (coverage)

Q10. How would you rate the care you receive through your health plan? If fair or poor, why?

Q11. Demographics (age, gender, income, zip code)

FIGURE 17–14 General Public Survey Questions

Surveys of referring physicians comprise a third source of valuable marketing information. These surveys can be conducted in writing or by telephone, and the respondents are frequently office managers or nurses rather than the physicians themselves. Figure 17–15 shows a sample referring physician survey questionnaire that was developed for a cardiology practice.

Step 4: Performing a S.W.O.T. Analysis

Analyzing the demographic data and information obtained from key audience surveys enables a practice to prepare an analysis of its strengths, weaknesses, opportunities, and threats (S.W.O.T.). The purpose of a S.W.O.T. analysis is to list the revenue opportunities available to the group and to estimate the likelihood of succeeding if those opportunities were to be pursued. A review meeting should be held with all practice principals to focus attention not only on goal setting for the

Q1. How were you referred to our practice?   (circle as appropriate)
    Friend/family member   1
    Physician referral   2
    Yellow pages   3
    Company medical plan   4
    Saw your advertising   5
    Recommended by the hospital   6
    Other   7

Q2. What was it about us that attracted you?
    Your reputation for quality medical care   1
    You are convenient to my home or work   2
    You have convenient hours   3
    Your cost is low   4
    Other   5

Q3. Which physician did you visit?

Q4. How satisfied are you with the following: (circle)

	Very Satisfied	Somewhat Satisfied	Somewhat Dissatisfied	Very Dissatisfied
Appointments scheduled at times that are convenient for you	1	2	3	4
Normal waiting times acceptable to you				
In the doctor's reception area	1	2	3	4
In the exam room	1	2	3	4
Being informed of your test results within a reasonable amount of time	1	2	3	4
Your phone calls handled promptly and courteously	1	2	3	4
Our after-hours answering service prompt and courteous	1	2	3	4
Our receptionists friendly and courteous	1	2	3	4
Our nurses sympathetic to your problems and concerned about you as a person	1	2	3	4
Our answers to your questions about insurance forms and payment	1	2	3	4
Our staff members' willingness to assist you	1	2	3	4
Our ability to solve your problems quickly	1	2	3	4
Your doctor seeing you in a reasonable amount of time after you arrive for your appointment	1	2	3	4
Your doctor taking time to answer your questions	1	2	3	4
Your doctor's interest in you as a person	1	2	3	4
Your doctor returning your calls within a reasonable amount of time	1	2	3	4
Your doctor spending enough time with you	1	2	3	4
The comfort of our facilities	1	2	3	4
Adequate parking	1	2	3	4
Reasonable charges	1	2	3	4
Our hours convenient for you	1	2	3	4
Our office convenient to your home or work	1	2	3	4

Q5. What is your overall rating of our practice?
    Excellent   1
    Good   2
    Fair   3
    Poor   4

Q6. Would you recommend our office to a family member or friend?
    Yes   1
    No   2
Why/Why not?

Q7. What other services would you like the clinic to offer?
Your health insurance coverage:
If you are dissatisfied with any aspect of our services, please tell us about it.

THANKS VERY MUCH FOR YOUR HELP!

FIGURE 17–13 Sample Patient Survey Questionnaire

Hello, I'm_____, and I'm calling on behalf of Dr. (name). We've been asked to conduct a brief survey of physicians who refer to Dr. (name) to learn their thoughts about his policies, procedures, and the quality of care (he or she) provides to your patients. The survey will take about eight minutes.

1. Approximately how many patients do you refer to Dr. (name) each month?_____In the last 6 months?_____In the past year?_____
2. What is the most frequent health consideration you refer to Dr. (name)?
3. What criteria do you use to decide which cardiologist to refer to? I'll read some representative criteria. Please tell me on a scale of one to five (five being the highest) how important each is to you:
   Proximity of office to patient's home
   Personal relationship with physician
   Professional relationship with physician
   Physician's communication regarding patients
   Feedback from patients
   How quickly patient can get an appointment
   Competence of physician
   Other
4. How do you actually make the referral to the patient?
   Provide one name
   Provide options with considerations (location, skill, proximity)
5. What other people in your office refer patients to cardiologists?
6. Who makes the appointment with Dr. (name)'s office for your patients?
   Your office_____Patients_____
7. Have you ever had a problem scheduling a patient with Dr. (name)? If yes, what was the problem?
8. Would you say that Dr. (name)'s staff is courteous and helpful? Yes_____No_____ If no, please tell us why.
9. Have you heard any positive or negative comments from patients regarding our practice? If yes, what were they?
10. Is there anything you'd like to see changed in our practice? If yes, what?
11. Does our location influence your decision to refer patients to us? Yes_____No_____
12. Would you be able to use cardiac education materials with your patients if we sent them to your office? Yes____No____

Thank you for your time. Your input will be of help to us in tailoring Dr. (name)'s practice to be more responsive to you and your patients.

FIGURE 17–15 Sample Referring Physician Survey Questionnaire

coming year(s), but also on the structural and operating changes necessary to reach the goals.

Step 5: Organizing the Marketing Plan

At this point, all the data and the S.W.O.T. analysis should be organized into a summary. The summary should recommend a set of achievable business objectives and present a road map of marketing activities. Figure 17–16 shows the general outline of a typical marketing plan.

Step 6: Obtaining Physician Involvement

The marketing plan must be presented to the decision makers in the practice, and they must be asked to help set priorities for each of the objectives. This allows activities to be planned and time to be organized. The plan also must be coordinated with other elements of the strategic planning process. Figure 17–17 contains a sample set of recommendations.

Title Page
Table of Contents
Executive Summary
• Limit to one page
• One-paragraph summary of situation analysis
• One paragraph on conclusions
• Bulleted list of recommendations
• Page numbers for extended discussion
Demographic Projections
• Areas currently served
• Communities targeted for expansion

Internal Analysis
• Practice assessment
• Patient survey
• General public survey
• Referral source survey
S.W.O.T. Analysis
Marketing Objectives Statement
Recommended Programs Description
• Activities
• Timetables
• Budgets

FIGURE 17–16 Marketing Plan Outline

Project

Internal Recommendations	Objective	Cost	Timetable
Prepare patient brochure	Educate patients regarding all clinic services	$ 2,500	1st quarter
Develop patient relations program	Improve customer service attitudes among staff	12,000	1st quarter
Extend office hours	Increase patient access	—	2nd quarter
External Recommendations			
Develop new logo	Enhance clinic image	1,500	1st quarter
Establish referral thank-you program	Increase referrals from community physicians	1,000	1st quarter
Develop health tips column	Improve community awareness of practice	—	2nd quarter

FIGURE 17–17 Sample Marketing Recommendations

The progress of each program toward the objectives must be monitored and strategies modified as appropriate. The progress of all marketing programs should be reported at periodic management meetings to keep all decision makers fully aware of and involved in the process. It is important to measure the success of each program against its objectives. Tracking can take a variety of forms, including monitoring new patient visits, making telephone inquiries, tracking patient complaints, monitoring requests for records transfer, tracking physician referrals, and other forms of tracking.

THE IMPORTANCE OF MARKETING

Today, marketing is an essential function of all medical groups and their administrators. The central role of marketing to practice viability, strategic planning, and thoughtful management cannot be overstated.

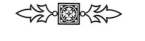

PART SIX

STRATEGIC MANAGEMENT ISSUES

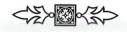

CHAPTER

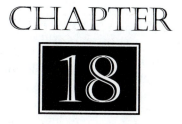

Institutional Issues

Austin Ross

LEARNING OBJECTIVES

Upon completing this chapter, the reader should be able to:

- Explain the new complexity of health care delivery
- Identify key issues facing executives in ambulatory care
- Describe new developing organizational models
- List important decision-making risks

It is obvious that the health care system has entered a state of chaos. The system is highly competitive, hospitals and systems are struggling to capture market share, and different tensions are surfacing between physicians and hospitals. Managed care as a means of practice is growing very rapidly. In addition, there is a rush under way to develop data-based information systems in order to improve the measurement of clinical outcomes and to merge clinical and financial data systems. Many of these trends are creating confusion for the patient. Ambulatory care executives and their management staffs should become familiar with these trends, because their success depends on the level of their understanding and their willingness to incorporate new concepts and methods into their practice life.

Some time ago Dr. Paul Ellwood noted that, "The mischief that began before the health care crisis of the 1970s is progressively disabling the vast machinery of medicine" (Ellwood, 1988). This chapter addresses some of this mischief.

THE EXTERNAL ENVIRONMENT

In the foreseeable future, practices will be market driven and highly competitive, and there will be little relief from these competitive pressures. These forces will create a need to effectively address such issues as the excess capacity of hospitals and professional services. There also will be dramatic decreases in the utilization of health services. In addition, the creation and entry into the health care market of giant, well-run, integrated delivery systems will change forever the way medicine is practiced and how professionals function within that practice.

The system will also experience further consolidation of insurance carriers, and this will drive medical care decision making. Employers, as purchasers of health care, will have more interest in declining premiums than in the finer points of service and quality for the patient. These market-driven forces will only worsen the probability that the underinsured or uninsured will find access to needed health care.

THE PRACTICE OF MEDICINE AND THE LIFE OF THE PHYSICIAN

Physicians will experience income reductions and turn increasingly to organizations capable of providing some economic protection, such as group practices, hospitals, insurance companies, and integrated health care delivery systems. In the face of these pressures, there will be renewed and vigorous efforts by organized medicine to "take back medicine" from the third parties in control. This will polarize the conflicts between these entities. Cutbacks in federal funding of research and education will have a significant impact on the development of new technology and result in substantial curtailments in traditional medical education programs based in both universities and the private sector. For the first time in recent memory, physicians will be laid off as a consequence of declining demand for services and the excess capacity of the system. Analyses of physician and system performance through sophisticated data bank comparisons will be a regular occurrence. There will be more involvement by physicians in management and strategic decision making. Physician insecurity, because of the changing environment, will be of great concern and may affect physicians' political clout and visibility.

THE PATIENT'S VIEWPOINT

As physicians and other health professionals focus increasingly on the needs of groups and patients, there will be less responsiveness to the needs of the individual patient. This represents the further industrialization of medicine. However, there will also be more emphasis on services being delivered by the appropriate professionals, with the roles and responsibilities of care givers being defined more clearly. This may result in healthier population groups. Patients also will tend to be better informed about the status of their health, and there will be an emphasis on wellness. This surge of interest in health will be at least partly driven by the new economics of health care. Consequently, the paternalistic medicine of the past will disappear as patients demand more involvement in health care decision making. In time, a different kind of medicine will surface. There will be greater rationing of care as an economic expediency. In addition, much greater reliance by physicians on real-time computer input into medical decision making will allow patients to be much better informed about health care decisions.

KEY ISSUES

The environment is volatile, and the key issues are in a constant state of flux. These key issues include the gamut of concerns experienced by health care executives as they address the political pressures to reduce health care costs while at the same time meeting patient expectations concerning the advancement of medical technology and quality of care. Meeting these challenges will require innovative and proactive leadership at all levels within the institution. Key concerns/initiatives are included in this chapter.

Physician Practice Patterns

Undoubtedly, the major institutional issue facing group practice physicians and administrators in this decade relates to the question of whether or not physicians will successfully modify practice patterns in response to competition and pricing pressures without diminishing the quality of care provided. To this end physicians and administrators must support the use of outcome measurements. They also must be willing to take the lead in developing new data base systems that help measure the relationships among effectiveness in the practice of medicine, true value for the patient, and the appropriate consumption of resources.

The following data illustrate the need for professionals to address practice patterns. The frequency of surgical procedures differs substantially among western nations, with the United States consistently showing the highest incidence. However, there does not appear to be evidence that this increased frequency of surgical procedures results in improved patient outcomes. Physicians also differ greatly in their prescription of services such as laboratory tests, radiology examinations, and the use of pharmaceuticals, and many of the services that are prescribed may be unnecessary. In one study of 173 patients, for which 8,000 services were ordered, reviewers considered 21 percent of the services to be unnecessary (Bernstein, 1988). Similarly, a review of reports from selected teaching hospitals showed that as few as three to five percent of the diagnostic tests that were ordered were actually used in the management of patient care. In addition, most current utilization studies focus on overutilization rather than underutilization of services, which reflects on an emphasis on costs rather than what is best for the patient. An example of this is the underutilization of mammography in the early detection of breast cancer.

Physician Payment Systems

The hospital payment system initiated by the federal government (that is, diagnostic-related groupings for Medicare hospital patients) slowed the rate of increase in hospital costs because it gave hospitals incentives for containing resource expenditures. It also encouraged an increase in the use of ambulatory services as an alternative to expensive hospital care. The fee-for-service mechanism for physician payment failed to provide similar incentives for cost containment. As a result, fees for physician services continue to increase.

The resource-based relative value system (RVS) resulting from Hsiao's study at Harvard led to the development of a national fee schedule that provided some parity in the relationship between physician payments (Hsiao et al., 1988). The new methodology was designed to address the discrepancies in charging patterns from one region of the nation to another and even within the same area. It also addressed the problem of fees being charged on the basis of traditional relationships and not necessarily on the basis of complexity of the procedures or the resources consumed. Another approach to standardizing care involves the development of medical protocols to help physicians allocate resources according to a specific medical condition. The use of carefully designed statistical and database systems to measure outcome or test protocol decisions is an absolute requirement of standardization.

Executives should take time to acquaint themselves with these and other developing methods. They may reduce costs and improve the quality of care and, thus, ultimately impact physician income.

New Medical Technology

The development of new medical technology is a significant contributor to costs. One of the problems in assessing technology as it enters the practice market is that decisions are driven by competition. Hospitals and group practices often attempt to gain market share by providing the very latest in medical technology instead of sharing new technologies, which promotes efficiency.

Generally speaking, health executives are not technically equipped to understand the details of new medical technology and must rely on experts for evaluation of effectiveness. Such experts have been known to have biases. The reimbursement system also tends to reward the provider with higher fees or higher cost reimbursements, which raises costs. New technology creates specialized jobs, and the expertise is often held only by a few. It takes time to assimilate information on new techniques, and by that time, the users of the new technology have acquired a vested interest in maintaining or expanding it. Technology itself tends to create new infrastructures within the organization. The computer is a good example of this. Existing processes tend to be adjusted to meet the needs of new technology, which can result in a patchwork approach to systems development.

The education of practitioners to understand better the appropriate use of technology, combined with improved data collection, offers some promise for the more appropriate selection and use of new medical technology.

Relationships with Hospitals and Integrated Health Care Delivery Systems

The character of relationships between group practices, on the one hand, and systems and hospitals, on the other, traditionally has been wary. Clinic executives and hospital administrators have not found many common areas of agreement. The clinic executive often has viewed the hospital structure as bureaucratic, resistant to change, and threatening to the group practice's financial well-being. The hospital administrator often has been equally suspicious and has seen the clinical executive as being focused on finances at the expense of social and patient needs. However, times have changed. The rapid growth of managed care has created incentives for hospitals and their medical staffs to concur on contracting arrangements. The ambulatory care administrator capable of viewing the big picture is learning to collaborate with management counterparts in the hospital or health delivery system.

Integrated delivery systems (IDS) are characterized by the formation of organizations with a common set of goals and with shared resources and management to provide a continuum of care to a selected patient population. The IDS operates with a single vision and set of objectives relating to patient care, education, and research. Executives of the IDS are selected to identify with the broader organizational mission, and department heads are discouraged from playing one organization or department against another. Executives typically move around to gain broader experience. With multiple boards, care is taken to achieve some level of overlap in board membership to enhance communication and joint decision making.

Creating success within the IDS is not easy. Failure or lack of achievement of system goals can be attributed to the following problems:

- Lack of a common mission and vision
- Divergence in scope of services, (due, for example, to different patient constituencies)
- Antitrust concerns that hamper integration strategies in achieving their full potential
- Absence of compatibility among the boards (including disagreements about board control and voting)
- Unresolved questions about merging of identities and assets
- Differences between the medical staffs (for example, in compatibility, quality, and involvement in decision making)
- Differences between corporate culture and management styles
- Historic differences between the employee staff (such as differences in unionization)

Medical Ethics

Medical ethics issues relate not only to questions regarding the prolongation of life but also to questions regarding the care of seriously ill newborns and responses to other catastrophic events. The rationing of health care resources for certain groups of patients will increasingly involve the ambulatory care administrator. The pressures of cost containment raise the inevitable question of how much society can afford to spend on the terminally ill. This is an ethical issue of great importance.

But medical ethics issues are not limited to the catastrophic. There are many smaller yet still important issues. An example might be how far the emergency room physician should go in ordering tests to protest against possible malpractice action. The issue of medical ethics is undoubtedly a new dimension in the inventory of concerns for the ambulatory care administrator of the year 2000.

THE ANGUISH OF DOWNSIZING

Downsizing involves pain, persuasion, and performance. Pain stems from the need to make tough choices and live with those choices. It requires the development of cultural and practice patterns of caring for those individuals who are released during downsizing as well as those who survive the downsizing process. Persuasion is needed to convince individuals that it is worth staying with the organization, to help rebuild broken communication lines, and to strengthen organizational confidence. Performance involves establishing new checks and balances to assure that a backwash does not occur. Once the immediate crisis is over, there may be a tendency to fall back into old ways, and this can lead to a cyclical pattern of crisis. Performance also involves the longer-range process of rebuilding morale and corporate culture.

Warning Signs

In volatile times, group practice managers and their staffs need to develop warning systems to alert them in advance of the need for downsizing. They must be able to determine when a cycle has turned into a trend. They must also monitor symptoms of impending disarray.

Month-to-month variations in the financial reporting systems may reflect simple cycles. However, when the variations persist over a long period of time, they may reflect a long-term trend. Executives sometimes aggravate negative trends by addressing them with short-range solutions. An example of a short-range solution to a long-term trend is reliance on price increases rather than expense reductions to achieve budget goals.

There are several signs of impending disarray that a manager must monitor. One is the failure to track cumulative commitments. A physician and support staff may be added in one specialty, several pieces of expensive high-technology X-ray equipment may be purchased, a contract may be let for a building addition, and other commitments may be made. Carelessness in tracking the cumulative financial effects of such commitments is a dangerous practice. Another is allowing cash reserves to shrink and borrowing to meet monthly expenses. Repeated borrowing to meet current commitments is a cause for serious concern.

Another sign of impending disarray is the occurrence of a series of unrelated problems that deflect the manager's attention from routine business. As the pace quickens, the manager may become consumed by specific projects or problems and, in the process, lose track of the basic operation of the practice, leading to a crisis situation. For example, failure to pay sufficient attention to accounts receivable because the manager is busy with unrelated problems can precipitate a genuine cash crisis for the overstressed manager and his or her organization.

Behavioral Responses

When an organization is faced with a financial downturn, leaders tend to behave somewhat predictably. The first stage is typically outright denial of the problem. Usually, executives react initially to economic downturns by believing them to be self-correcting cycles and denying that there is a real problem. In this denial stage, they may look for evidence to support this point of view. All types of excuses may surface, such as "We miscalculated concessions but that has now been corrected," or "Our receivables are up temporarily but we can get them down in another 60 days," or even "That snowstorm last February affected volume more than we thought." When the situation gets worse instead of better, everyone wonders why steps to correct the problem were not taken earlier, and the pessimists in the organization start predicting that the practice will be unable to recover. This may lead to widespread depression.

Depression is like a virus, and it affects employees, managers, and physicians alike. Some may begin to think that it is time to bail out. Unfortunately, if panic sets in, some of the organization's best people are likely to leave first. A feeling that nobody is in charge may start to pervade the organization, and quality and capacity of leadership may be challenged. Board members may begin to propose solutions which, if adopted precipitously, could add to the problem.

Then, leaders dig in and start to tackle the problem. As decisions are made, attitudes begin to change. Now creeping into conversations is such talk as "We've experienced rough times before; why is this so different?" or "Look at how the department managers are responding to the crisis; we have some real capacity in hand to turn this thing around." During this process, stories of similar challenges faced by other organizations begin to filter through the organization. If leaders monitor the outside environment, it may help physicians and others to understand that some of the internal problems may be related to external environmental conditions.

As leadership reasserts itself, the healing process is under way. Morale improves, and the practice begins to move down the road to recovery.

Making Those Tough Decisions

One of the most difficult challenges facing any organization is the need to deal with members of the staff who are not capable of change. As the organization grows, careful monitoring is required so that individuals who cannot cope with change can be eased aside before damage occurs, either to the individuals or to the organization. Chief executive officers sometimes assume that everyone always strives for promotion. This is not the case. An individual who is overextended in terms of performance and responsibility and shows signs of losing effectiveness does not necessarily want to be promoted into a position requiring additional responsibility. Such an individual may perform better and more comfortably in a lower level position. Chief executive officers of integrated organizations also must keep in mind that it takes more than chiefs to run an organization. Team members are critical.

Fixing the Problem

Fixing problems in a medical practice often involves a strategy of improving marketing and services while reducing expenses. Basically, this means convincing a lot of people that they will have to work harder with less support. If department managers cannot cut budgets enough, employees may have to be terminated, especially if unfilled positions have already been frozen. Choosing individual employees within the organization to be terminated creates great anxiety. Personnel may be laid off by seniority or by level of competency, although, if the organization is heavily unionized, there may not be a choice. The impact of laying off senior employees should not be underestimated, because this tears at the culture of the organization and undermines the implied contract with the employee that tenure means something. To minimize the level of anxiety, an organization should:

- Cut budgets more deeply than is believed necessary to avoid asking for a second or third cut, which lowers confidence in decision making
- Be generous with separation packages to help sustain employee morale and maintain essential standards of fairness and equity
- Plan the sequencing of events carefully and work out placement arrangements ahead of time, and rehearse with supervisors how to present information to those who must leave
- Make cuts cleanly and compassionately without delaying implementation
- Help those being separated with references and job assistance
- Be sure administrators and managers remain highly visible and executives are honest and open in communicating tough decisions
- Preserve core administrative competency so the organization can respond to new threats

- Realize that time is usually needed in order to rebuild teams and confidence

Communicating with Physicians During a Crisis

During a crisis, management must continue communicating with physicians, who otherwise may feel left out of the cycle. However, communication with physicians may lag as the focus at the time of layoff turns to the employees. As a result, it may be the physician's office assistant who brings news of his or her own layoff to the physician. This should not occur; news of this nature should not reach physicians secondhand. However, communications take staff time, which may not be easy to find, particularly with a thinned-down administrative staff. Engaging in crisis management requires energy to assure success. These programs require careful planning to assure management credibility.

Board Interaction

When crises occur, board members are inclined to want more involvement and information, which tends to translate into more frequent meetings. The major problem with increasing the frequency of meetings is that it increases the risk of making spur-of-the-moment decisions without adequate study. When pressure begins to build, decision making may become sloppy as the urgency to take action increases.

Crisis Leadership

A crisis is a time when administrators kick into high gear and either excel or burn out. It is not easy to predict how members of the management team will respond to a crisis. Some are flattened by it and find it difficult to cope. Others rise to the occasion and are positively challenged by the circumstances. The latter managers need to be nurtured and supported, because they represent an asset of great value.

Three factors aid immensely in the turnaround of the organization. The first is to always do right by people. When times are tough, organizations sometimes become shortsighted in how they deal with staff being separated, or they can do poorly in working with those who remain. The second is to base the organization on human value, as reflected by service to patients. Retrenchment matters can then be dealt with more easily, and the organization as a whole can recover more quickly.

The third factor concerns the quality of the relationships between physicians and administrators. Administrators who are solo performers and who build administrative turfs, believing that physicians should have little to do with management, are likely to fail in times of crisis and be doomed to short tenure. Administrators who survive volatile times are those who understand the importance of involving physicians in decision making. A synergistic relationship between physician leaders and executive administrators is needed to provide solutions to difficult problems and permit the organization to be proactive in meeting current and future challenges.

THE CHALLENGE

The health care environment is undergoing revolutionary change. Therefore, it is important to prepare for tough times ahead, and such preparation must include maintaining an external environment surveillance system. It is also essential to work harder than ever before to build the strongest possible management team. Knowing supervisors, socializing with them, taking inventory of their strengths and weaknesses, and hiring only people who are very capable is more important then ever. It is also important to keep an eye on the mission and culture of the organization, because the reason for the organization's existence, service to patients, flounders in an environment that seems to reward only the financial aspects of performance.

Finally, the amount of energy required to turn an organization around once it is in trouble should not be underestimated. If an organization thinks that it can simply "increase production" without addressing expense reductions, it is likely to fail. Also, reducing expenses is not a one-time event. From here on out it will be the routine and not the exception. Those who survive when confronted with such challenges will do so because they chose the right course of action and demonstrated, even in the midst of crisis, some optimism for the future. Optimism is crucial because it provides the source of stability for the organization. Leaders do not lose hope. They display courage, consistency, compassion, and competency, minute by minute, hour by hour, and day by day.

REFERENCES

Bernstein Research: The future of health care delivery in America. (1988, July 9).

Ellwood, P. (1988, June 9). Shattuck Lecture. *New England Journal of Medicine, 318*(23), 1549–1556.

Hsiao, W.C., Braun, P., Becker, E., Dunn, D., Kelly, N., & Yntema, D.B. (1988, September 27). *A national study for resource-based relative value scales for physician services* (Final report to the Health Care Financing Administration, Department of Health Policy and Management, Harvard School of Public Health and the Department of Psychology, Harvard University, under HCFA Contract No. 17–C–98795/1–03. Cambridge, MA: Harvard University.

CHAPTER

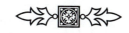

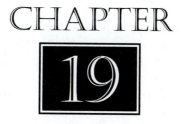

Managed Care

Frederick J. Wenzel

LEARNING OBJECTIVES

Upon completing this chapter, the reader should be able to:

- Describe and discuss the evaluation of the health care delivery system
- Explain the emergence of managed care
- Describe the impact of managed care on the group practice of medicine
- Discuss positioning to take advantage of the move from fee-for-service to managed care and capitation

Writing about history as it is being made, during a period of rapid change, is a most difficult task. So it is with managed care, medical practice, and reimbursement systems at a time when there exists neither a clearly stated public policy for health nor a consensus statement on how health care should be managed. The public debate, however, continues. It has led to a number of process changes, one of the most recent of which is the advent of managed care and all that is associated with it (Relman, 1996; Abramowitz, 1988; Schraeder, 1994; Dunn, 1994).

Managed care means different things to different people. Prior to the 1980s, most physicians would have defined it as "care for patients requiring close supervision at each step of examination, diagnosis, and treatment." At the same time, the public might have defined managed care as "care in which a physician leads a team of providers in a complex case." Since the 1980s, there are a number of new definitions of managed care, cast in the light of alleged excessive increases in health care costs and the need to control physician and patient behavior:

- "A system designed to control the utilization of health care and to place the provider at financial risk" (Ross, Williams, & Schafer, 1991)
- "Systems or techniques that are used to affect access to and control payments for health care services"
- "Systems that integrate financing and delivery of appropriate health care through arrangements with selected providers to furnish comprehensive service to members, with explicit standards for selecting providers, have formal ongoing quality assurance and utilization review programs and have financial incentives to use plan providers and procedures" (Gradison, 1995)
- A system that "integrates the financing and delivery of care" (Puma & Schiedermayer, 1996)

This notion of managed care has become so popular that for-profit companies have been formed to provide health maintenance organizations (HMOs) and insurers with the tools to control utilization and manage care. At the same time physician organizations (POs) and physician/hospital organizations (PHOs) are springing up to assure that physicians and physician groups are not left out of managed-care contracting.

This current state of affairs will prevail for quite some time. Abramowitz (1988) suggested that by 1997, fully 90 percent of all care would be delivered through a managed-care system, be it HMO, preferred provider organization (PPO), or conventional indemnity insurance. Weiner (1994) reported a growth in managed-care enrollment from 12.5 million persons in 1988 to 45 million in 1993. While the percent suggested by Abramowitz (1988) may be high, most authors believe between 60 and 90 percent of all care will be managed care by the year 2000.

The importance of managed care and its influence on the group practice of medicine is the subject of this chapter. An analysis of the present state of managed care and its historical roots is presented. Stress is placed on understanding how health care financing developed during the latter half of the twentieth century and on financial arrangement's practical application to the practice administrator. Finally, the next phase of managed-care system development is described, in which a rational approach is brought to the delivery of health services.

RECENT CHANGES IN THE HEALTH CARE SYSTEM

World War II accomplished two things. It spawned a GI educational benefit that sent thousands of young men to medical school who otherwise might not have found their way into the health care system. These students, strong in the Protestant work ethic, have since had a great influence on the development of the health care system in general and on group practice in particular. In addition, technological developments of the war were later transformed into medical diagnostic and treatment tools. For example, ultrasound technology developed out of sonar technology.

The technological focus of the 1950s gave way to a focus on access in the 1960s. Congress sought to remedy problems in access at least in part, by passing Medicare and Medicaid legislation in 1965. With the passage of this legislation, a new socioeconomic experiment was under way for the aged, disabled, and indigent, and for children in economically disadvantaged families. Medicare and Medicaid also brought previously unknown controls and oversight mechanisms to providers of medical care. The roots of many current managed-care programs are found in Medicare and Medicaid, such as preadmission certification and professional review organizations (PROs) (Schraeder, 1994).

The decade of the 1970s witnessed a wave of health care system development unmatched by developments at any other time in this century. The HMO Act of 1973 marked the beginnings of managed care under the guise of health maintenance and preventive medicine. Although at that time cost was not a great concern, early in the 1980s health economists predicted that the Medicare Trust Fund would be bankrupt by 1987. Congress issued a call to action, and the real era of cost containment began. HMOs were poised to take part in this new trend in the health care system, and the indemnity health insurers jumped on the bandwagon. Business and industry, not wishing to be left out, formed coalitions and round tables whose objectives were to control health care costs by limiting utilization and placing providers at risk.

Out of these events and the ensuing race for the health care dollar, managed care was born. It spread quickly in the early 1990s without a widely accepted definition as to what it really was. That uncertainty persists to this day. It is still unclear, for example, what the difference is between a managed-care contract and an HMO or indemnity contract. However, there does seem to be a strong relationship between the HMO of the 1970s and managed care of the 1990s. The managed-care movement is so popular today that Herschberg (1994) described a physician manual for managed care, which he advised should be a "living document," with frequent review and updating.

Before embarking on an in-depth discussion of the relatively new phenomenon of managed care, a brief review of the major past and current reimbursement methods used in the health care system is valuable. It is through some of these reimbursement methods that most managed-care systems operate.

History of Reimbursement

For decades, health care was financed on a fee-for-service basis. The first major change came when the Health Care Financing Administration (HCFA) introduced the notion of cost-based reimbursement as a means to pay for inpatient hospital services for Medicare enrollees. The theory was that the cost-based approach would yield a rational system that could be controlled. Eventual disappointment with that system led to the introduction of diagnostic related groupings (DRGs) in 1983. Sandwiched by these developments, in the 1970s, was the idea of capitation, or payment-per-person-per-time-period, irrespective of the quantity of services provided. Capitation remains the principal reimbursement method used by HMOs.

The concept of relative values was introduced in the 1960s, along with fee schedules reflecting relative values. Originally, relative value scales were thought to violate antitrust provisions of federal law, but these arguments were swept inside with the publication of the resource-based relative value scale (RBRVS) by Hsiao and associates (1988). Hsiao stated that the new system would "level the economic playing field for physicians," but it contained no provision to control utilization, costs, or, more precisely, reimbursement. The volume performance standards, which came along with the Medicare fee schedules, have proven to be a poor substitute for any type of cost control.

A new body created by Congress, the Physician Payment Review Commission (PPRC), used the Hsiao study to recommend sweeping reform in reimbursement for physician services to the Medicare population. In contrast to Hsiao's report, the PPRC recommended ways to control cost through geographic reimbursement caps. These caps are as close to universal capitation as any system advanced thus far. At the same time, Robert Fetter (1987), the father of DRG, continued his work on ambulatory visit groupings (AVGs), another method for reimbursing physicians that would have, implicit in its structure, ways to control reimbursement once the system was established. To accomplish this task, Fetter advocated utilizing lessons learned in administering the DRGs.

In the 1990s, capitation is rapidly replacing fee-for-service and discounts as part of managed-care systems. The growth in capitation in group practice is evidenced by a recent report. Robinson and Casalino (1995) studied six large medical groups in California where capitated enrollees increased 91 percent from 1990 to 1995. In this group of 759,474 enrollees, patient hospital days per 1,000 for nonMedicare enrollees were 120 to 149, compared to 232 for all of California and 297 for the United States as a whole. For enrollees covered by Medicare the days were 1,337 compared to 1,698 for the United States as a whole. The average annual number of visits to physicians in the six groups, for both Medicare and nonMedicare patients, was slightly below state and national averages. The capitation model appears worth pursuing, and it has been predicted that capitation will be the reimbursement method of the future (the Governance Committee, 1994).

The outcome of all this activity on the reimbursement side is yet to be determined, but one thing is certain: managed care and capitation will play key roles in whatever system or systems predominate in the next decade. Accepting this fact and understanding the principal elements of managed care, utilization control, and risk will provide a good perspective on where we are today and a useful preview of the health care system of the future.

Managed care has at its roots control over the utilization of health services using financial incentives or penalties. On the positive side, from the standpoint of patient welfare, managed care could provide a basis to more critically define needed clinical services. On the negative side, managed care could significantly alter professional judgment, intrude on the physician-patient relationship, cause shifts in physician specialization, and tempt the physician to see more patients. It almost certainly would produce a resentful medical professional chafing at subservience to the for-profit managed-care company (Kahn, 1987). Contracts with managed-care entities may even strip the physician of the legal rights found in a traditional private practice.

Control Mechanisms in Managed Care

Managed care utilizes a host of methods to control utilization and to shift risk to the provider. These include preadmission certification, concurrent review of hospital stays, second surgical opinions, and individual management of high-cost cases. The first two control methods have been around for a long time and have been used effectively by HMOs to reduce admissions and the length of hospital stays. Second surgical opinions are meant to counter abuses such as excessive numbers of tonsillectomies and coronary vein bypass operations. However, there is no clear agreement that the second opinion method really works (Bayliss, 1988), and it has virtually disappeared.

A variety of methods to reduce utilization and costs have also been developed. All result in managing care by changing the culture, or the way things are done. Included in these cultural changes are outpatient surgery, same-day admission surgery, hospices, formularies, non-duplication of services, generic prescription drugs, home health care, step-down units, nursing homes as an alternative to long-term hospitalization, and co-payments and deductibles. A number of these methods have caused a marked shift in care from the inpatient to the outpatient setting, making it possible for multispecialty clinics to expand the scope of services they provide. Each of these methods seeks to change the behavior of the provider and/or the patient. In some cases, the provider can still make a decision about how care is delivered. However, with increasing frequency there is not a choice but a mandate. The price for noncompliance is reduced and no payment for services or cancellation of contracts.

The shift from inpatient to outpatient surgery has a great impact on the cost of surgical procedures. It has been speculated that more than 60 percent of all surgeries in the next few years will be done on an outpatient basis. Although some may not see this as managed care, it is probably one of the more dramatic, positive examples of it. The result of these changes will be hospitals that are basically intensive care units and clinics where individuals with even significant illness will be treated as outpatients.

No formal methods, except for capitation, benefit limitation, and co-payments, have been introduced to control the volume of outpatient visits and ancillary services. However, some insurers limit the number of laboratory studies and radiologic exams that may be done in a given period of time. There will be significant activity in this area in the near future as resources become scarcer. There will also be an increased emphasis on standards of practice, prior authorization, protocols for expensive diagnostic exams or treatments (such as preoperative examinations, lithotripsy, and magnetic resonance imaging), and outcome studies. The government will exert its influence by freezing fees, establishing expenditure caps, or not paying for the services at all. Clinics and physicians will be left to find a way out of this dilemma.

The Role of HMOs and PPOs in Managed Care

Managed-care systems, in one form or another, have been around for the better part of this century. However, it was the growth surge in HMOs in the 1970s that heralded the real emergence of managed care. The HMO was originally envisioned as a vehicle for preventive medicine and health maintenance, goals that have not been realized. Instead, HMOs moved to capitation, and this alternate financing system was to remain relatively pure during the 1970s and early 1980s, with attractive consumer features such as open enrollment and community rating. Few HMOs had deductibles and copayments. Then the walls came tumbling down in the early to middle 1980s, and most HMOs succumbed to the pressures of competition and abandoned the characteristics by which they were once defined. They have, however, stressed utilization controls, especially on the hospital side, where they have been effective in reducing both admissions and the length of stays (Miller & Luft, 1994). In this regard, group practice models appear to be more effective than independent practice associations (IPAs) (Marion Laboratories, Inc., 1988). In fact, most IPAs look more like traditional indemnity systems. Fee-for-service, although discounted, persists. Utilization controls and provider risk are virtually absent, although there are some exceptions found among the more highly organized, large-scale IPAs. However, this has been disputed by Miller and Luft (1994) and Gold et al. (1995), who found group practice HMOs to be no more effective than IPAs.

The consumer is still interested in more choice than is offered by closed-panel HMOs. This consumer preference factor gave rise to the PPO in the early 1980s. A PPO operates largely through a system of discounts from providers, with a substantial payment for services when the enrollee seeks care outside the designated panel of physicians. Typically, the patient bears 20 percent of the cost when care, other than emergent care, is provided outside the system. Elden (1989) suggested that "the sophisticated segments of the marketplace have selected the PPO as the vehicle for the transition to actual managed care." The PPO concept is also supported by a point-of-service option in many managed-care plans.

Managed care of the future will include the use of diagnostic and treatment protocols. First used by the HMOs, such protocols will be expanded to PPOs and, in all likelihood, will become a hallmark of managed indemnity programs as well. Specialty medical and surgical societies and the HCFA are focusing significant effort on developing standards of care and protocols for both diagnosis and treatment. Thus far, however, there has been strong resistance to this move. Many physicians believe that no two patients are alike and that they therefore cannot be treated alike. In *A Physician's View of Managed Care,* Kahn (1987) stated that "a serious moral and economic hazard exists when the physician serves as economic gatekeeper under contracts now imposed by commercial health care companies." Many of these companies have made significant moves toward the mandatory use of protocols in the care of their insureds, but the involvement of physicians and other professionals has been minimal. (Clancy & Brody, 1995).

Managed Care and Integration

It would appear that managed care and managed-care contracting can best be dealt with through the development of an integrated system for delivering health care services. The integrated system can develop its own managed-care product (that is, an HMO or other vehicle), or it can strengthen itself to provide a significant resource for managed-care contracting. There are a number of multispecialty clinics that are part of, or have acquired, hospital systems. When it comes to contracting for care, they are in an enviable position. The tighter the integrating bond, the more successful these organizations can be when they contract with managed-care insurers. It would appear that the most effective and efficient system would be one in which the physician group, the hospital, and the insurance, or risk function, are all under one roof.

Another factor that can strengthen these organizations is that they offer physicians an opportunity to work together as a collegial professional group to lay down criteria for managed care. The medical director can work with the medical and surgical departments to increase their efficiency. The medical group can work with the hospital, with which they share risk and with which they have their incentives aligned, to assure quality, while at the same time making the system as efficient as possible. They can also establish measurable benchmarks to provide the efficiencies needed to survive under a managed-care system. If managed care is to have a real future, the integrated system is most likely where it will lie. This is true whether the system has its own plan or operates primarily as a contractor.

A word of caution should be noted. Managed-care contracting is a complex business, and physicians especially should not enter this arena unless they have special training and experience. The road to poor financial performance and even bankruptcy is paved with inexperienced contractors. Let the seller beware.

The Managed Care Company

Business enterprises, whose sole product line is the management of utilization of nonemergent care, have moved onto the stage. Although these firms typically are engaged to serve as gatekeepers for large insurance companies, they are increasingly managing care for self-insured firms. A physician who sees the patient and recommends treatment is required to call the managed-care company for approval. Most often, a battery of questions is asked by a staff nurse, and a decision is made by phone. Questions are related to symptoms, need for service, cost, length of treatment, appropriateness of hospital admission, length of stay, and complication rates.

Software is now available to compare the physician's fee for the service with the fees charged by other physicians. Many self-insured corporations are taking certain benefits, such as mental health, from their indemnity programs and using a managed-care approach to administer them. Managed-care companies are following the same denial process used by Medicare for "medically unnecessary" services, except that they operate on a prospective basis. This trend causes great concern in the medical community because it is not clear how the criteria and standards were developed in the first place.

Managed Care: Legal and Ethical Issues

The legal and ethical issues surrounding managed care have actually been around for several decades. The HMO Act of 1973 raised the question of whether an HMO could be party to a malpractice suit. The issue has been discussed, but little has been found in the courts, and certainly there have not been enough cases to establish a legal foundation. It is axiomatic in malpractice cases that "everyone in sight gets sued," but this has not been the case with HMOs or managed-care plans. However, that may change in the future.

The ethical issues related to managed care have raised more concerns than the legal. Denial of access, infringement on the physician-patient relationship, the temptation to undertreat, and the replacement of the ethics of medicine with the ethics of business are but a sampling of the ethical arguments against managed care (Jecker, 1994). Other objections to managed care include erosion of the physician's freedom to practice medicine and constraint of the patient's freedom to chose a provider and ask for the services he or she desires.

Jecker (1994) also cites a number of ethical arguments that support managed care. They include:

- Overtreatment can harm the patient as much as undertreatment
- Health care businesses are increasingly held to high ethical and societal standards
- The process of managed care with its focus on gatekeepers improves rationalization
- Outpatient care is emphasized to reduce costs
- Decisions on whether tests are cost effective are critically assessed

Some limits on professional autonomy may not be all bad. The patient's trust in the physician may sometimes be appropriately tempered. Choice under managed care may be made on a more informed and reasoned basis. These arguments, although interesting, seem weak in the light of experience in managed-care systems. The fact that managed care can actually improve the efficiency and effectiveness of the system, if the standards are set by the profession, answers virtually all the ethical arguments against managed care.

Jecker (1994) proceeds to define guidelines that might be considered, including:

- Require frank disclosure of economic and resource constraints when these infringe upon treatment decisions
- Separate physicians' incomes from treatment choices
- Guarantee a basic set of health care benefits
- Maintain a closed system within which resource tradeoffs can occur
- Educate physicians in cost-containment measures, including both positive methods that reduce unnecessary procedures and negative methods that should be avoided because they might lead to inappropriate withholding of necessary services
- Provide patients with the option of remaining with traditional, fee-for-service medicine
- Enable physicians to participate in establishing the standards used to evaluate cost containment within their respective managed-care groups

The ethical arguments will most likely go on unabated as managed care continues to mature. These arguments will surely be tested in society's court of public opinion. Until that time the arguments will be made in the professional literature without resolution.

Managed Care: Government Programs

Experimentation with both Medicare and Medicaid began in the late 1970s and early 1980s. The results were varied, and it was not until the cost crunch of the late 1980s that managed-care programs, characterized by contracting, became popular. A number of states have adopted Medicaid managed-care capitation contracts as a standard way of doing business. Whether or not these contracts have dealt effectively with the cost concerns of the Medicaid program is open to question. Some programs, such as California's Medicaid program, have been successful, but others, such as Tennessee's Tencare pro-

gram, have had more questionable results. Perhaps the real question is whether or not socioeconomic problems in this population can be solved using managed care. It seems only logical that health care problems cannot be solved with managed care unless the socioeconomic aspects, such as poverty, can be dealt with effectively.

More recently it has been suggested that the survival of Medicare is dependent on re-engineering the program, with managed-care programs as the basis for change. Even though the managed-care program would be optional for Medicare recipients, political liberals cried "foul." They stated that this approach would disenfranchise senior citizens and raise barriers to access, thus denying needed care. As long as the programs are optional, however, enrollees still have a choice.

While there have been abuses of managed-care-like programs in some states, including Florida, there have also been positive experiences with Medic-Gap supplemental coverage. In most, seniors prepay on a quarterly basis and have their Medicare benefits assigned. The satisfaction rate in these plans is high. However, most plans also do not have stringent managed-care controls at this time. Only time will tell how managed care can work with government programs, but the experiment is worth the risk in attempting to provide better services for reasonable costs.

THE IMPACT OF MANAGED CARE ON THE GROUP PRACTICE OF MEDICINE

Planning a successful future for the medical group practice is dependent on many assumptions, including the economics related to revenues and expenses of the organization. In the fee-for-service environment of the 1960s and the 1970s, that was not difficult. One only had to know the projected volume and calculate the fee increase needed to cover expenses. Those salad days are gone forever. Now it is necessary not only to predict volume, but also to predict the percent of charges that will be paid by the different payers in the mix of payers. This implies a comprehensive understanding of reimbursement methods as well as of the rules implemented by the managed-care systems.

This has a profound effect on the future financial health of the group practice and its compensation system. Multispecialty groups depend on making up re-imbursement shortfalls in one specialty or service by shifting costs from one area to another. However, the rules of managed-care systems do not accommodate this approach. Because of this, there are great pressures to change the way physicians practice medicine.

These systems go far beyond simply rationing hospital utilization and curbing the use of expensive technology. For example, the emphasis on primary care gatekeepers has had some influence on the technically related specialties by reducing such referrals. However, as indicated below, group practices are in an excellent position to deal with managed-care issues and to turn what has been identified, to this point, as a problem into a significant opportunity.

To be successful, it is necessary for the group to manage its resources carefully. Efficient utilization of non-physician staff will be critical. This obviously takes an in-depth evaluation of the culture of the organization and an understanding of the way it does business. As discussed elsewhere in this text, sophisticated financial information systems are becoming critical to managing managed care.

Groups need an accrual-basis accounting system in order to be knowledgeable about its financial status in detail on a monthly basis. Income statements, balance sheets, financial ratios, such as current, quick, debt to equity, and return on equity, and receivable time, encounter rates, practice-days, and costs per encounter, are important information for decision-making managers. Shifting resources based on these reports and ratios, although difficult, is critical. When managed care dictates how much may be paid for a given illness, diagnosis, or service, it is necessary to allocate the resources necessary so that significant financial losses will be avoided. To do this, it is obvious that more sophistication in information gathering, storage, and retrieval is necessary.

The ability to model for predictive purposes is becoming part of the everyday life of the successful group. More than one clinic started an HMO, either on its own or with an insurance partner, only to find that in order to offer a competitive premium in the market-place, the clinic had to accept fee-for-service equiva-lents as low as 40 to 60 percent. These are levels at which losses mount rapidly unless something changes in the practice system.

Prepayment mandates significant changes in practice habits. For the clinic that has its own plan, capitates itself, and has affiliated providers outside the group, if these outside providers are reimbursed at rates of 85 percent or greater, with no risk or built-in controls, the clinic and its plan are headed for troubled times.

These changes, along with increased competition, have already pushed groups toward regionalization and involvement in other ventures. A number of authors have suggested that clinics of any size should be involved in regional networks, mergers, acquisitions, joint ventures, the establishment of ambulatory surgery centers, regional services, and consultation programs (Studin & Grennel, 1988; Bermas, 1985; Bohlmann, 1987). Although these approaches have great attraction for building volumes and creating efficiency in the managed-care environment, they are not without risk. For example, joint ventures, mergers, and acquisitions can have unsettling consequences for the groups involved as the different organizational cultures clash during the integration process. Great care must be taken to assure that adequate attention has been paid to studying the cultural differences between the organizations as each prepares to become part of the other.

The antitrust implication of mergers and acquisitions must also be considered. The rush to make the systems more efficient in order to cope with the managed-care environment will place many organizations at risk of becoming too significant a force in the marketplace, and thus attracting the attention of their competitors or the Federal Trade Commission (FTC). The case of Blue Cross/Blue Shield of Wisconsin vs. the Marshfield Clinic is a case in point (McDonald & Troupis, 1995). As groups attempt to cope with declining reimbursement as a result of the influences of managed care, there is no doubt that they will incur financial, competitive, and legal risks. There are enough cases of significant problems and some outright failures to suggest that management should evaluate the risks in new ventures (Proger & Miles, 1988).

CASE STUDY 19–1

THE FINANCIAL PERILS OF HMO RELATIONSHIPS

Jane Smith is the administrator of a 225-physician clinic in a community with a population of 150,000. Two-and-one-half years ago, the clinic decided to establish an HMO in cooperation with a major insurance company. This action was partially motivated by the activities of a competing clinic that was discussing the start-up of an HMO. When the insurance company first approached Ms. Smith's clinic, they offered to be responsible for administering the plan in return for the clinic, through its ownership, paying the insurer 15 percent of premium. The insurance firm also offered to handle sales and marketing communications and monitor plan utilization. The deal seemed like a good one for the clinic. The insurance company estimated that the fee-for-service equivalent payments would be about 87 percent and that the clinic would be assured a captured population. Marketing was successful, and enrollment reached 40,000.

A week ago, the representatives of the insurance partner visited the clinic to present the annual report to the board of directors. The representatives explained that, because of insurance cycles, the plan had not done very well and that there was adverse selection, which caused significant losses. Furthermore, they believed that because of the need for more intensive management (that is, more managed care), their fee should be increased from 15 to 20 percent. At about this same time, Jane Smith received a report from the clinic's financial office showing that the reimbursement on a fee-for-service equivalency basis was 62 percent.

After the meeting, the president of the clinic called Ms. Smith into his office and asked, "Where were we while all this was occurring?" However, he also adds that he believed the board of directors was as responsible as clinic management and that it would take a team effort to recover from this substantial financial loss. He asked Ms. Smith to design a strategy that would cover not only the immediate problems but also those that would be likely to occur in the future.

Case Discussion Questions

1. How should Ms. Smith begin to design such a strategy?
2. What are the managed-care implications?
3. What information would she need to be able to get the board to understand the origin of the problem, its seriousness, and the alternatives for returning the clinic to profitability?
4. The president also asked Ms. Smith's advice in explaining the situation to the membership at large. What should she suggest?

THE PHYSICIAN IN THE MANAGED-CARE SYSTEM

The physician is inexorably bound up in the net of managed care from both the professional and the financial perspectives. As a professional, he or she must honor the social contract with the patient. In doing so in the managed-care environment, significant financial disincentives and controls introduced by managed-care companies place the physician at serious risk of violating principles of sound medical judgment (Kahn, 1987; Clancy & Brody, 1995). These disincentives and controls may be found both in solo practice and in multispecialty groups. The opportunity for a managed-care

---

CASE STUDY 19–2

THE MANAGED CARE COMPANY RESPONDS

A physician from a group, who ordinarily is calm and cool in tense situations, went storming into the group administrator's office with the following story. He had examined a patient under age 65 who needed a transurethral prostatic resection. In discussing arrangements for admission to the hospital, the patient stated that he had an insurance plan requiring the physician to call a number listed on his insurance card. The physician dutifully followed the instructions, and once the insurance company had been reached, he was asked the following questions: What is your charge for the surgery? What is the average length of stay? What is your complication rate? What symptoms is the patient having at the present time? How long have these symptoms persisted? Are the symptoms causing great inconvenience to the patient?

At that point, the physician became irate and told the person on the other end of the line that it was none of her business, that he was not going to answer the questions, and that it was his medical judgment. The person on the other end of the phone said, "Well, that's fine, doctor, you do not have to answer the questions; I will simply send our client to another physician." In frustration, the physician stated that the managed-care company would get a call from the group's administrator. After hanging up the phone, the physician went to the administrator's officer to explain what had happened.

Case Discussion Questions

1. What should the administrator's immediate response to the physician be?
2. What should the administrator's approach to the managed-care company be?
3. Should the administrator bring cases such as this one to the general staff, or should she deal with them on an individual basis?

---

company to dictate the way medical practice is conducted is great. Today, it is not unusual for a physician to be required to call a toll-free number to discuss elective surgery or treatment with a representative of a managed-care company. Not all of these encounters have had good outcomes for either the physician or the patient. Case Study 19–2 illustrates the frustration of the physician and the dilemma faced by the administrator.

In the all-out effort to contain cost, there can be serious intrusions on the care system, intrusions that interfere with the critical relationship between physician and patient. The implications of this are obvious. There may not be a direct relationship between all managed-care systems and quality of care, but the opportunities for adverse results are great.

What role can the physician play in the managed care-environment? Kahn (1987) suggests that "physicians must manage physicians." To do that, physicians must know and understand how health care institutions, insurance companies, and managed-care programs operate. They must understand insurance principles, including the actuarial basis for premium setting, benefit design, claims processing, and contracting. They must participate in developing criteria for quality assurance, utilization controls, and outcome studies. Physicians also must "establish in clear terms their obligations to their patients" (Kahn, 1987). If there are to be standards of care and protocols for diagnosis and treatment, they should be established by physicians. If a vacuum exists, the government and third parties will rush in and establish standards and protocols, which will not necessarily be in the interest of good medical care.

Maurer (1988) suggested that managed care include incentives and disincentives for providers, appropriate care protocols, claim reviews and audits, initial and periodic screening of providers, and control of access to care. He also emphasized choice by patients in coordination with providers and streamlined coordination of benefits and subrogation.

Ideally, managed-care programs directed by physicians would establish an effective and efficient care environment that would operate on the basis of providing the best care rather than on the basis of compensatory punishment. Managed-care programs established solely on financial incentives or disincentives, on the other hand, are bound to affect quality adversely. The insurer may gain, but the patient will lose.

THE MANAGER'S ROLE IN THE MANAGED-CARE SYSTEM

To live in the world of change, the manager—whether physician or nonphysician—must understand the importance of the culture of group practice organizations. More specifically, he or she must understand the culture of his or her own organization.

If managed care is to be physician-organized and effectively developed, this effort must come from within the organization. The underpinning of each clinic's unique delivery system must be well understood, because its roots are likely to be as deep and old as the clinic itself. Managers must understand the mission of their organization if they are to prepare it for the changes that are already underway. They must help their colleagues understand the need for change and prepare them for the medical care system of the next decade and, more importantly, the next century.

Physicians have always "managed" care in the traditional sense. Now it has become necessary to define that concept more clearly and to adapt to systems for managing care in an environment of increasingly limited financial and human resources. Multispecialty group practices have significant advantages, because most have already begun to address managed-care issues

1. Trust in the relationship between negotiators
2. Understanding of the elements of the proposal or contract
3. Open sharing of information
4. Willingness to compromise
5. Understanding that neither individual nor group could do the job better alone
6. Desire of both groups for a win-win outcome

FIGURE 19–1 Principles of Successful Negotiations

through integrated practice patterns and consultations, their own HMO's, or affiliations with outside HMOs. Successful group practices already possess the outstanding leadership and management, discretionary income distribution systems, and sophisticated information systems that are imperative for survival in the new managed-care environment.

It will become necessary for many clinics to negotiate managed-care contracts (King & Topping, 1987). Strong leadership and management, with the knowledge necessary to negotiate, are critical. Successful negotiations are based on a defined set of principles that clinic management must know and observe. These principles are listed in Figure 19–1.

Successful negotiations can be either hard or soft, depending on the nature of the proposition under negotiation, the positions of the principals, and the importance of the perceived outcome. Hard and soft negotiations have the characteristics outlined in Figure 19–2. Managers must be aware of these characteristics and decide before negotiations start which path they wish to pursue. It is apparent that the opening of the

Hard
- Open with high demands
- Make a few trivial concessions and reduce even these as negotiations proceed
- Appear unconcerned about the threat of deadlock
- Emphasize winning
- Make threats

Soft
- Open with modest demands
- Be flexible and make many large concessions
- Be terrified of deadlock and show it
- Emphasize maintaining good relationships
- Make more concessions

FIGURE 19–2 Characteristics of Hard vs. Soft Negotiations

negotiations will, for the most part, dictate which path is followed. The circumstances surrounding the negotiations should provide managers with the information they need to decide whether to pursue the hard or soft route or something in between.

Managers must be prepared to deal with government agencies, HMOs, PPOs, managed indemnity insurers, and large self-insured industries or businesses. Thus far, many groups have allowed the payer to dictate the terms of the benefits and payments. Clearly, if there are to be negotiations, they must be two-way. To negotiate such contracts, managers must understand the elements that make negotiations for HMO, PPO, or managed-care contracts successful. Numerous questions must be raised and answered in order to develop a base of knowledge with which to address the practicality of signing with an HMO. A list of such questions is given in Figure 19–3.

The questions in Figure 19–3 shape the direction of the decision-making process when evaluating the pros and cons of linking with a managed-care plan or organization. A carefully constructed management information system should help determine a fair-market practical capitation fee that fits the clinic's historical practice patterns. The clinic should negotiate the capitation rate from a position of strength based on data. Indeed, it will soon be apparent that claims data are the key to managed care.

It is safe to say that if the group is to survive and do well, it must be in a position to turn problems into opportunities. It must have strong physician leaders and competent, alert management who have good general, financial, legal, and information system management skills and credentials. Success or failure will not be based on which reimbursement program is adopted or which managed-care company is strongest. Instead, it will be based on the quality of the practice and the strength of the management team.

CAN A CLINIC BE ITS OWN MANAGED-CARE COMPANY?

Any group wishing to establish its own HMO, PPO, or managed-care system should study not only success-
ful programs but also those that have failed. An insurance-related business requires a knowledge and appreciation of approaches to the market that are quite different from those relating to group practice.

Understanding this aspect of the business and building a staff with appropriate expertise in the insured side of the care system are critical. Even then, clinic leadership and management must pay close attention to the program from the outset to monitor the influence managed care will have on the group. If the way the care is provided cannot be changed to provide efficiency without affecting quality, the clinic's own HMO program can lead to extremely poor financial performance.

Another essential strategy that must be considered is the integration of the management and financial systems of both the clinic and the HMO or managed-care system. Without such integration, the clinic may lose sight of its central mission, and the HMO may prosper to the disadvantage of the clinic. The premium may cover hospital management, and other services well but leave clinic services at a disadvantage, with a low rate of reimbursement. At this point, HMO advocates in the group may want to take the HMO outside the clinic, an entrepreneurial move that seldom helps the clinic. In short, "the tail may begin to wag the dog." Integration should exist at all organizational levels so that the goals of the medical, general management, financial, marketing, and information systems can be coordinated fully. For example, the president of the clinic also should be the president of the HMO.

For those clinics interested in the managed-care business, the elements that must be in place to implement a successful program are listed in Figure 19–4. Roovers (1989) reviewed the special considerations important in designing software for managed-care applications. He emphasized the elements listed in Figure 19–4 and added other features that also should be included. These are shown in Figure 19–5.

Lack of strength in any one of these elements spells trouble for the group. It takes the knowledge and skills mentioned throughout this chapter to compete successfully in the managed-care business. However, the integration of a strong multispecialty clinic, a hospital, and HMO or PPO is an ideal way to prepare for the

- Is the risk sharing being done totally by the physicians who contract with the MCO? Could the risk be shared more fairly with the patients, the hospitals, and the MCO? What role do physicians play in management and case review of the MCO?

- What are the withholds and what is their history for being paid? Are primary care physicians and specialists assuming unequal shares of the withholding risks? What percentage of withholding risks are the MCO and hospitals assuming?

- How large is the membership of the MCO? How fast is it growing? Is it growing too fast for management to operate it effectively? How is it faring with respect to its competitors? Does it have contracts with any large firm or population group that might seriously affect patient volume for the clinic?

- How does the MCO track utilization? What are its methods for changing physician practice patterns? How are its cases reviewed? What percentage is reviewed? What data collection system does it have in place? Has it been in place for some time, or is it new and untried? Is the system effective in tracking global and individual panelist costs? Can cost-effective physicians be identified? What methods are in place for disciplining cost-ineffective physicians? Have any physicians been dropped from membership after yearly reviews?

- What is the history of the management of the MCO? Has it undergone recent changes? Does its structure allow it to operate efficiently and effectively? Does it have major shareholders who would compromise its working with the clinic?

- Are there any incentives to undertreat? If so, what are the organizational arrangements to avoid undertreatment?

- How does the MCO determine its capitation rates? Will the MCO share the actuarial data that were used in determining the capitation? Are the rates consistent with the clinic's past cost for patient care?

- What is the potential for adverse selection? How are new members selected? Are there age, sex, welfare, or chronic illness standards?

- How long after the end of the fiscal year are the withholds paid?

- What will the clinic's responsibilities be if the MCO fails?

- What is the management fee for the MCO that sponsors the plan? Should it be lower?

- Is a quality assurance program in place? What is its organizational structure?

- Is preadmission certification required? Who does the certification? How knowledgeable is this individual or group?

- What are the MCO's utilization rates (bed-days per thousand members)? How do these rates compare with those of other MCOs in the area and across the nation?

- Does the MCO have binding contracts or arrangements with hospitals that might create travel distance problems for the physicians? Would clinic physicians be free to admit to any hospital without withhold penalties?

- What is the MCO's profit and loss record? How does the financial statement hold up when analyzed by the clinic's accountant or business office?

- Using financial modeling techniques, what will be the total number of patients for whom the clinic will have to assume risk if it accepts the new contract and how will financial variables be impacted?

- Can the clinic remain profitable with a possible drop in revenue per patient? Does it have an effective cost-accounting system in place to predict whether it can be profitable under this capitation plan?

- Will the increased volume of potentially low-revenue-producing patients from the new MCO stress the overall quality and completeness of care by the clinic?

- Does the clinic have an effective system in place for tracking utilization practices? Will the clinic be able to cut costs if necessary to remain profitable with the capitation rate? Can the number of physicals per year, number of laboratory and X-ray tests ordered, number of emergency room and hospital admissions, and hospital lengths of stay all be monitored?

- What is the overall percentage of MCO-discounted revenues that the clinic receives? Is this figure getting so high that the clinic is becoming too dependent on discounted pricing, thus eliminating the possibility of raising prices when necessary, or becoming unable to invest in new services and technology when needed? How many contracts does the clinic want, and how has this been evaluated during the strategic planning process?

- How competitive is the local MCO market? Are premiums based on reality, or are they so market-driven that they are unrealistically low?

- Is the clinic large enough to refer internally to its own specialists to gain some control of costs?

- How often will the contract be renegotiated, and will the clinic be hurt if it has to pull out of the contract in the future?

FIGURE 19–3 Questions To Guide the Decision Whether To Sign with a Managed-Care Organization (MCO). Source: Carey (1989).

CASE STUDY 19–3

NEGOTIATING IN THE BEST INTEREST OF THE CLINIC

A national HMO, which has a reputation for a strong managed-care program, recently decided to begin marketing in the geographic area served by a large clinic. The clinic has 180 physicians and is located in a college community with a population of 175,000. The HMO, the only multispecialty group in town, decided to discuss its plans with the clinic's president and board of directors.

The HMO indicates that the clinic is an important provider and that the HMO would be most interested in negotiating a contract with the clinic to provide services to its enrollees. In fact, a contract has already been prepared for the clinic administrator and board to consider. The following seven provisions appear in the contract:

1. The contract will be exclusive, and the clinic may not participate in any other HMO in the community
2. The clinic will accept the managed-care program outlined by the firm
3. The HMO plan, which will include an estimated 40,000 enrollees, will have a member of the clinic as its (uncompensated) medical director
4. The clinic will be capitated and serve as the main focus for the new plan; the clinic may add affiliated providers, if it wishes, under its capitation contract
5. A board of directors will direct the activities of the HMO; of the nine board members, two will be from the clinic
6. All providers will sign a "hold harmless" agreement under which, should the HMO fail, the providers may not bill the enrollees for any services rendered
7. The clinic will negotiate with local hospitals for rates

Case Discussion Question

1. Prepare a brief response to each of these contract provisions, indicating whether the clinic should agree, disagree, or suggest new contract language.

- Sophisticated delivery systems
- Utilization review
- Quality assurance
- Membership/enrollment/eligibility expertise
- Claims processing
- Knowledgeable management
- Strong financial systems
- Understanding of capitation
- Premium billing
- Clinical support practice
- Marketing
- Support for providers
- Information systems support

FIGURE 19–4 Elements of a Managed-Care Business

- Enrollment/eligibility
- Document registration
- Claim entry/processing/adjudication
- Referral authorization and tracking
- Claim tracking—paid, pend, deny
- Premium billing
- Utilization review
- Cost-effective analysis
- Quality assurance
- Health delivery performance evaluator
- Correspondence generator
- Administrative reporting
- Integrated word processing

FIGURE 19–5 Elements of Software Design for Managed-Care Applications

challenging economic environment of the next decade. The combination becomes a competitive model that has the opportunity to look to the health of its own patient population and in addition negotiate services with other providers, thus extending the influence of a particular clinic and strengthening its referral base.

WHERE WILL IT ALL END?

Managed care is here to stay. For some, this is a problem; for others, it represents an opportunity. As we look to the year 2000, it is apparent that the issues will begin to sort themselves out and become clearer. According to Kerns and Ockers (1995), we are well into an evolutionary process that began in the 1970s, in which phase one saw the birth of the HMO movement. In that phase, the negotiation of discounts was a key factor in containing health care costs. Volume discounts on a unit of service were not very effective, and controlling utilization became a driving force. Phase two, in the 1980s, brought the gatekeeper concept. Enrollment growth potential was limited, however, because a majority of the population wanted, and in many areas continues to demand, freedom of choice of provider and free access to the system. Phase three, in the 1990s, brought further modification of managed-care plans to meet the access demand. Companies developed point-of-service (POS) options to provide unrestricted access to providers, principally specialties, under an indemnity arrangement with increased out-of-pocket payments. Today, we are moving toward phase four, in which costs will be reduced principally by medical management. Payment will most likely be through capitation. This phase will depend on the development of effective and efficient medical delivery based on sophisticated information systems. Successful practices of the future will depend on these systems, which will promote outcome matched with input through the use of the economic, rather than the accounting, model for evaluating health care.

There will also be a stronger demand to articulate a public policy for health. There will be continued insistence on high quality, and strong emphasis will be placed on outcomes. High tech will be coupled with high touch. Genetic engineering and "spare parts tech-

nology" will become a routine part of medical services. There will be an increased focus on chronic diseases and diseases of aging, and there will be renewed emphasis on the influence of behavioral factors in health care. Poor nutrition, lack of proper exercise, and the abuse of drugs and alcohol will be appreciated better for their contribution to increasing health care costs. Physicians will have to set priorities, make choices, eliminate bad or questionable medical care, stop practicing defensive medicine, and reestablish incentives that are clinical first and financial second. Relman (1996) stated recently that, "In the long run, physicians must be in charge of medical care, but they must live within budgets and be accountable to payers and their patients. The only solution that makes sense to me is one based on multiple local physician networks, organized on a not-for-profit basis. I predict that staff and group model HMOs will be the mainstay of the medical care delivery system within a few decades."

If Relman's prediction is not correct or goes unmet, a brand of managed-care that will punish both the system and the physicians will prevail. If, however, his challenge is met by using the opportunities offered by multispecialty group practices, a new health care organization will be developed that, at its center, will have a strong physician-organized and managed system (Wenzel, 1988). Under the new organization, the current definition of managed care, "punishment by economic means," will be changed to a definition that speaks of high-quality, efficient, and coordinated services. A system can be built in which it can truly be said that care is managed and the patient is number one.

REFERENCES

Abramowitz, K.S. (1988, October 26). HMOs—Past/present/future, the future of health care delivery in America. Paper presented at the national meeting of the Medical Group Management Association, Dallas, TX.

Bayliss, R. (1988, March 19). Second opinions. [Editorial] *British Medical Journal, 296* (6625), 808–809.

Bermas, N.F. (1985). Joint ventures in ambulatory care. *Journal of Ambulatory Care Management 8*(4), 79–87.

Bohlman, R.C. (1987, Jan/Feb). Minimergers. *Medical Group Management 34*(1), 24–25.

Carey, T. (1989, May.) Major issues in health care. Unpublished exam answer, XMHA Program, University of Colorado Graduate School of Business, Denver, CO.

Clancy, C.M., & Brody, H. (1995). Managed care: Jeckyll or Hyde? [Editorial]. *Journal of the American Medical Association, 273,* 338–339.

Dunn, L.J., Jr. (1994). Beware: Managed care is gaining the upper hand in the law. *American Medical News, 37*(31), 16–17.

Elden, D.L. (1989, January) The trend is toward managed care PPOs. *Commerce Magazine,* 8–9.

Fetter, R.B. (1987, December). *Development of an ambulatory patient classification system* (Final report to Yale University under HCFA Grant Nos. 18–P–98361/1–01 and 18–C–98361/1–02). New Haven, CT: Yale University.

Gold, M.R., Hurley, R., Lake, T., Ensor, T., & Berenson, R. (1995, December). A national survey of the arrangements managed care plans make with physicians. *The New England Journal of Medicine, 333*(25), 1678–1683.

The Governance Committee Advisory Board. (1994). Capitation strategy. Washington, D.C.: Author.

Gradison, W.D. (1995, April 2). The future of reimbursement. Paper presented at the 12th Annual Legislation Conference of the Medical Group Management Association, Washington, D.C.

Hsiao, W.C., Braun, P., Dunn, D., & Becker, E.R. (1988). Resource-based relative values: An overview. *Journal of the American Medical Association,* 260(16), 2347–2353.

Herschberg, S. (1994). A manual for the managed care physician: Why needed, how developed, and how used. *Physician Executive 20,* 37–41.

Jecker, N.S. (1994, August). Managed competition and managed care: What are the ethical issues? *Clinics in Geriatric Medicine, 10*(3), 527–540.

Kahn, L. (1987, Fall). A physician's view of managed care. *Health Affairs, 6*(3), 90–95.

Kerns, E.H., & Ockers, N.T. (1995, May 5). *Managed care industry overview.* New York: Alex, Brown & Sons, Inc.

King, M.M., & Topping, T.T. (1987, June). The hidden cost of contracting with managed care plans. *Trustee, 40*(6), 27–30.

McDonald, K., & Troupis, J.R. (1995). Point/counterpoint. *Antitrust Health Care Chronicle, 9*(3), 6–9.

Marion Laboratories, Inc. (1988). *Marion managed care digested, update 1988.* Marion Laboratories, Inc., 9300 Work Parkway, Kansas City, MO 64114.

Maurer, W.J. (1988, December). Understanding managed care. *Wisconsin Medical Journal, 87*(12), 31–32.

Miller, R.H., & Luft, H.S. (1994). Managed care plan performance since 1980: A literature analysis. *Journal of the American Medical Association, 271,* 1512–1519.

Proger, P.A., & Miles, J.J. (1988, October). Recent cases cloud price-setting issues for managed care. *Contract Health Care,* 30–31.

Puma, J., & Schiedermayer, D. (1996). *Pocket guide to managed care.* New York: McGraw Hill.

Relman, A.S. (1996, January). The future of medical practice. *Physician Executive, 22*(1), 23–25.

Robinson, J.C., & Casalino, L.P. (1995, December 21). The growth of medical groups paid through capitation in California. *The New England Journal of Medicine, 333*(25), 1684–1687.

Roovers, T. (1989). Managed care: When, where and why. *U.S. Healthcare, 6*(2), 32–33.

Ross, A., Williams, S.J., & Schafer, E.L. (1991). *Ambulatory care management* (2nd ed.). Albany, NY: Delmar Publishers, Inc.

Schraeder, S.A. (1994). The latest forecast: Managed care collides with physician supply [Editorial]. *Journal of the American Medical Association, 272,* 239–240.

Studin, I., & Grenell, B. (1988, July/August). Strategic and business planning for physician owned networks. *Group Practice Journal, 37*(4), 28, 30.

Weiner, J.P. (1994, July). Forecasting the effects of health reform on US physician workforce requirement. *Journal of the American Medical Association, 272*(3) 222–230.

Wenzel, F.J. (1988, April). Grouping together is the answer. *Consultant, 28*(4) 105–107.

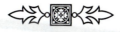

CHAPTER

20

Integrated Health Care Systems

Dean C. Coddington and Suzanne S. White

CHAPTER TOPICS

What Is Integrated Health Care?
Strategies of Integrated Health Care
Issues Facing Integrated Health Care Systems
Summary

LEARNING OBJECTIVES

Upon completing this chapter, the reader should be able to:

- Define integrated health care
- Summarize the strategies of integrated health care systems
- Discuss major challenges for the future of integrated health care

The closer we look at integrated health care systems, the greater the variety of organizational forms, objectives, and implementation strategies we observe. There was a saying in the mid-1980s, when preferred provider organizations (PPOs) first came into common use, that if you had seen one PPO, you had seen a single PPO (in other words, they were all different). In many respects, the same could be said of integrated health care organizations. How, then, can we identify patterns or common themes for analysis?

The recent transition and restructuring of the health care industry has gone beyond the wildest predictions of most industry observers. In 1994, many people, both in and out of health care, waited for the latest pronouncements coming out of the Clinton health care task force about a standard benefits package, accountable health plans, and health insurance purchasing cooperatives (HIPCs). While health care policy development on a national level has stood still, many employers, payers, physicians, and hospitals have moved ahead to implement a new vision of health care. In this new vision, the focus is on improving quality and access, measuring outcomes, reducing costs, increasing value added, and accepting responsibility for the health status of a defined population.

One health care industry trend that has been evident for a decade or longer is the growing proportion of employees and their dependents included in managed-care plans, mainly health maintenance organizations (HMOs) and PPOs. As HMOs have become increasingly important, approaching the 50-million mark in terms of number of subscribers (or covered lives) in the mid-1990s, physicians and hospitals have become increasingly aware of the fact that they are not in a position to accept the risk for caring for all these patients. As a result of the growth of capitation, a new buzz phrase, single-signature contracting, has come into being, usually meaning that a single entity could take responsibility for a defined population for a fixed amount of money (capitation).

Growing recognition of the trend toward capitation, and a desire, often bordering on panic, to avoid being locked out of the delivery system has led to the formation of a number of physician/hospital organizations (PHOs). By some estimates, there were as many as 1,500 PHOs in existence in the mid-1990s, and nearly all of them came into being since 1990.

In the 1993–1994 national debate about the Clinton health care reform plan, many industry experts favored an approach that would encourage the states to try their own reform experiments, and, indeed, many states have done just that. The argument was that if we had a number of experiments under way in various states, we could learn from the process and use the experience in designing a truly effective national approach. Although not on the scale visualized in 1993–1994, state experiments are taking place, primarily through the introduction of managed-care approaches in the Medicaid program and through legislation authorizing provider-controlled networks that can accept risk.

However, most of the innovation in reorganizing health care financing and delivery is not the result of government action. Rather it is the result of entrepreneurial experiments taking place throughout the country, as physicians, hospitals, and health plans actively search for new ways to work together. A steadily increasing number of physicians, hospitals, and health plans have come together into previously unheard-of organizational structures that are enabling them to work as single entities.

The factors driving this movement are as diverse as the organizational structures. In some communities such as the Twin Cities and communities in southern California, employers are forcing fundamental changes. In other communities, such as Albuquerque and Phoenix, the competitive environment is driving change: previously independent physicians and hospitals are organizing to meet the challenge of a group- or staff-model HMO or other competitor that offers a more seamless system of care. In many market areas, the possibility of more managed care, particularly the capitated variety, has motivated physicians and hospitals together to take on risk.

In many other locations where there is no immediate competitive threat and little managed care, visionary physicians, hospital leaders, and health plan managers are seeing the potential benefits to customers of integration, and they are moving in this direction.

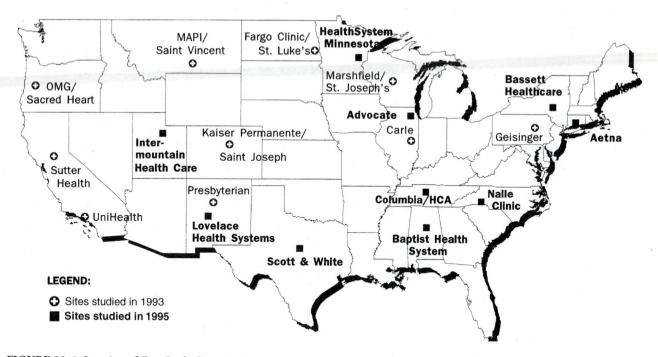

FIGURE 20–1 Location of Case Study Organizations

One of the popular themes in these markets is "controlling our own destiny." Physician leaders often refer to the advantages of "having a seat at the table," and they say that "change is coming whether we want it or not, so we might as well try to influence it."

This chapter addresses these issues regarding integrated health care. It defines integrated health care, summarizes the strategies of integrated health care systems, and discusses major challenges for the future of integrated health care. The findings reported in this chapter are based on two major studies of integrated health care organizations, both sponsored by the Medical Group Management Association (MGMA) (Coddington et al., 1994; Coddington et al., forthcoming). The research involved the preparation and analysis of case studies of 20 organizations. A map showing their locations is given in Figure 20–1.

WHAT IS INTEGRATED HEALTH CARE?

There are numerous approaches to defining integrated health care. For purposes of the research pre-

sented here, however, three approaches were relied on. First, integration was viewed as a matrix or as part of a continuum. A more formalized definition, based on mission statements and other material provided by several integrated systems, was also developed. The third approach to defining integrated health care was based on the common characteristics of such systems.

Integrated Health Care Matrix

Using a matrix such as the one in Figure 20–2 sometimes helps in understanding the various stages of integration for physicians and hospitals.

The figure shows two trends: one in the direction of the integration of physicians into larger medical groups and physician organizations, and the other in the direction of hospitals purchasing physician practices and generally increasing their economic ties with physicians. These two trends are shown on the horizontal and vertical axes, respectively, of Figure 20–2.

The third dominant trend is an increasing number of organizations moving in the direction of becoming fully

CASE STUDY 20–1

CAN ADMINISTRATORS AND PHYSICIANS WORK TOGETHER?

George Johnson has been CEO of 150-bed Saint Vincent's Hospital for 17 years. Over that long period of time, he has become known as a strong leader and a person not to be crossed.

When several physicians approached George two years ago about establishing a task force to look into starting an integrated system, little did they know that George had been attending conferences and studying the literature on this subject. He had been told to be patient, to not take the lead or get ahead of the physicians. He has thrilled that physicians wanted to proceed, and a task force was formed.

During the six months of meetings of the physician-dominated task force, George seldom spoke. In fact, there were meetings where he uncharacteristically never said a word. However, George and his staff were active in the background, providing information to the consultants and suggesting strategies for getting physicians to buy into the process. The process resulted in the formation of a for-profit limited liability health plan. Although it was not the organizational model George had envisioned, it worked to move the organization into integrated health care.

Case Discussion Questions

1. What were the strengths of the process described in the case study?
2. If George had taken a more active role, would the same result have been accomplished?
3. Who was leading the process? Explain your answer.

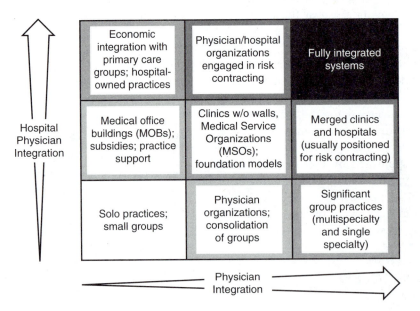

FIGURE 20–2 Integrated Health Care Matrix

CASE STUDY 20–2

ALIGNING INCENTIVES

The president of a statewide Blue Cross/Blue Shield system meets with the leaders of the state medical society and hospital association to discuss the double-digit rates of increase in hospital and physician costs the plan is experiencing. The head of the medical society says, "I can't tell my members to cut their charges so that you can make more money. They already believe that you are getting rich at the expense of the people in this state." The hospital association president adds, "You have over 40 percent of the market and are making good profits. Over half of my members lost money last year. If they hadn't received a subsidy from the counties where they are located, they couldn't have survived." He also points out that, because of shortfalls in Medicare payments, some of the hospitals had to raise their rates for private payers, including Blue Cross/Blue Shield.

The president of the Blue Cross/Blue Shield organization responds, "How can we ever get a handle on health care costs when both of your organizations are doing everything they can to increase their members' revenues and profits? Because of that, we have no choice but to pass the costs along to employers and patients."

Case Discussion Questions

1. Is there any way these leaders can work together to resolve these issues?
2. Is there a common interest among the participants of this discussion?
3. What are some possible solutions to the discussion?
4. How would an integrated system begin to address these issues?

integrated systems. In the figure, they are shown moving diagonally from the lower left to the upper right corner. The center box in Figure 20–2 identifies a number of organization forms (for example, clinics without walls and management services organizations) that are often used to bring physicians and hospitals together.

This is not to suggest that every physician and hospital should strive for a position in the upper right corner of the matrix—the fully integrated system. Only a few organizations have the capability or desire to move into this position. On the other hand, most health care organizations in the United States are moving in this general direction.

Integrated Health Care Systems

An integrated health care system can be defined as follows:

An integrated health care system combines physicians, hospitals, and other medical services with a health plan (or the ability of the system to enter into risk contracts) to provide the complete spectrum of medical care for its customers. In a fully integrated system, the three key elements—physicians, hospital(s), and health plan memberships—are in balance in terms of matching medical resources with the needs of purchasers and patients.

This is not meant to imply that an integrated system must own all of the key elements. For example, some of the case study organizations described in this chapter do not own a health plan; however, many of them have strategic relationships, or partnerships, with one or more health plans. This is often referred to as *virtual integration,* and it is an approach that meets the definition given above.

It should also be noted that very few integrated systems are in balance in terms of matching medical resources with needs. Most have excess hospital capacity and too many specialists. However, more fully integrated systems often have plans in place to achieve such a balance.

Common Characteristics of Integrated Health Care Systems

In the authors' research, 10 characteristics of integrated health care systems were identified. These are summarized in Figure 20–3. The 10 characteristics are useful in defining the extent of integration of various health care systems. For example, a later-stage integrated health care system can be defined as one that earns 75 to 100 points on the BBC Integration Index (Coddington et al., forthcoming). Similarly, a midstage integrated system can be defined as one that earns 50 to 74 points, and an early-stage system as one that earns 25 to 49 points.

Figure 20–4 shows many of the most common forms, or models, of integrated systems and relates them to their degree of integration. The broad categories of integration models listed in the left-hand column range from those that integrate physicians with one another (first row of figures) to those that integrate all three major components—physicians, hospitals, and health plans (last row of figures). Across the top of Figure 20–4, the three major levels of integration are identified. The purpose of this figure is to show, in general terms, how well several of the models of physician and hospital organization meet the mission of integrated health care.

STRATEGIES OF INTEGRATED HEALTH CARE

When case study participants, especially physician leaders, were asked about the most important decisions made and implemented over the past decade, two were mentioned most often: developing a primary care network and starting (or growing) a health plan. These and other strategies used by case study participants are reviewed next.

Strategy 1: Geographic Coverage/Accessibility

One strategy adopted by some health care systems is making themselves more convenient to their customers by offering extended hours or adopting other approaches (for example, greater use of minor emergency centers). As a physician who had once competed against Lovelace Health Systems said, "We noticed that when Lovelace opened a large outpatient facility in the northern suburbs of Albuquerque, patients loved the convenience. They flocked to this new place. As we look back, it seems like such an obvious move, but we certainly didn't get the picture at the time it happened."

Recently there has also been an accelerating national trend for hospitals, multispecialty groups, and health plans to acquire primary care practices to expand geographic coverage and for systems control integration. The authors share the view of many that this may eventually present problems to hospitals and health plans that have engaged in this practice. It may add to fixed costs, decrease flexibility, and reduce the productivity of primary care physicians. At the same time, it is a critically important strategy for integrated systems, especially those moving more aggressively into managed care.

1. Physicians play key leadership role
2. Organizational structure promotes coordination
3. Primary care physicians are economically integrated
4. Practice sites provide geographic coverage
5. System is appropriately sized
6. Physicians are organized
7. System owns a health plan, offers single signature contracting, or has a strategic relationship with a health plan
8. Financial incentives are aligned
9. Clinical and management information systems tie the elements of the system together.
10. System has access to capital and ability to shift financial resources

FIGURE 20–3 Ten Common Characteristics of Integrated Health Care Systems

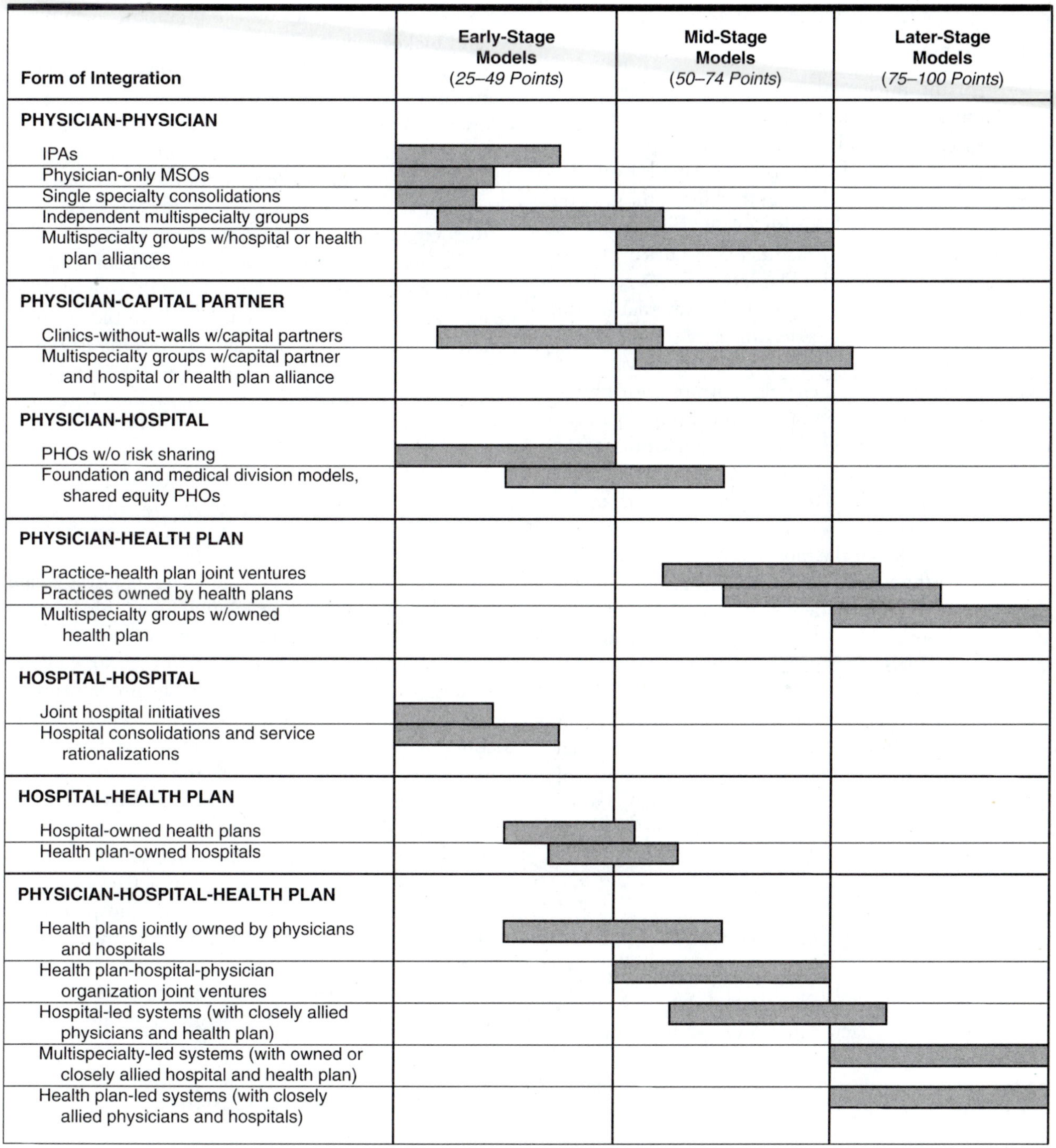
Form of Integration
Early-Stage Models (25–49 Points)
Mid-Stage Models (50–74 Points)
Later-Stage Models (75–100 Points)
PHYSICIAN-PHYSICIAN
IPAs
Physician-only MSOs
Single specialty consolidations
Independent multispecialty groups
Multispecialty groups w/hospital or health plan alliances
PHYSICIAN-CAPITAL PARTNER
Clinics-without-walls w/capital partners
Multispecialty groups w/capital partner and hospital or health plan alliance
PHYSICIAN-HOSPITAL
PHOs w/o risk sharing
Foundation and medical division models, shared equity PHOs
PHYSICIAN-HEALTH PLAN
Practice-health plan joint ventures
Practices owned by health plans
Multispecialty groups w/owned health plan
HOSPITAL-HOSPITAL
Joint hospital initiatives
Hospital consolidations and service rationalizations
HOSPITAL-HEALTH PLAN
Hospital-owned health plans
Health plan-owned hospitals
PHYSICIAN-HOSPITAL-HEALTH PLAN
Health plans jointly owned by physicians and hospitals
Health plan-hospital-physician organization joint ventures
Hospital-led systems (with closely allied physicians and health plan)
Multispecialty-led systems (with owned or closely allied hospital and health plan)
Health plan-led systems (with closely allied physicians and hospitals)

FIGURE 20–4 Forms and Stages of Integration

Strategy 2: Health Plan Development, or Partnering

Most of the integrated systems studied have their own health plan, and it is an important part of their strategies to grow this plan and increase the proportion of patients coming to physicians and hospitals from the system-owned plan. Based on our tracking of the growth of these system-owned health plans (for example, Geisinger Health Plan, Marshfield's Security Health Plan, Scott & White Health Plan), they are succeeding.

There are also major changes in the way that health plans, especially the venerable Blue Cross/Blue Shield systems operating in every state and most metropolitan areas, are restructuring their relationships with physicians and hospitals. Some of the case study organizations, such as Bassett Healthcare and HealthSystem Minnesota, are involved in strategic partnership relationships with health plans, and this appears to be working well.

On the other hand, the movement toward establishing physician/hospital organizations (PHOs) is slowing. There is increasing skepticism about the desire of large employers and health plans to enter into single-signature contracts. As a physician-consultant said, "I sat in a two-hour meeting with the leaders of a PHO where they discussed and argued over the wording of their contracts. I finally asked them how many covered lives they had; the answer was zero. What a waste of time and energy!" However, there are two major studies suggesting that many PHOs are meeting their objectives (Ernst & Young, 1995; Gorey, 1994).

Strategy 3: Quality Improvement

Integrated systems in the middle and later stages of integration are taking continuous quality improvement (CQI) seriously. In fact, some organizations consider this to be one of their core business strategies. Several of the case study organizations provide concrete evidence that physicians are not only involved in CQI but are taking leadership positions in this process. There is also evidence in several case studies of attainment of one of the long-terms goals of CQI—changing the culture of

the organization in terms of how it empowers employees and makes decisions.

As physicians have become more involved in CQI, many of the previous efforts have evolved into the development and implementation of clinical guidelines to reduce clinical variation, improve service, and cut costs. This may be one of the most important recent developments in health care.

Reducing clinical variation is an important concern. Doctors come from dozens of medical schools and residency programs, and they have different ways of diagnosing and treating various medical problems. It is generally agreed that some standardization, especially in high-cost procedures requiring inpatient hospitalization, has the potential for major cost savings, better patient service, and increased quality of care.

Strategy 4: Clinical and Management Information Systems

Most midstage and later-stage integrated health care systems believe that the development of information systems is important. Indeed, the investment in information systems exceeds that of any other single category of investment (other than establishing a primary care network), and by a wide margin. It is not unusual to find these integrated systems investing $5 to $10 million per year in building their information systems.

The development and implementation of an electronic medical record is an important step for most integrated systems. Related to this, most mature integrated systems are linking up physicians' offices in remote locations with the health plan, hospital, and central clinic where most specialists work. Information systems are frequently described as the glue that holds the organization together, or as the central nervous system of an integrated health care organization.

Strategy 5: Corporate Culture

Developing a tight culture among physicians and between physician groups and administrators continues to be important, especially for early-stage and midstage integrated health care systems. A tight corporate culture facilitates progress on other strategies as well as improving value. Several individuals who were interviewed in the research, especially in organizations such as Scott & White in Texas, HealthSystem Minnesota, and Advocate in Chicago, said the development of a strong corporate culture was a top priority. The importance of developing a corporate culture is discussed in more detail later in this chapter.

Strategy 6: Alignment of Incentives

How can incentives be aligned when most integrated systems serve both fee-for-service and capitated patients? How can incentives be aligned when physicians and hospitals do not own their own health plans? How can employed physicians be given the financial incentives to be more productive? How can for-profit and not-for-profit organizations share the same incentives?

Clearly, the alignment of incentives is a complex subject and beyond the scope of this chapter. However, alignment of financial incentives may increasingly be the key to success of health care organizations of all types. (Problems of making the transition from a fee-for-service environment to capitation are discussed later in this chapter.)

Strategy 7: Reducing Costs

Every case study organization—indeed, every integrated health care system—is focusing on reducing costs. One concern is that integrated systems, especially those that employ large numbers of physicians and operate multiple practice sites, have high fixed costs. Of course, the trend toward paying primary care physicians more and reducing compensation for specialists continues to be a key issue.

Several of the organizations studied had gone through a downsizing (often referred to as "right sizing") over the previous 12 months. Opportunities to reduce duplication of facilities and services were receiving more attention, and re-engineering efforts were in full swing.

Strategy 8: Access to Capital

Anyone associated with health care knows that the capital required to develop an integrated health care system can represent tens of millions of dollars. These funds are needed most often for primary care networks and information system development, starting a health plan, and positioning the system to be successful.

At the same time that the capital needs of integrated systems have become better defined, there have been significant changes in the potential sources of financing of integrated health care organizations, especially those that involve physicians. For-profit practice management firms, including PhyCor, Pacific Physician Services, and Coastal, represent new money, primarily for primary care physicians and multispecialty clinics. Columbia/HCA has become a more important source of capital for hospitals.

ISSUES FACING INTEGRATED HEALTH CARE SYSTEMS

Despite the many advantages of integrated health care systems in terms of gaining competitive advantage for participants and creating value added for payers and patients, these systems face many unsettled matters, or issues, which vary in importance from one stage of integration to another. Later-stage systems face somewhat different issues than those in the middle stage, and both middlestage and later-stage systems face substantially different issues than those in the early stages of integration. In the remainder of this section, three important issues, out of ten that were identified in the research, are presented for each stage of integration (Coddington et al., forthcoming).

Issues Facing Early-Stage Integrated Health Care Systems

Three important issues facing health care organizations in the start-up phase of integration are getting physicians to buy into the concept of integration, developing commitment to a common vision, and physician leadership.

Getting Physicians To Buy into the Concept of Integration

Physicians often fail to see the advantages of becoming integrated. Particularly specialist physicians tend to feel threatened by integration and all that it entails. They often dislike the concept of a primary care gatekeeper and fear that their access to patients may diminish. A typical physician comment is, "Why should I participate in an organization that will speed along changes that I don't want to see come to this community?" Hospital managers and board members, on the other hand, tend to buy into the concept of integration more readily. They usually view integration as a logical step for a hospital.

It was revealed many times during the case study research that the presence of an external threat helps tremendously in getting the attention of physicians and motivating them to work together with a hospital to form a PHO or some other type of early-stage integrated organization. In situations where an external threat does not exist, most physicians seem to respond well to arguments that participating in an integrated system gives them their best opportunity to control their own destiny. They may feel that if they don't do it themselves, someone else will do it for them. As noted earlier, physicians like the idea of "having a seat at the table." Physicians are also taking notice of the trend toward the purchase of primary care practices, even in rural areas. As evidence mounts that physician-driven integrated systems can achieve measurable success, many more doctors are likely to be open to the concept.

Commitment to a Common Vision

Developing a common vision is one of the first tasks of any group of physicians and hospitals interested in taking steps toward integration. An example of a vision developed by a group of physicians and two hospitals is the following:

> Our vision is a medical community aligning its efforts toward a common goal of delivering the highest quality health care in the most cost-effective manner. We can best accomplish this by developing a physician-led and

locally controlled network of providers, an integrated delivery system.

The authors' experience in consulting with emerging integrated systems and lessons learned from the research reported on here reinforce the importance of developing and embracing a common vision. It is especially important for not-for-profit systems. Without a widely accepted common vision, this type of entity tends to lose its sense of direction.

Although developing a vision statement and gaining approval for it from physicians and hospital boards is difficult, obtaining a long-term commitment to the ideals expressed in the statement is even harder. It often boils down to stating words versus accepting meaningful core values, and a willingness on the part of physicians to move ahead in committing their energy and resources to an integration effort.

Early-stage integrated systems can learn a lesson about the importance of a common vision from later-stage integrated systems, such as Scott & White and HSM. Executives in these mature organizations believe it is critically important to have a common vision, to live by it, and to constantly reinforce it. The benefits of widespread acceptance and understanding of a strong vision include alignment of incentives (because everyone is working toward the same goal), better decision making, and greater job satisfaction.

Nearly every newly established organization has developed a vision or mission statement. Our greater concern is the use of such statements in resolving conflicts, achieving buy-in, especially among doctors, and keeping the organizational efforts moving forward. There is a great tendency in organizing a PHO or other early-stage integration organization to lose sight of the target and to focus too much time and interest on internal issues.

Physician Leadership

There are three important aspects that relate to the role of physicians in start-up integrated systems: recognizing the critical nature of physician leadership, finding physician leaders, and keeping doctors involved in governance. Regardless of the extent of integration, strong physician leadership is the single most important characteristic of a successful integrated health care system. There is unanimous agreement on this issue among successful leaders and experts in the field. Strong physician leadership in all aspects of the organization is likely to be the most important factor differentiating integrated health care from situations in which physicians and hospitals continue to follow the fragmented traditional approach.

Nonetheless, some early-stage integrated organizations still try to form without adequate recognition of the essential role of physicians. One executive in charge of a 10-hospital system in the Midwest commented that physicians have too many conflicts of interest and too much interest in their own pocketbooks to be able to provide leadership. This is contrary to the experience of nearly every successful integration effort.

From the author's experience and that of later-stage integrated systems, it seems likely that many physicians in every community, organization, and specialty possess innate leadership skills. Potential physician leaders usually can be identified by the respect they have earned from their peers, their perspective on their own practice versus the medical community as a whole, their previous involvement in medical staff activities, and their willingness to participate in forming a new venture—a physician organization, a PHO, a health plan.

Most of the later-stage integrated systems that were studied have a culture that encourages physicians to participate in different aspects of the organization. Younger physicians often begin by serving on medical staff or hospital committees or on task forces. This allows physician leaders to quickly identify doctors coming up through the ranks who have the potential to take on greater responsibilities. This process occurred in nearly every case study, and it is observed in the author's consulting practice. Early-stage systems should learn from these experiences.

Most of the leaders in the mature integrated systems studied were specialists who continued to practice on a part-time basis in their specialty. However, medical specialty is not important as a criterion for leadership. In addition, regardless of their medical specialty, successful physician leaders are strong proponents of primary care.

But when health care is organized in the traditional fragmented manner, primary care physicians are defensive and find it necessary to promote their own cause. Specialists are reluctant to articulate the importance of primary care and sometimes raise questions about the quality of care provided by family practice doctors.

Issues for Midstage Integrated Health Care Systems

The issues facing midstage integrated systems are quite different. They include managing the transition from fee-for-service to capitation, maintaining or improving physician productivity, and developing core values and corporate culture.

Managing the Transition from Fee-for-Service to Capitation

For midstage organizations, managing the transition from fee-for-service to capitation—referred to as the *new paradigm*—is often an unresolved but extremely important and challenging issue. Among the case studies, there were a number of organizations that had committed themselves to operating as if all of their business was on a fixed price contracting (capitated) basis. Lovelace Health Systems and HealthSystem Minnesota had made this kind of decision as had UniHealth America in Los Angeles and Geisinger. Whereas physicians and managers recognized that this decision might lead to lower short-term earnings, leaders of the systems were convinced that it was a step they had to take. As one manager put it, "If we don't decide which way we are going on this issue, we are schizophrenic. How can we convince physicians that we are serious? We can't have it both ways."

Positioning the organization in a dual payment system is definitely one of the most complex issues facing most integrating health care systems and other health care providers as well. None of the case study organizations, even the most fully integrated, operated in a 100 percent managed-care environment. Lovelace Health Systems, with a large health plan, reported that 70 percent of its patients originated from its own plan. However, 30 percent of Lovelace's patients were covered by

Medicare or other fee-for-service arrangements. None of the other systems we studied had as high a percentage of capitated patients as Lovelace.

There may be a point, say, when capitation grows to 35 to 50 percent of all revenues, when the time is ideal for a midstage integrated system to commit itself to a different approach. In several organizations, Medicare and Medicaid are viewed as the key to this paradigm shift. The physician leader of one integrating system said, "As long as these two government programs, especially Medicare, pay on a fee-for-service basis, it is difficult to make the change to functioning as a capitated system with full alignment of incentives. But when these programs begin to change, you will see substantial movement by integrating systems."

The leaders of many midstage integrated systems are strong supporters of changing the way physicians and hospitals are paid for Medicare patients. They would like to see more risk contracting, but on a basis where there is a reasonable chance of making money. However, the primary reason for wanting more Medicare beneficiaries under managed-care arrangements is to speed up the paradigm shift to capitation.

Maintaining or Improving Physician Productivity

Although physician productivity is a critically important issue for all types of integrated systems, midstage organizations face the greatest challenges in terms of physician compensation and productivity. Midstage organizations have recently acquired a cadre of primary care physicians and are in markets that are increasingly moving toward managed care, especially capitation. Most early-stage integrated systems have yet to face this issue, although they know it is on its way, and later-stage systems already have mechanisms in place to deal with it.

The strong trend toward acquiring primary care physician practices and small- to medium-sized multispecialty clinics raises a host of issues about maintaining or improving the productivity of doctors. Many organizations experience a drop in productivity when physicians go from being at risk for their own income to having guaranteed income. As one hospital trustee reported, "Physicians are human beings, and they respond to the same incentives the rest of us do."

Nearly every organization studied was trying to get away from two extremes: productivity-based compensation (where productivity is measured in dollars generated) and straight salaries with limited financial incentives. A top manager of one case study organization said, "When we purchase a practice, we guarantee compensation for a year or two. We want to get these doctors on a different basis as soon as possible."

One of the important distinctions in assessing the financial performance of system-owned primary care practices is whether or not the network is growing and adding new physicians. Average physician productivity is likely to be lower when new offices are being opened and physicians recruited. The executive in charge of primary care clinics at the Baptist Health System (BHS) in Birmingham said that if the system stopped adding physicians to its primary care network, it would reach breakeven within two years. He also said that BHS was moving away from physician salaries toward financial incentives based on productivity, as measured by numbers of patient encounters.

Maintaining and improving physician productivity is one of the most important challenges facing midstage integrated systems. As noted above, most of these organizations have the majority of their patients in discounted fee-for-service payment plans and have not yet met a full commitment to the new paradigm, involving the provision of health care within a fixed monthly budget.

Developing Core Values and Corporate Culture

This is an especially important challenge for midstage integrated health care systems. By the later stage, most integrated systems, and especially those coming from the culture of a multispecialty clinic, usually have made significant progress in developing a meaningful culture. Recent research has shown that, for visionary companies, a strong corporate culture and core values that are embraced by every member of the organization are critical for the future. Thus, it is important for midstage integrated systems to quickly develop cohesiveness among physicians.

There are different approaches to developing a meaningful and sustainable corporate culture, as illustrated by several later-stage or close-to-later-stage systems, including Lovelace Health Systems, Intermountain Health Care, HealthSystem Minnesota, and Scott & White. In these and other organizations, terms of physicians, as well as other clinical and administrative personnel, work together to develop practice guidelines for episodes of care. Most of these teams include both primary care physicians and specialists.

The increasing emphasis on communicating through greatly expanded clinical information systems should help physicians get to know one another and speed the flow of information. This should be especially helpful in developing a culture between physicians in geographically separated locations and between primary care doctors and specialists.

Physician leaders of midstage integrated systems realize that development of a strong culture is a long-term proposition, and they are approaching it patiently. A major part of the process is developing trust among various medical specialists and between physicians and health care executives (of both hospitals and health plans). No one expects this to happen quickly. At the same time, the challenge is to pay attention to all of the details that make people want to continue to work together toward the achievement of a common vision.

Issues Facing Later-Stage Integrated Health Care Systems

Even the most mature, and many would say most successful, integrated health care systems face many issues. Three that are especially important are developing clinical and management information systems, reducing fixed costs, and maintaining consistent throughput.

Developing Clinical and Management Information Systems

The development of clinical and management information systems is a major issue because of the costs in-

volved and the importance attached to these systems by nearly all integrated health care systems regardless of their stage of integration. Despite the huge sums that continue to be invested, the results to date have not led to large-scale implementation. There are just a few pilot programs, in organizations such as HealthSystem Minnesota, Intermountain Health Care, Scott & White, and Kaiser Permanente in Colorado.

A physician leader at Scott & White said that information will be a major point of competitiveness in the future. "We have to know our outcomes. I am still not convinced we have an electronic medical record that lends itself to the kinds of analysis we need to be doing. For example, in order to manage care, we need to know what percentage of the members who join our health plan each year have hypertension. Right now we have no idea." Most leaders of integrated systems would agree with this physician, but the information systems are not yet capable of providing the kinds of information required.

With many different information system initiatives under way among integrated systems, one of the issues they face is whether they will be able to maintain a competitive advantage over those physician groups and hospitals that adopt a wait-and-see strategy in terms of committing significant dollars to information system development. Organizations that go slowly and allow others to be innovators or that purchase software from vendors may end up with superior information systems at significantly lower costs. The issues for many are how fast they should pursue information system development and whether they really want to be the pioneers.

Quality improvement in integrated systems appears to be picking up momentum. More and more physicians are becoming involved, and in several systems, such as Intermountain Health Care, HealthSystem Minnesota, and Scott & White, doctors are taking strong leadership positions. There is increasing evidence that quality improvement is positively impacting the cultures of many later-stage and midstage integrated systems.

There is also increased emphasis on the development of clinical guidelines. Although the efforts go by many different names (for example, practice guidelines or care process models), physicians are coming together to develop practice protocols in an effort to reduce clinical variation. These efforts are often closely tied to clinical information systems and the perceived need to have practice guidelines easily accessible on computers in physicians' offices. This is a promising development that should give a competitive advantage, at least in the long run, to integrated systems making this kind of investment.

Payers continue to demand information on medical outcomes to give them an edge over their competitors. Physician leaders also value information on medical outcomes, but they tend to see this information as feedback data to be used to continuously improve clinical guidelines or other systems. They do not appear interested in using the information to increase members, as payers are interested in doing.

The potential for published clinical outcomes information to impact health care purchasing decisions appears limited. The serious efforts of many organizations to reduce clinical variation will result in less variation in medical outcomes. As the differences in outcomes shrink, consumers and payers will have even more difficulty than they do today in differentiating among health care organizations on the basis of quality. In addition, there are too many ways to manipulate the data and too many complexities and explanations for outcomes data to lead to the shifting of huge blocks of patients from one health care delivery system to another.

These are the authors' opinions, and they certainly are not shared by all. It is likely, however, that later-stage integrated systems will continue to monitor outcomes and other measures of performance, but for the primary purpose of improving quality of care and service. In the authors' view, this is where the emphasis should be.

Reducing Fixed Costs

Lowering fixed costs is a close second, after clinical information system development, as an important challenge for later-stage integrated systems. In several case study organizations, top management expressed the concern that fixed costs were too high and that the cost structure increasingly would inhibit the ability of the system to compete. System leaders anticipated that many of their more loosely knit competitors, especially those that do not employ physicians and are able to price some of their services at the margin (that is, to not recover all of their overhead), may be able to gain competitive advantage, at least in the short run.

Later-stage integrated systems see their efforts to reduce clinical variation as a key part of becoming more cost effective. Many physicians believe that reducing clinical variation in specialist procedures and lowering inpatient hospitalizations can lower physician and hospital costs by 20 to 30 percent. Research into the factors driving health care costs indicates that this estimate is realistic.

Maintaining Consistent Throughput

One of the classic issues facing integrated organizations in a variety of industries—whether they are large oil companies, automobile manufacturers, or telephone systems—is maintaining a consistent throughput over long periods of time. Later-stage integrated systems are not designed to react quickly to changes in volume, especially when those changes are on the downside. For example, in 1993 Lovelace Health Systems received a jolt that threw the organization into an unprofitable position for several months when it lost 20,000 covered lives from the state of New Mexico. It took some time for Lovelace to downsize and adjust its cost structure, and many physicians were upset by the layoffs and what they perceived as a threat to the quality of care. This experience sensitized Lovelace to the importance of limiting its fixed costs and maintaining a steady volume of covered lives in its health plan.

Goldsmith (1994) raises a similar concern when he questions whether it is good strategy for an organization to own everything, including its own health plan, physician network, and hospital beds. In his words:

> Contemporary strategies such as physician-hospital organization development or physician practice acquisition are, for many organizations, really no more than exceptionally risky efforts to prop up excess capacity and fixed cost by buying utilization or market share wholesale.

Goldsmith considers these efforts risky because they increase fixed costs and require constant throughput in order to be cost effective. As a result of these risks, he favors virtual integration, in which the various components of an integrated system are tied together with operating agreements and contracts rather than common ownership.

Concerns about maintaining constant throughput are well placed, especially for later-stage integrated health care systems. The possibility of significant variations in volume places a burden on integrated systems to control variation in health plan membership through careful pricing and excellent service. It suggests that later-stage integrated systems should consider opportunities to subcontract more services, in other words, to think about converting fixed expenses to variable costs. It is also extremely important to maintain flexibility in physician compensation arrangements so that doctors can bear a portion of the risk of fluctuations in demand.

SUMMARY

In summary, integrated health care appears to offer the potential for increasing value added of health care for both payers and patients. Integrated organizations that deal with these and other issues are likely to be successful.

REFERENCES

Coddington, D.C., Moore, K.D., & Fischer, E.A. (1994). *Integrated health care: Reorganizing the physician hospital and health plan relationship.* Englewood, CO: Center for Research in Ambulatory Health Care Administration.

Coddington, D.C., Moore, K.D., & Fischer, E.A. (forthcoming). *Making integrated health care work.* Englewood, CO: Center for Research in Ambulatory Health Care Administration.

Ernst & Young LLP. (1995, February). *Market-driven health care reform: Physician-hospital organizations profile.* New York: Author.

Goldsmith, J.C. (1994, September/October). The illusive logic of integration. *Healthcare Forum Journal,* 20–31.

Gorey, T. (1994). *Case study analysis of physician hospital organizations* (Sponsored by the American Medical Association, Illinois State Medical Society, Indiana State Medical Association, and Michigan State Medical Society). Chicago, IL: American Medical Association.

CHAPTER

21

Research in Service to Ambulatory Care Management

Barry R. Greene and Jeanine L. Barlow

CHAPTER TOPICS

Health Services Research As an Applied Field of Inquiry

The Fundamental Issue in Ambulatory Care Research

The Complexity of Measurement Issues in Ambulatory Care

Ambulatory Care Research and Strategies for Assuring Quality Health Care

Organizing for Ambulatory Care Research

Conceptual Issues and Agendas

The Challenge of Research

LEARNING OBJECTIVES

Upon completing this chapter, the reader should be able to:

- Define health services care research
- Discuss reasons for the importance of ambulatory and primary care research
- Explain important methodological issues in ambulatory care research
- List important areas of ambulatory care research
- Discuss basic issues in primary care and managed-care research

Ambulatory care is receiving a lot of research attention at the present time, and there are some basic reasons for this. The primary reasons relate to costs, quality, and access, which, in one form or another, have guided health services research since the research field began prior to the 1930s. Anderson (1966) indicated that social definitions of issues surrounding the organization, financing, and quality of health services shaped the direction of health services research. More recently Ginzberg (1991) pointed out that there was a direct relationship between the passage of Medicare and Medicaid in 1968 and the development of health services research. Escalating costs of health services stimulated interest in understanding the demand, organization, financing, and use of those services.

In 1968, the National Center for Health Services Research was created within the United States Public Health Service to stimulate and give direction to these research areas. Then, in 1989, Congress created the Agency for Health Care Policy and Research, with expanded funding for patient outcomes research, clinical effectiveness research, and the development of practice guidelines.

Clearly the objectives of health services research change over time as they are influenced by the changing social milieu. Currently, social, political, and economic forces are leading to an increased need for better understanding and managing of the role of primary care services in the context of an increasingly managed-care environment.

Ambulatory care services and the accompanying technology costs are rising, but existing research in this area sheds little light on how to identify or manage the cost/quality questions surrounding this increase in services and costs. The strong movement toward the systemic approach provided by continuous quality improvement (CQI) remains. In this chapter, the role of ambulatory care research is examined as it relates to the broad context of CQI activities. In the first section, an overview of health services research as an applied field of inquiry is considered.

HEALTH SERVICES RESEARCH AS AN APPLIED FIELD OF INQUIRY

Shortell & LoGerfo (1978) defined health services research as:

> . . . research concerned with studying the relationships between consumers and providers as they affect and are affected by health care organizations, technology, financing and payments systems.

In 1979, the Institute of Medicine (IOM, 1979: 34) defined health services research as an applied field of inquiry with a problem-oriented focus. The IOM report stated:

> By definition, applied fields are problem oriented. Their questions are drawn from the work of practical affairs, and their theoretical and methodological approaches are more diverse than any of the individual disciplines that contribute to the field. Research on why people use different types of health services, for instance, may draw upon concepts and methods of economics, psychology, and sociology, using administrative or clinical definitions to categorize types of health services.

The IOM report pointed out that in such applied research, social problems and expectations shape research priorities and agendas.

An important difference in health services research, as compared to research in the behavioral or social sciences, is the difficulty of working with very large data sets. The problem is one of selecting the appropriate data reduction technique and formulating meaningful categories that are statistically significant. In ambulatory care research this is a very significant challenge.

THE FUNDAMENTAL ISSUE IN AMBULATORY CARE RESEARCH

The role of CQI is very well known throughout the health services field. This analytic tool is even being discussed as the basis for survival of health service organizations. A key dynamic in CQI is the primary role of consumers in the determination of process improvement. In the rapidly developing managed-care environment, consumers and corporate purchasers of health services are working together to define choices among health plans, negotiate financial incentives, and contract for products (Gold et al., 1995). These activities are a source of unrelenting pressure on health service organizations for low-cost/high-quality products, and organizational survival is at stake.

Griffith (1994) pointed out that the annual rate of growth of health care expenditures since 1970 was 11.6 percent as compared to an 8.8 percent growth rate for the gross domestic product. Based on this relationship in growth rates, Griffith suggested that the long-term solution to cost control rests on the ability of health service organizations to reduce expenditures by at least 3 percent.

The ability of an organization to survive will also depend on continuous productivity improvement, as measured by capitation cost per member per year and at interim levels as cost per episode of care, as in diagnosis-related groups (DRGs) and bundled outpatient services. This statement draws attention to other important areas for research in ambulatory care management. Currently, research in ambulatory care does not provide a precise specification of the systemic processes that can explain resource consumption. This means that, at present, many of the basic concepts and tools of management, such as cost-control techniques, cannot be applied to ambulatory care services. This predicament is driving much of ambulatory care research.

THE COMPLEXITY OF MEASUREMENT ISSUES IN AMBULATORY CARE

Evaluation and management of health care services is dependent on measuring system operations. But measurement is a complex issue, as will be discussed in detail in this section.

Measurement Problems in Ambulatory Care Research

The research framework in ambulatory care can be considered in system terms as a problem of process identification and management. System inputs must be identified, and the transformation of these inputs into specified outputs, which are useful and clinically cogent, is the primary objective. This is a very difficult challenge for ambulatory care researchers, and the overall process is similar to the pursuit of the outputs of hospitals that began in the early 1970s and resulted in the current prospective payment system for inpatients.

Classification Systems: Relating Diagnostic-Related Group Methodologies to Ambulatory Care Research

The highly significant research that resulted in diagnostic related groups (DRGs) classified hospital inpatients into administratively meaningful and clinically cogent (that is, both meaningful and of practice utility for use by physicians) groups for the systematic analysis of hospital outputs. DRGs as hospital products are the accepted case-mix measure for the inpatient prospective payment reimbursement system. It is important to point out that this research process and the DRG system taught analysts, administrators, payers, and policy makers to think in system terms when trying to understand, organize, and finance health services. Trying to identify the inputs, throughout processes, and outputs of ambulatory care services are the basic challenges for researchers in this field. Traditionally, providers of services have not thought of the services as product lines. DRGs and the resulting pressures to contain costs and understand resource use have pushed providers into a product-line frame of reference employing the system perspective. The discussion now turns to why this is so complicated.

Complex Process Identification

In hospitals, the organizational system being studied quite literally has walls that enable organizational designers and researchers to determine when someone enters or leaves the system. In contrast, ambulatory care ranges from very simple primary care to high-tech and invasive care, and it is difficult to determine when someone enters, participates in, or leaves the system. The objective must be process identification, but where does one draw the boundaries of the organization in order to derive the properties of the system? This problem makes it difficult to classify people, processes, and events to permit valid and meaningful comparisons.

Case-Mix Methodologies

There are several ambulatory care case-mix methodologies under development that are somewhat analogous to DRGs for hospital inpatients. The development of these methodologies is one of the most important areas of ambulatory care research.

Researchers have tried to classify different categories of care, such as patient visits/encounters (Fetter et al., 1984; Schneider et al., 1986). Patients or populations are the analytic units for ambulatory care groups (ACGs) (Starfield et al., 1991). This type of visits or use classification is based on a person's demographic characteristics and his or her pattern of disease, and it is used over an extended period of time, such as a year. There are 51 mutually exclusive ACG categories. Such a classification reflects the illness burden of a patient population, and it has the potential to predict, and thus permit risk adjustment of, the defined patient population.

Diagnostic clusters also have been used to construct physician profiles and analyze the content of physicians' medical practices. Schneeweiss et al. (1983) found that 21 diagnostic clusters accounted for about 70 percent of the episodes treated by primary care physicians. The diagnostic cluster methodology consists of 125 groups that are supposed to account for the great majority of ICD–9 codes used in ambulatory and hospital settings.

Obviously, different groups and grouping methodologies can be developed for different reasons, which may include the study of resource consumption, service quality, or both. At the present time, however, these methods are still in the developmental stage and do not offer much assistance to ambulatory care managers.

AMBULATORY CARE RESEARCH AND STRATEGIES FOR ASSURING QUALITY HEALTH CARE

In its 1994 *Annual Report to Congress,* the Physician Payment Review Commission (Physician Payment Review Commission, 1994) discussed basic strategies for assuring high-quality health care. The report pointed out that quality performance reporting is improving because of the rising pressure on health plans to demonstrate their quality to purchasers. They are attempting to do this through CQI, and the performance reports of leading plans and managed-care organizations are contributing to the knowledge base in this important area. Some strategies for this are discussed below.

A definition for and basic elements of CQI are presented in Figure 21–1. The key elements of the CQI process are illustrated in the case studies. Strategies for examining quality are discussed next.

Quality Performance Measurement and Reporting

The National Commission on Quality Assurance (NCQA) is continuously developing its Health Plan Employee Data and Information Set (HEDIS) that can be applied to managed-care plans, and NCQA is establishing performance measures of quality, access, member satisfaction, and financial integrity. NCQA also is involved in a demonstration project that is using HEDIS as the basis of performance reporting for 21 health care plans. Through the efforts of the CQI

---

1. The definition of CQI is: an ongoing, organization-wide framework in which Health System Organizations (HSO) and their employees are committed to and involved in monitoring and evaluating all aspects of the HSO's activities (inputs and processes) and outputs in order to continuously improve them
2. The important elements of CQI are that it:
   • is organization wide
   • Is process focused
   • uses output or inspection measures
   • is customer driven

FIGURE 21–1 Definition and Elements of Continous Quality Improvement

process, major health plans, such as United HealthCare of Minneapolis and Kaiser Permanente of northern California, have issued reports of quality of care in their plans.

Joint Commission for Accreditation of Healthcare Organizations (JCAHO)

JCAHO is an organization that accredits a wide variety of health care organizations. Its traditional focus has been hospital accreditation, but in the late 1980s JCAHO began accreditation of a broader variety of organizations, such as surgicenters, home health agencies, and medical practices. JCAHO accreditation is required in many states for hospitals and in an increasing number of states for surgicenters and other organizations. Whereas medical practice accreditation is not yet required, some managed-care plans and employer groups are asking for practice accreditation as a condition of contracting. Organizations are surveyed on site. Functional areas, for example, environmental issues or leadership, are reviewed. Increasing emphasis is placed on demonstrated competencies at functional levels, such as use and maintenance of an X-ray machine, as well as on systems for quality improvement.

Developing and Evaluating Methods To Promote Ambulatory Care Quality (DEMPAQ)

DEMPAQ was a research project funded by the Health Care Financing Administration (HCFA) starting in 1990. DEMPAQ used medical records information and Medicare claims to assess the quality of care given to Medicare beneficiaries in physicians' offices. Claims and records representing thousands of beneficiaries and physician practices in Maryland, Alabama, and Iowa were studied.

Key DEMPAQ concepts included quality review, development of performance measures with interaction between physicians, the research team and peer review organizations (PROs), and a profiling approach to practice patterns. Communication with physicians (feedback) and education were emphasized

rather than the simple reporting of performance data. The measures used focused on specific clinical conditions such as diabetes. The project focus emphasized using the information for nonpunitive education and continuous quality improvement. Several of the profile indicators used in DEMPAQ mirror those used as HEDIS measures. Although DEMPAQ did not describe individual physician behavior, its concepts have major implications for communicating with physicians about profiled practice patterns (Lawthers et al., 1995 & 1993).

Feedback is critical to affecting change in human behavior. Physicians are no exception to this rule. Often systems are put into place for monitoring quality that do not achieve the desired result. What can be done to effectively feed back information from the natural experiments that occur in medical practice? Designing key elements of the data collection/feedback effort is essential. These elements include:

- Buy-in from those involved in the measurement, as to its credibility, prior to the data collection
- Confidential information, including comparison of the individual with a valid peer group (for example, some specialty, same type of patients, or similar percent of managed care in their practice), provided to the individual
- Opportunities for individual, confidential discussion with an appropriate supervisor and/or a respected opinion leader on the issue
- Data without individual identifiers presented to a group in a nonpunitive educational manner
- Data presented in concise, easy-to-read summary form, using graphs to the greatest extent possible
- Time for both individuals and groups to absorb, consider, and respond to information

The manner in which data, such as that of Drs. Welch and Sanders in Case Study 21–1, are presented has a significant impact on other practice physicians. Perceptions, such as those in Table 21–2 drawn from Case Study 21–1, override intentions and ineffective communications. Therefore, all performance measurement data, whether specific to quality or not,

CASE STUDY 21-1

USING INFORMATION FEEDBACK TO ADDRESS QUALITY CONCERNS: THE ANNUAL RETINAL EXAM FOR DIABETIC PATIENTS

Dr. Joseph Welch is a 47-year-old general practitioner with Willowdale Internal Medicine, a 10-physician general internal medicine practice. Medicare beneficiaries make up about 40 percent of Dr. Welch's patient panel. A year ago, Willowdale implemented a new quality measurement initiative. The initiative included three major components:

1. Work toward JCAHO accreditation (required by area's major employers)
2. Track data needed for HEDIS measurements (in cooperation with its major health plan partner, Options Plus, but tracked for all Willowdale patients)
3. Use CQI principles and tools (for example, brainstorming, process flowcharts, cross-functional teams, and run-and-control charts to study any issues flagged by higher-level data)

One of the HEDIS criteria focuses on an annual fundoscopic, or retinal, exam as a tool for improving the health status of its diabetic patients. The exam is connected to early detection of retinal changes that can greatly decrease the risk of blindness in diabetic patients (Lawthers et al., 1993).

Diabetes is, overall, a frequent diagnosis among Willowdale patients, as the practice sees predominantly Medicare beneficiaries. Willowdale's diabetic population appears slightly above the 13.4 percent found in the DEMPAQ study of the retinal exam in a similar population (Weiner et al., 1995). While the practice has not studied it specifically, it is estimated that about one-third of Willowdale diabetic patients have other diseases (comorbidities) concurrent with their diabetes.

The 10 Willowdale physicians reached consensus on the HEDIS diabetes criteria as well as the other quality initiatives prior to their implementation. Information system upgrades necessary to conduct more extensive quality measurement are progressing fairly close to schedule and budget. The practice culture has always been one of consensus, because all of the physicians are equal partners.

Willowdale physicians understand that HEDIS measures require that all persons enrolled with a health plan be counted in the denominator of HEDIS rates. However, managed care compromises only 10 percent of the Willowdale total, and member enrollment (eligibility) is not tracked electronically. Therefore, as the basis of the study, the practice is using claims data for patients with a diagnosis of diabetes or who had received insulin or oral glycemics in 1994. The data base also includes patients who have a prior diagnosis of diabetes but do not have 1994 claim. Table 21–1 shows the general frequency of diabetic patients among the 10 physicians at Willowdale.

More specifically, Willowdale uses the claims billing system and a small data base to:

- Review claims for all patients in the data base with the diagnosis of diabetes or who received insulin or oral hypoglycemics; procedure codes related to ophthalmic exams, services, or ophthalmoscopy are included
- Load selected claims data elements into diabetes data base, which includes previously diagnosed diabetics who do not have a 1994 claim
- Link each patient with a referring physician, as indicated in the claims system

CASE STUDY 21–1 (continued)

TABLE 21–1   Identified Diabetic Patients in the Willowdale Practice, by Physician, 1994

Physician	Approx. total number of patients per physician	Number identified as diabetic per physician (% of total panel)	% of diabetic patients for whom an annual retinal exam was billed in 1994
Dr. 1 (Welch)	1500	180 (12%)	20
Drs. 2 and 3 (Sanders and Brown)	750	100 (13%)	20
Drs. 4, 5, 6, 7, 8 (each physician)	1000	140 (14%)	45
Dr. 9 (Smith)	1000	180 (18%)	60
Dr. 10(Jones)	1500	250 (16%)	75
All 10 physicians	10,500 patients	1,510 diabetics (14.3% of total)	Range: 20–75%

After one full year of study, Dr. Welch's 1994 diabetes criteria profile shows that 80 percent of his 180 diabetic patients have not received the retinal exam. Two other physicians, Drs. Sanders and Brown, have similar profiles. Dr. Brown has been with the practice for two years, Dr. Sanders for just six months.

Dr. Jackson, who founded Willowdale 20 years ago, serves as medical director and leads discussion about quality issues in medical staff meetings. He is annoyed that clinical criteria are not being met by all physicians after going through the consensus process. In his authoritative style, he plans to insist that this change at the medical staff meeting in two weeks. For their part, Drs. Welch, Sanders, and Brown are uncomfortable that they will be confronted at the meeting by questions from Dr. Jackson about their diabetic patient management.

Case Discussion Questions

1. What might be some reasons for variation in clinical practice patterns, both at the upper and lower ends of the scale?
2. What are some ways that the physicians could assess these reasons?
3. How should Dr. Jackson approach this variation among practice physicians?
4. How might what is learned about the practices of Dr. Welch and Dr. Sanders impact the other physicians? How might it affect the practice's quality initiatives?
5. How might the relative successes of Drs. Smith and Jones be shared with the other physicians?

TABLE 21–2   Physician Variation Issues with Methods for Further Study, Annual Diabetic Retinal Exam

Issue	Study Method
Physician is new to the practice	Review criteria, related guidelines, and processes with individual; clarify any questions or misperceptions. Example: physician believes only those aged 65+ should receive exam, but HEDIS recommends all diabetics ages 31+ be screened.
Physician states test is being done but not showing up in claims data: physician performing test his/herself	Review medical records for tests documented but not billed. Advise HEDIS recommends the test be done by ophthalmologist or optometrist; dilation required.
Physician states test is being done but not showing up in claims data: physician referring out of practice for the test	Review medical records for documentation of tests done by other physicians: notes, letter, etc. Contact referral specialists to improve communication flow of notes, etc.
Physician does not feel test is necessary	Review practice decision to adhere to criteria; review supporting evidence (guidelines, DEMPAQ, other literature). Address physician's concerns; ask for any evidence contradicting test. Are there other indicators that the physician believes the group should reevaluate as measures of diabetic care quality? Example: this review was of retinal exam, but additional DEMPAQ measures of diabetic care included glycosylated hemoglobin and total cholesterol measurement. Review cases: do some contraindicate the test, e.g. already blind? Are there more Type I or Type II diabetics in the population?
Physician states he or she sees more diabetics than colleagues	Assure data have been adjusted for differences in panel size before reporting to physicians. Facilitate discussion of how test is handled.
Patients referred for test but non compliant; they don't go for test	Reviews medical records to assure referral is documented. Contact referral specialists to determine no-shows. Contact no-shows personally to emphasize need for test. Coordinate with patient education, transportation, etc. to assure patients can access the test facility. Patient/physician discussion reveals patients are receiving tests through a source other than Willowdale or its referral specialists. Contact other providers indicated by the patient for documentation.

must be shared using the "three Cs" of information feedback:

1. Clarity: presented using terms, formats, and media that are easy for the receiver to grasp and interpret
2. Confidentiality: presented without individual identifiers in a group and with the opportunity to discuss the data privately with an appropriate person
3. Cooperation: presented with opportunities for interaction and involvement before, during, and after the communication

Performance data at the level of raw information are a first-cut tool to flag issues for further study. They should not be used to single out individuals for action without further information. Whatever data are collected and reported, they are but key pieces in the puzzle.

Quality Improvement

Another improvement strategy is to provide physicians with feedback. This approach is illustrated by the Maine Medical Assessment Foundation (MMAF), which began its activities as the Maine Medical Assessment Program in 1980, and is based on previous epidemiologic analyses done in Maine. The original studies found that hysterectomy rates varied widely by 31 hospital service areas. The service areas were comparable geographically. The variations were "statistically significant, persisted over time and were unexplained by illness, demographics, or referral patterns of the residents" (Maine Medical Assessment Foundation, 1994). The variations were due instead to local physician practice patterns and beliefs. A series of nonpunitive, confidential, and interactive educational sessions in subsequent years brought the number of procedures within the expected range by 1981, where it has since remained.

Case Study 21–2 also illustrates the use of physician feedback to improve quality.

ORGANIZING FOR AMBULATORY CARE RESEARCH

The establishment of organizations, topics, and approaches to research in ambulatory care settings is addressed in this section. Research that is applicable to practice is also emphasized.

An Organizational Model for Ambulatory Care Research

The Center for Research in Ambulatory Health Care Administration (CRAHCA) provides one organizational model for ambulatory care research. Figure 21–2 depicts some of CRAHCA's elements. The relationship of CRAHCA to the flow of information is presented in the figure. Information flows are identified as input variables to CRAHCA, or the center. These input variables are the basis of center functioning. Obviously, information flows go in both directions, but it is the

conversion of the information into useable knowledge by CRAHCA that is represented by the model. This role is achieved through the refinement of the input variables for the process.

The input variables shown in Figure 21–2 are basic to the understanding of the structure and function of group practice and ambulatory care in today's changing health services environment. Each of them is discussed below.

Ambulatory Encounters

The research initiatives in this area constitute an important set of inputs for the study of ambulatory care. It is very likely that something similar to one of the case-mix methodologies outlined earlier will become the direct analogue of DRGs and serve as the basis for a modified prospective payment system. The development of innovations in resource management and quality assessment will follow the specification of the processes in ambulatory care just as it did in DRGs.

Provider Performance

Measures of the provider performance input variable include resource-based relative value scales, which will comprise the basic building blocks for changes in the Medicare fee schedule. Physician and administrator teams need this baseline information to work more efficiently and effectively together. Measuring work in this way can facilitate performance comparisons across organizational and geographic boundaries. Such profiles of physicians and practices form the basis of the CRAHCA Robert Wood Johnson Physician Profiling Project, which was funded in March, 1994, and continued through August, 1997. The national data base that will result from this project will enable CRAHCA and other research teams to frame an important series of research agendas.

Group Practice Organizations

The group practice organizational input variables indicated in Figure 21–2 include complexity, size, governance, and specialty mix, and they are of major importance to any research effort in ambulatory care.

CASE STUDY 21–2

THE ROLE OF PHYSICIAN PROFILING AND EDUCATIONAL FEEDBACK IN THE UTILIZATION OF HEALTH SERVICES.

The State X Hospital Association just released a new report, given in Table 21–3, showing that asthma admission rates for pediatric patients vary widely among the state's 20 hospitals. The highest rate is over three times that of the lowest rate (205 per 100,000). The report has received a lot of attention because the press linked the variation to cost issues. For a variety of professional reasons, but motivated by the recent report, a number of the state's pediatricians recently formed a new organizations, the XYZ Pediatric Study Consortium. Several large medical group practices, a major area payer, and a professional association have committed to cosponsoring consortium work over the next three years.

TABLE 21–3   State X Hospital Association Report: 1993 Pediatric Admission Rates for Asthma

Hospitals	*Pediatric (age 18 or less)* *Asthma Admission Rate/100,000*
A. Hawkins Community Hospital, Jackson Center (2)	645
B. St. Peter, Jamesville Community (2)	460
C. Louisville West Medical Center, Health Center One, St. Joan (3)	345
D. Frankfort West, Methodist Center, Children's Hospital, Baptist Clinics (4)	310
E. Louisville Medical Center, Lutheran Center (2)	290
F. St. Matthew, Gospel Medical, Louisville East, Carrolton Community (4)	215
G. Appleton Medical, Percy Community, Wesley Teaching Hospital (3)	205

The consortium formed to improve the health care status of the state's pediatric patients. They decided to begin by learning more about why state pediatric admission rates for asthma vary. They think inappropriate admissions can be reduced, but more information must be gathered before they begin a physician education process. The rationale for reducing admissions is that "many, if not most, inpatient admissions for the care of asthma are thought to be preventable if [health plan] enrollees receive optimal outpatient care (Health Plan Employer Data and Information Set, 1995)." The consortium agreed that children should be "hospitalized for treatment of these conditions as infrequently as possible (Keller, 1992)."

As a guide to target rates, the consortium used the United States Public Health Services's (1990) *Healthy People 2000: National Health Promotion and Disease Objectives.* The objective for pediatric asthma admissions, as adopted also by HEDIS, is (per 100,000 population, for children 14 years or younger):

1987 Baseline	2000 Target
284	225

The consortium leaders and its research analyst began working to understand the variation using small-area variation analysis. First, they organized the hospitals by geographic

CASE STUDY 21–2 *(continued)*

location using metropolitan statistical areas (MSAs). The consortium's pediatric asthma admission rate classifications were:

High 400+

Moderate 399–249

Low 249–99

Table 21–4 shows clusters of high, medium, and low admission rates for various geographic locations.

TABLE 21–4   1993 Pediatric Asthma Admission Rates by State X Geographic Area

Geographic Region Rural Designation/MSA	Hospitals in Region	Rate	Rate Category		
			High	Moderate	Low
Rural areas 1, 2	Louisville Med., Lutheran (2)	290		X	
Rural areas 3, 4	St. Peter, Jamesville (2)	460	X		
Suburban areas 6–10	St. Matthew, Gospel Med., Louisville E., Carrolton (4)	215			X
Urban areas 11–12	Appleton, Percy, Wesley (3)	205			X
Urban area 13	Frankfort W., Methodist, Children's Baptist (4)	310		X	
Urban area 14	Louisville W., Health Center One, St. Joan (3)	345		X	
Urban area 15	Hawkins, Jackson (2)	645	X		

The data were further adjusted for patient demographics to remove variation attributable to patient age, sex, and race. Some data elements were not collected by the hospital association, so further data collection was needed. The hospital association also allowed additional analyses of its data to remove cases of children aged 15–18 years so as to be consistent with the *Healthy People 2000* definition (children 14 or younger). These adjustments took an additional five months for record review, data collection, and analyses.

The consortium now felt confident that differences were due mainly to physician decisions and not other factors (Maine Medical Assessment Foundation, 1994). The consortium was particularly interested in addressing the high rates found in rural areas 3 and 4 and urban area 15. However, they decided to address all areas with the same information. Materials explaining small-area analysis were carefully developed for presentation to physicians. Information about pediatric outpatient management was developed using specialty association guidelines and other resources. It was time for the first educational session about the variation, seven months after the hospital association report was released.

Case Discussion Questions

1. How might the consortium gain credibility among the state's pediatricians?
2. What are important points to address in the first educational session?
3. How should change in variation be measured?
4. How might changes and advancements in pediatric asthma care be monitored and communicated to the pediatricians?

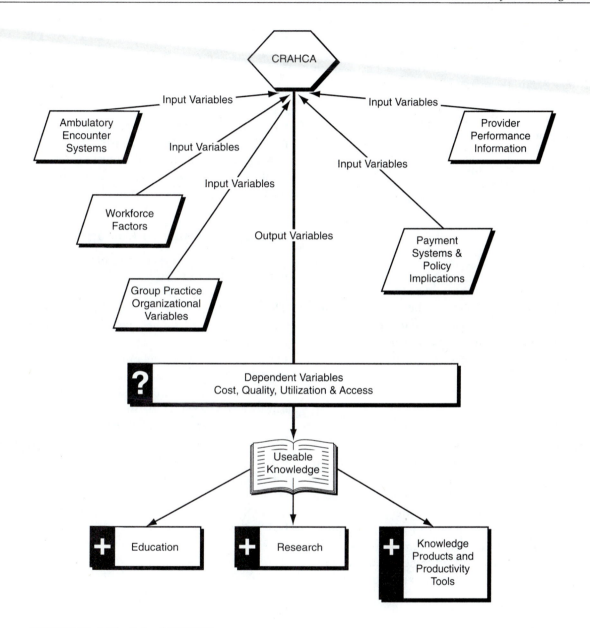

FIGURE 21–2 The Role of CRAHCA

Clearly, the group practice organization has become a primary analytic unit for understanding the health system of today and the foreseeable future. The context of this analysis is the patient populations and those communities served by the practices. The incentive structure surrounding hospital inpatient status and the management implications of that paradigm are not likely to guide group practice managers of the present or future. There is much to be learned in understanding how group practice organizations work and what role they might play in the new managed-care environment.

Payment Systems

CRAHCA has a primary responsibility to participate in and monitor the grants and contracts that underlie payment system reform. The fundamental importance of payment mechanisms is so great that all managers must be concerned with any proposed or studied changes.

Workforce Data

Another input variable indicated in Figure 21–2 is workforce data. This input variable refers to changes in the number, mix, and distribution of health care professionals in the workforce. There is very little research in this area that is helpful for forecasting purposes. Research is needed to examine human resource requirements under different workforce assumptions related to the supply of physicians and other health service professionals engaged in the delivery of ambulatory care.

Global Dependent Variables

The global dependent variables of cost, quality, and access form the basis for the ambulatory care research agenda. In a research development organization such as CRAHCA, there is the added objective of the development of useable knowledge. This type of knowledge serves to support practitioners through ambulatory care research.

CONCEPTUAL ISSUES AND AGENDAS

Understanding and predicting first require the ability to classify, which is exactly where much of the research in ambulatory care is today. Classification systems are needed to specify the full range of system properties in ambulatory care. Both the processes surrounding the content and delivery of services and the very organizations that make up the participants must be identified. Managed care provides a good example of the need for such classification systems.

Conceptual Issues in Managed Care

Managed care has evolved to mean an increasing variety of activities to improve the performance of the health care system (Hornbrook & Goodman, 1991). This broad and inclusive definition of organizations and processes does not help researchers in their attempt to understand precise and controlled phenomena. Health services researchers make the case for developing a taxonomy of managed-care systems, rather than forcing restrictive definitions on research activities. Enthoven's (1988) work in health maintenance organizations, provides a framework for the study of managed-care systems, leading to the development of lists of managed-care structures and processes that outline an agenda for future research on managed care. Bell et al. (1990) concur with other analysts that managed care logically should lead to "control of utilization, effective management of contracts of purchased services, expansion of benefits, and innovation in both quality of care and cost controls." Their model for managed-care research includes both the patient and the provider, with the physician-patient relationship as the ultimate focus.

A Primary Care Research Agenda

This focus on the physician-patient relationship is also found in a recent research agenda in primary care. Paul Nutting (1991) presented the framework for a research agenda in primary care that is presented in Figure 21–3. The agenda focuses on the doctor-patient

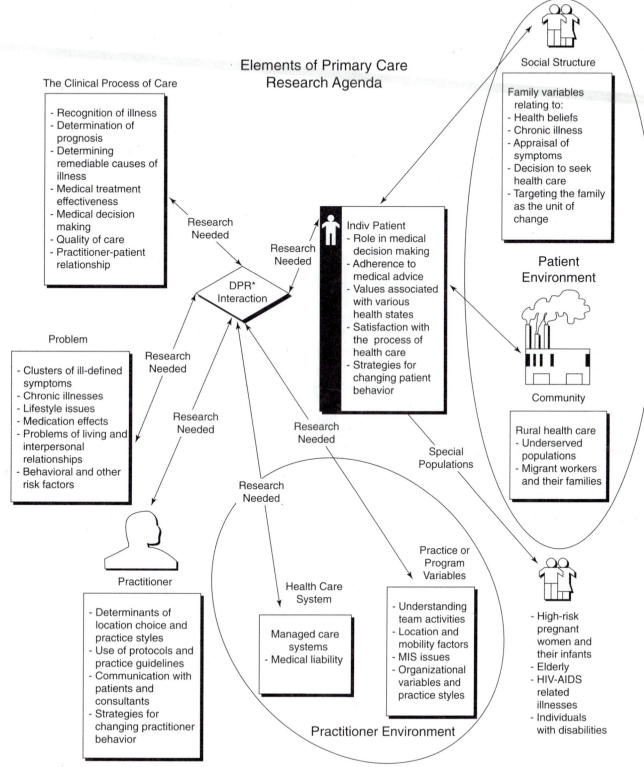

Elements of Primary Care
Research Agenda

The Clinical Process of Care

- Recognition of illness
- Determination of prognosis
- Determining remediable causes of illness
- Medical treatment effectiveness
- Medical decision making
- Quality of care
- Practitioner-patient relationship

Research Needed

DPR* Interaction

Research Needed

Indiv Patient
- Role in medical decision making
- Adherence to medical advice
- Values associated with various health states
- Satisfaction with the process of health care
- Strategies for changing patient behavior

Social Structure

Family variables relating to:
- Health beliefs
- Chronic illness
- Appraisal of symptoms
- Decision to seek health care
- Targeting the family as the unit of change

Patient Environment

Problem

- Clusters of ill-defined symptoms
- Chronic illnesses
- Lifestyle issues
- Medication effects
- Problems of living and interpersonal relationships
- Behavioral and other risk factors

Research Needed

Research Needed

Research Needed

Research Needed

Special Populations

Community

Rural health care
- Underserved populations
- Migrant workers and their families

Practitioner

- Determinants of location choice and practice styles
- Use of protocols and practice guidelines
- Communication with patients and consultants
- Strategies for changing practitioner behavior

Health Care System

Managed care systems
- Medical liability

Practice or Program Variables

- Understanding team activities
- Location and mobility factors
- MIS issues
- Organizational variables and practice styles

Practitioner Environment

- High-risk pregnant women and their infants
- Elderly
- HIV-AIDS related illnesses
- Individuals with disabilities

*Doctor Patient Relationship (DPR)
Source: Adapted from Nutting, 1991.

FIGURE 21–3 Primary Care Research Agenda

interaction and considers the many factors of the practitioner environment and the patient environment. These elements and the areas of needed research illustrate very well the basic tasks ahead of much of the important work in the ambulatory care area. The social structure, community factors, patient environment, and health care system and clinical practice environment show the true complexity of the many variables that enter into and determine the form and structure of the doctor-patient interaction.

THE CHALLENGE OF RESEARCH

This chapter began with a general definition of health services research and explained how social and economic changes in the health care system have focused this research into an applied and problem-oriented field of inquiry. The data in this multidisciplinary field often come from secondary sources and very large data sets. These, in turn, require sophisticated data reduction techniques. Health services programs are shaped by economic and social incentive systems. As a result, researchers are constantly analyzing different organizational structures and processes through social and economic determinants.

Unfortunately our health and social policies tend to precede definitive solutions to important social and economic problems. The drastic change from the institution-based system to the community-based system, with its emphasis on ambulatory and managed care, is the latest illustration of this evolving situation. More sophisticated research in the future will provide policy and management guidance throughout the health care system.

REFERENCES

Anderson, O.W. (1966). Influences of social and economic research on public policy in the health field: A review. In D. Mainland (Ed.). *Health Services Research,* (pp. 11–48, 56). New York: Milibank Memorial Fund.

Bell, C.W., Lewis, B.E., & Zelley, M.O. (1990). Managed care: Update and future directions. *Journal of Ambulatory Care Management, 13,* 15–26.

Enthoven, A.C. (1988). Theory and practice of managed competition in health care finance. *Professor F. De Vries Lectures in Economics, 9.* Amsterdam: North-Holland.

Fetter, R.B., Averril, R.F., Lichtenstein J.L., & Freeman, J.L. (1984). Ambulatory visit groups: A framework for measuring productivity in ambulatory care. *Health Services Research, 19,* 415–437.

Ginzberg, E. (Ed.). (1991). *Health services research: Key to health policy.* Cambridge, MA: Harvard University Press.

Gold, M., Nelson, L., Lake, T., & Hurley, R. (1995, September). Behind the curve: A critical assessment of how little is known about arrangements between managed care plans and physicians. *Medical Care Research and Reviews, 52*(3), 307–341.

Griffith, J. (1994). Reengineering health care: Management systems for survivors. *Hospitals & Health Services Administration, 39*(4), 219–242.

Hornbrook, M.C., & Goodman, M.J. (1991). Managed care: Penalties, autonomy, risk, and integration. In *Primary Care Research: Theory and Methods.* Agency for Health Care Policy and Research Conference Proceedings. Institute of Medicine (1979) *Health Services Research.* Washington, DC: National Academy of Sciences.

Keller, R.B. (1992, July/August). Physicians and profiling. *Group Practice Journal, 41*(4), 63–67.

Lawthers, A.G., Palmer, R.H., Banks, N., Garnick, D.W., Fowles, J., & Weiner, J. P. (1995, January). Designing and using measures of quality based on physician office records. *Journal of Ambulatory Care Management, 18*(1), 56–72.

Lawthers, A.G., Palmer, R.H., Edwards, J.E., Fowles, J., Garnick, D.W., & Weiner, J. P. (1993, December). Developing and evaluating performance measures for ambulatory care quality: A preliminary report of the DEMPAQ project. *The Joint Commission Journal on Quality Improvement, 19*(12), 552–565.

Maine Medical Assessment Foundation (1994). *Annual report.* Augusta, ME: Author.

Moller, J.H., Powell, C.B., Joranson, J.A., & Borbas, C. (1994, December). The pediatric cardiac care consortium—revisited. *Joint Commission on Accreditation of Healthcare Organizations, 20*(12), 661–668.

National Committee for Quality Assurance. 1995. *Health Plan Employer Data and Information Set (HEDIS)* [version 2.5]. (1995) Washington, DC: Author.

Nutting, P.A. (1991). *A research agenda for primary care: Summary report of a conference.* Rockville, MD: Agency for Health Care Policy and Research.

Physician Payment Review Commission (1994). *Annual report to Congress.* Washington, DC.

Schneeweiss, R., Rosenblatt, R.R., Cherkin, D.D., Kirkwood, C.R., & Hart, G. (1983). Diagnosis clusters: A new tool for analyzing the content of ambulatory medical care. *Medical Care, 21,* 105–122.

Schneider, K.C., Lichtenstein, J.L., Fetter, R.B., Freeman, J.L., & Newbold, R.C. (1986). *The new ICD–9–CM ambulatory visit groups classification scheme: Definitions manual.* New Haven, CT: Yale University.

Schoenbaum, S.C. (1993, March). Feedback of clinical performance information. *HMO Practice, 7*(1), 5–11.

Shortell, S.M., & LoGerfo, J.P. (1978). *Health services research and public policy: Definitions, accomplishments, and potential* (Paper prepared for the Institute of Medicine Steering Committee on Health Services Research) (Winter).

Starfield, B., Weiner, J., Mumford, L., & Steinwachs, D. (1991). Ambulatory care groups: A categorization of diagnoses for research and management. *Health Services Research, 25,* 990–1015.

U.S. Public Health Service. (1990). *Healthy people 2000: National health promotion and disease objectives.* Washington, DC: Author.

Weiner, J.P., Parente, S.T., Garnick, D.W., Fowles, J., Lawthers, A.G., & Palmer R.H. (1995, May). Variation in office based quality—a claims-based profile of care provided to Medicare patients with diabetes. *Journal of the American Medical Association, 273*(19), 1503–1508.

APPENDIX: SOLUTIONS TO SELECTED CASE STUDIES

⬚

Case Study 3–1
Allocating Service Department Costs

1. Direct method of allocation:

Responsibility Centers	Direct Costs	Occupancy	Support	Total
Occupancy	$ 240,000	$(240,000)		0
Support	120,000	0	$(120,000)	0
Operating	300,000	112,800	19,200	$ 432,000
Outpatient	900,000	127,200	100,800	1,128,000
Full Cost	$1,560,000	$ 0	$ 0	$1,560,000

2. Step-down method of allocation (occupancy allocated first):

Responsibility Centers	Direct Costs	Occupancy	Subtotal	Support	Total
Occupancy	$ 240,000	$(240,000)	$ 0		$ 0
Support	120,000	36,000	156,000	$(156,000)	0
Operating	300,000	96,000	396,000	24,960	420,960
Outpatient	900,000	108,000	1,008,000	131,040	1,139,040
Full Cost	$1,560,000	$ 0	$1,560,000	$ 0	$1,560,000

3. Contribution to profit–direct method cost allocation:

	Operating	Outpatient	Total
Revenues	$800,000	$2,400,000	$3,200,000
Direct Costs	432,000	1,128,000	1,560,000
Contribution	$368,000	$1,272,000	$1,640,000
% of revenue	46.0%	53.0%	51.3%

Case Study 3–2
Determining the Cost of a Procedure

1. Cost per sigmoidoscopic procedure:

Direct material	$ 5.75
Direct labor:	
Physician (40 hrs × 48 wks = 1,152 hrs	
$200,000 / 1,152 hrs = $173.61/hr	
$173.61 / 60 min = $2.89 × 15 =	43.35
Technician (24,000 / 1,800 hrs = $13.33/hr	
$13.33 / 60 min = $.22 × 60 =	13.20
Indirect overhead:	
$146,000 / 9,000 procedures = $16.22/procedure	16.22
Direct overhead:	
$12,000 / 4 yr = $3,000 per yr / 600 =	5.00
Total	$83.52

2. Patient profit per sigmoidoscopic procedure:

	Medicare	NonMedicare
Charge	$ 81.25	$110.00
Full Cost	83.52	83.52
Profit (Loss)	$(2.27)	$ 26.48

Case Study 4–1
Developing the Budget

1. Comprehensive budget for Catskill Clinic for 19X8
   A. Profit plan—Catskill Clinic profit plan for the year 19X8

	Per Visit	Total
Budgeted patient visits		30,000
Revenue from patient visits	$50.00	$1,500,000
Variable expenses		
Medical supplies	$ 6.00	180,000
Service bureau	1.00	30,000
Other operating expenses	3.00	90,000
Total variable expenses	$10.00	$ 300,000
Contribution margin	$40.00	$1,200,000
Fixed expenses		
Administrative and technician salaries		$ 228,000
Nursing salaries		216,000
Rent		48,000
Service bureau		24,000
Other fixed expenses		72,000
Depreciation expenses		16,000
Total fixed expenses		604,000

Net income before distributions	596,000
Physicians' salaries	594,000
Net income	$ 2,000

B. Computation of cash flows

	Profit Plan Amount	+	Beginning Balance	−	Ending Balance	=	Cash Flows
Cash receipts							
Gross charges*	$1,500,000						
Patient receivables			$240,000		$220,000		$1,520,000
Cash disbursements							
Medical supplies	$ 180,000						
Increase in balance	12,000						
Supplies purchased	$ 192,000						
Accounts payable			$ 6,000		16,000		$ 182,000
Service bureau	$ 30,000						
Accounts payable			$ 4,000		2,500		31,500
Other variable expenses	90,000		—		—		90,000
Fixed expenses	588,000		—		—		588,000
Depreciation expense	16,000		—		—		0
Physicians' salaries**	594,000		—		—		594,000
Total							$1,485,500
Net cash flow							$ 34,500

*Billings to patients = Population × Percentage × Visits per year × Billing rate
= 24,000 × 25% × 5 × $50
= $1,500,000

**Physicians' salaries
Number of physicians = Patient visits/(600 × 12)
= 30,000/7,200
= 4.17 = 4.5 physicians
Physicians' salaries = 4.5 physicians × $11,000 × 12 months
= $594,000

C. Cash budget

Catskill Clinic cash budget for the year 19X8

Cash flow from operations	
Collections from patients	$1,520,000
Cash payments for expenses	(1,485,500)
Cash from operations	34,500
Cash flow for investing	
Purchase of equipment	(80,000)
Cash flow from financing	
Increase in line of credit	35,500
Change in cash	(10,000)
Beginning cash balance	20,000
Ending cash balance	$ 10,000

D. Projected statement of financial position

Catskill Clinic projected statement of financial position end of 19X8

Assets		
Cash		$ 10,000
Patient receivables		220,000
Supplies		20,000
Equipment	$ 80,000	
Less accumulated depreciation	(16,000)	64,000
Total assets		$314,000
Equities		
Accounts payable: supplies		16,000
Accounts payable: other		2,500
Line of credit		35,500
Total liabilities		$ 54,000
Beginning partners' equity	$258,000	
Budgeted income (loss)	2,000	260,000
Total equities	/	$314,000

E. The clinic is showing a small net income at this level of operations, with the average billing rate of $50 per patient visit and the cost structure of $10 per patient visit and $604,000 fixed cost per year. With the contribution margin of $40 per patient visit, any change in the activity level will have a significant impact on income. The administrator should examine the costs closely. Given the large contribution margin, the clinic may generate additional income by increasing the number of patient visits, increasing productivity, reducing expenses, or increasing the billing rate.

The objective, as stated in the flexible budget and productivity data, is being met. Cash flow from operations is positive, in part because of increasing the collection rate. Because collections are delayed over one month and most expenses are paid in the month of incurrence, any increase in activity may result in a cash shortage.

Case Study 4–2
Clinic Performance Evaluation

1. Evaluation of performance of Catskill Clinic for 19X8:

A. Income statement

Catskill Clinic income statement for the year 19X8

				Variances	
	Performance			Due to Activity	Due to Price, Spending and Efficiency
	Profit Plan	Budget	Actual		
Patient visits	30,000	28,000	28,000	(2,000)	0
Revenue from patient visits	$1,500,000	$1,400,000	$1,344,000	$(100,000)	$(56,000)

Variable expenses					
Medical supplies	$ 180,000	$ 168,000	$ 159,000	$ 12,000	$ 9,000
Service bureau	30,000	28,000	24,000	2,000	4,000
Other operating expenses	90,000	84,000	88,000	6,000	(4,000)
Total variable	$ 300,000	$ 280,000	$ 271,000	$ 20,000	$ 9,000
Contribution margin	$1,200,000	$1,120,000	$1,073,000	$ (80,000)	$(47,000)
Fixed expenses					
Administrative and tech. salaries	$228,000	$ 228,000	$198,000	$ 0	$30,000
Nursing salaries	216,000	216,000	195,000	0	21,000
Rent	48,000	48,000	48,000	0	0
Service bureau	24,000	24,000	24,000	0	0
Other fixed expenses	72,000	72,000	70,000	0	2,000
Depreciation exp.	16,000	16,000	16,000	0	0
Total fixed	$604,000	$ 604,000	$551,000	$ 0	$53,000
Net income before Distributions	$596,000	$516,000	$522,000	$(80,000)	$ 6,000
Physicians' salaries	$594,000	$594,000	$552,000	$ 0	$42,000
Net income	$ 2,000	$ (78,000)	$ (30,000)	$(80,000)	$48,000

B. Computation of cash flows

	Income Statement Amount	+	Beginning Balance	−	Ending Balance	= Cash Flows
Cash receipts						
Gross charges	$1,344,000					
Patient receivables			$240,000		160,000	$1,424,000
Cash disbursements						
Medical supplies	$ 159,000					
Decrease in balance	(4,000)					
Supplies purchased	$ 155,000					
Accounts payable			$ 6,000		10,000	151,000
Service bureau	$ 24,000					
Accounts payable			$ 4,000		2,500	25,500
Other variable expenses	88,000		—		—	88,000
Fixed expenses	535,000		—		—	535,000
Depreciation expense	16,000		—		—	0
Physicians' salaries	552,000		—		—	552,000
Total						$1,351,500
Net cash flow						$ 72,500

C. Cash flow statement

Cash flow from operations	
Collections from patients	$1,424,000
Cash payments for expenses	(1,351,500)
Cash from operations	$ 72,500

Cash flow for investing		
Purchase of equipment		(80,000)
Cash flow from financing		
Increase in line of credit		5,000
Change in cash	($	2,500)
Beginning cash balance		20,000
Ending cash balance	$	17,500

D. Statement of financial position

Assets		
Cash		$ 17,500
Patient receivables		160,000
Supplies		4,000
Equipment	$ 80,000	
Less accumulated depreciation	(16,000)	64,000
Total assets		$245,500
Equities		
Accounts payable: supplies		$ 10,000
Accounts payable: other		2,500
Line of credit		5,000
Total liabilities		$ 17,500
Beginning partners' equity	$258,000	
Net income (loss)	(30,000)	228,000
Total equities		$245,500

E. The income statement prepared for the Catskill Clinic shows both the profit plan and the performance budget for 19X8. The variances are computed to show the impact of the change in volume (profit plan minus actual) and the impact of changes in price, spending, and efficiency (performance budget minus actual). Losing 2,000 patient visits reduced income by $80,000. However, income was increased by $48,000 because of changes in price, spending, and efficiency.

Because a change in activity should not change fixed costs, the expected decrease in income (of $80,000) can be explained by multiplying the 2,000 change by the planned contribution margin of $40.00.

Variances due to price, spending, and efficiency show that the reduction in fees reduced total revenue by $56,000. The variances also show that only the other variable operating expenses were more than the performance budget. In fact, expenses were reduced by $62,000, supplies by $9,000, and fixed costs by $53,000.

Performance of the clinic was outstanding. The reduction in activity should have resulted in a reduction of $80,000 in income, but the price, spending, and efficiency effects increased income by $48,000. As a result, the loss for the year was only $30,000.

The clinic improved its cash position by increasing the collection of patient receivables. The clinic was able to purchase the new equipment and borrow less than planned because of the improvement in collections.

Case Study 5–1
Analyzing Operating Results

1. Operating results can be analyzed with a series of critical performance indicators that reflect relationships between key financial variables for the two years. These indicators include:

Critical Performance Indicators	19X5	19X0
Net earnings as percent of net revenue	17.57%	(12.79%)
Encounters per practice-day	20.11	20.98
Encounters per staff FTE	904	798
Encounters per physician FTE	2,129	1,660
Total revenue per practice-day	$4,025	$3,365
Percent change	20%	
Total revenue per encounter	$ 200	$ 160
Percent change	25%	
Total direct expense per encounter	$ 149	$ 160
Percent change	(7%)	
Discounts as percent of total revenue	9.58%	11.28%
Physician salaries as percent of revenue	43.70%	56.60%
Staff salaries as percent of revenue	18.58%	25.03%
Staff FTE / Physician FTE	2.35	2.08
Occupancy as percent of total revenue	7.58%	13.48%

Comments:

- Net earnings increased significantly from a loss to a profit
- Encounters per staff FTE went up 13 percent and per physician FTE 28 percent
- Total revenue per practice-day went up 20 percent and per encounter 25 percent
- Total direct expense per encounter went down 7 percent
- Improvement in discounts went down (from 11.28 percent to 9.58 percent)
- Salaries as a percent of net revenue went down for both physicians and staff
- Staff FTE went up relative to physician FTE
- The higher volume level spread occupancy costs over more encounters, yielding a lower occupancy cost as a percent of total revenue

Case Study 5–2
Using Relative Values in Cost Determination

1. Develop a relative value scale for each acuity level:

Acuity Level	Hours of Care	Relative Value Units
1	2.5	1.00
2	3.8	1.52*
3	5.1	2.04
4	7.3	2.92
5	9.4	3.76

*3.8 / 2.5 = 1.52

Calculate the total RVUs for all the patient-days at each acuity level during the last year:

Acuity Level	Patient Days	×	RVUs	=	Total RVUs
1	160	×	1.00	=	160.00
2	280	×	1.52	=	425.60
3	350	×	2.04	=	714.00
4	190	×	2.92	=	554.80
5	110	×	3.76	=	413.60
	1,090				2,268.00

Calculate the estimated cost of an RVU of nursing service

Total nursing costs / Total RVUs = Cost per RVU
$198,530 / 2,268 = $87.54 per RVU

2. The nursing cost for burn care for the average patient stay of nine days is:

Acuity Level	Patient Days	×	RVUs	×	Cost/RVU	=	Total Cost
1	2	×	1.00	×	$87.54	=	$ 175.08
2	4	×	1.52	×	87.54	=	532.24
3	2	×	2.04	×	87.54	=	357.16
4	1	×	2.92	×	87.54	=	255.62
5	0	×	3.76	×	87.54	=	0.00
	9						$1,320.10

Note: To establish a pricing strategy for prepaid contracting, the clinic must start with the current direct cost of nursing care of about $1,320 per average patient stay. The strategy must also reflect numerous factors besides direct costs of nursing care, but the direct costs provide an initial benchmark upon which to base the negotiation of an acceptable contractual arrangement for the clinic.

Case Study 6–1

Part A: Make or Buy Ancillary Services

1. To make the decision, the relevant costs to compare are those costs that differ between the two alternatives. These are shown in the following table.

	Test Inside	Purchase Outside
Variable costs:		
Conduct inside		
(7,200 × $12)	$ 86,400	—
Purchase outside		
(7,200 × $14)	—	$100,800
Fixed costs:		
Unavoidable	22,000	22,000
Avoidable	18,000	—
Total	$126,400	$122,800

The quantitative analysis shows that it will cost less to purchase testing services outside the clinic. Indeed, doing so will save the clinic $3,600 per month. However, Dr. Ballet must also consider qualitative factors, such as maintaining the internal capability to conduct tests, the lack of control over prices charged, the quality of testing done by the external source, and the possibility of reducing the variable costs internally to offset the cost advantage shown above.

Part B: Expanding the Practice with Prepaid Services

1. To make this decision, the relevant accounting information is the incremental revenue and costs that would occur if the HMO business were accepted versus the status quo. Because the practice has excess capacity, if it is assumed that additional patient treatments will not increase fixed costs, then the incremental revenue will be $375,000 (1,000 × $375) per year and the incremental costs will be $350,000 (1,000 × $350) per year. Thus, the clinic will be $25,000 better off per year with the HMO business. Average costs are irrelevant to the decision.

2. Other assumptions involved in this decision are:

   • The average severity of illness in HMO patients will be the same as in the current 6,000 patients. An increase in acuity would be likely to raise the average variable costs.
   • The current level of charges will be maintained. A reduction in charges might more than offset the benefit of the HMO patients.

Case Study 6–2
Analyzing Break-Even Points and Dealing with Practice Constraints

1. Break-even points for the three DRGs can be calculated using the following steps:

   (a) Find the weighted average charge and variable cost:

DRG			Charge						Variable Cost		
M	50%	×	$1,700	=	$ 850		50%	×	$1,000	=	$ 500
J	30%	×	$2,600	=	$ 780		30%	×	$1,200	=	$ 360
P	20%	×	$ 900	=	$ 180		20%	×	$ 600	=	$ 120
	Weighted average				$1,810						$ 980

   (b) The appropriate level of fixed costs is $1,720,000, because all fixed costs, both DRG-specific and joint fixed costs, must be covered before any profit can be realized.

   (c) Calculate the break-even point, in total treatments, as:

$$
\begin{aligned}
BE &= \text{Total fixed costs} & / & \quad \text{Wgtd. avg. contribution margin} \\
&= \$1,720,000 & / & \quad (\$1,810 - \$980) \\
&= \$1,720,000 & / & \quad \$830 \\
&= 2,072.29 \text{ total treatments}
\end{aligned}
$$

   (d) Distribute the total treatments among the three DRGs as follows:

M	50%	×	2,072.29	=	1,036
J	30%	×	2,072.29	=	622
P	20%	×	2,072.29	=	414

2.

DRG	Charge	Variable Cost	Contrib. Margin	Avg. Length of Procedure	Contrib. Margin per Hr.
M	$1,700	$1,000	$ 700	2 hrs	$350
J	$2,600	$1,200	$1,400	5 hrs	$280
P	$ 900	$ 600	$ 300	1 hr	$300

(a) If there is excess capacity, DRG J should be promoted because it has the highest contribution margin per treatment ($1,400).

(b) If the office is almost at maximum capacity in terms of available hours, DRG M should be promoted because it has the highest contribution margin per hour ($350).

Case Study 6–3
Deciding On an Alternative Investment

1a. Payback Method

Payback period = Investment / Annual cash flow (Labor cost savings)

Model A = $120,000 / $40,000 = 3 years
Model B = $110,000 / $32,000 = 3.4 years

b. Net present value

Cash Flows	Timing	Amount	Factor	Value
Model A:				
Investment	Year 0	$(120,000)	0.000	$(120,000)
Cash savings	Years 1–5	$ 40,000	3.352	$ 134,080
Net present value				$ 14,080
Model B:				
Investment	Year 0	$(110,000)	0.00	$(110,000)
Cash savings	Years 1–5	$ 32,000	3.352	$ 107,264
Net present value				$ (2,736)

c. Internal rate of return

Factor relationship of investment and cash savings = Investment / Annual cash flow (Labor cost savings)

Model A: $120,000 / $40,000 = 3.000

Referring to the PV of an ordinary annuity table, on the line in the table for five years, 3.000 lies between 18 percent and 20 percent; by interpolation, the internal rate of return is estimated to be about 19.8 percent.

Model B: $110,000 / $32,000 = 3.437

Referring to the PV of an ordinary annuity table, on the line in the table for five years, 3.437 lies between 12 percent and 14 percent; by interpolation, the internal rate of return is estimated to be about 13.9 percent.

Recommendation: All three criteria indicate that Model A is preferable to Model B; specifically:

- Model A's payback period meets the three-year criterion; Model B's does not
- NPV is positive for Model A, negative for Model B
- IRR for Model A is greater than the target rate of return; IRR for Model B is less than the target rate of return

2. Considering the effects of income taxes for model A: The cash savings would be reduced by the 40 percent income taxes assessed on it; thus, after-tax cash savings would be $24,000 ($40,000 less 40 percent of $40,000, or $16,000). In addition, there would be a tax shield of savings emanating from the tax deductibility of depreciation of $9,600 ($120,000/5 = $24,000 × 40 percent). Thus, the total after-tax cash flows would be $33,600, and their present value would be $112,627 ($33,600 × 3.352). With the investment of $120,000, the net present value becomes a negative $7,373 ($120,000 − $112,627).

   Considering the effects of income taxes for model B: The after-tax cash savings are $19,200 ($32,000 less 40 percent of $32,000, or $12,800) and the depreciation tax shield would be $8,800 ($110,000/5 = $22,000 × 40 percent). Total after-tax cash flows would be $28,000 ($19,200 + $8,800), and present value would be $93,856 ($28,000 × 3.352). The net present value becomes even more negative $16,144 ($110,000 − $93,856) than it was pre-tax.

   In conclusion, both models have a negative present value after taxes, indicating that neither model's return on investment meets the 15-percent-rate-of-return criterion established by management.

Case Study 8–1
Getting Started

1. They should address such questions as: How big will the building be? Will the clinic be the only tenant, or will other doctors or the hospital also occupy space? Does the hospital plan to impose restrictions on the practice? Who will own the new facility? What is the anticipated cost of occupancy? When will it be ready? Will there be expansion space? How will parking be controlled? What will happen to the existing building?

Case Study 21–1
Using Information Feedback To Address Quality Concerns:
The Annual Retinal Exam for Diabetic Patients

Dr. Jackson should speak privately and separately in a non-threatening way with Dr. Welch and Dr. Sanders. They should work toward agreement with Dr. Jackson on a way to validate their impressions for why they appear to differ.

Case Study 21–2
The Role of Physician Profiling and Educational Feedback
in the Utilization of Health Services

Data credibility and interpretation are major issues in physician profiling. Schoenbaum (1993) notes several factors related to profile content and feedback that increase physician acceptance:

Content	Process
• Derive measurement from evidence- or consensus-based guidelines • Data produced, provided it is accurate, auditable, and statistically stable • Adjust for case mix as appropriate • Supply actionable information	• Obtain physician participation in measurement development • Convene physicians, encourage physician participation to interpret data

The consortium illustrated in Case Study 21–2 should assure that the connection between target rates, the view that a lower rate is a better rate, and evidence-based guidelines are made clearly and often. Not all pediatricians will agree that lower is better (Keller, 1992). The best that can be presented is the scientific information, with back-up detail for those whose questions and concerns are not satisfied by basic information. Endorsement by a respected professional organization, such as a specialty association, the National Institutes of Health, a professional journal, or the state medical association, can increase comfort levels about the source and credibility of data.

At the first educational session, the consortium should be prepared for the following types of reactions to the information:

• The data are not credible
• My patients are sicker
• How I practice medicine is my business

Information about how the data were adjusted for case mix and patient demographics should be presented clearly and concisely. The educational, nonpunitive nature of the information must be emphasized—there is no right rate.

Perhaps the consortium could sponsor a state medical society program on the topic. Effort must be made to include both formal and informal physician leaders in each session. Sessions should respect physician time and schedules to the extent possible without giving short shrift to the information. This may mean linking with existing staff meetings or educational programs. Depending on the community's culture, the hospital, the medical practice, or a neutral setting such as a university campus may be the most effective session setting.

The consortium should establish clear agreements with the other organizations that will provide data to monitor whether practice changed after feedback. These include the data elements, reporting schedules, confidentiality statements, and type of medium on which data can be accepted.

The consortium plans to form study groups of physicians to examine any change over time and to communicate new issues and findings in the field relevant to pediatric asthma admissions (Keller, 1992). The groups can serve as an effective means of disseminating information (Moller et al., 1994; Lawthers et al., 1993).

INDEX